Towards a Contextual Psychology of Disablism

In recent years, disability studies has been driven by a model of disability primarily concerned with the material exclusions and inequalities experienced by disabled people. Although an important counterbalance to a pathologising medical model, the social model risks presenting an impoverished and disembodied view of disability, one that ignores the psychological nature of oppression and its effects.

This innovative work argues that a psychological framework of disability is an essential part of developing a more cohesive disability movement. Brian Watermeyer introduces a new, integrative approach, using psychoanalysis to tackle the problem of conceptualising psychological aspects of life with disablism. Psychoanalytic ideas are applied to social responses to impairment, making sense of discrimination in its many forms, as well as problems in disability politics and research. The perspective explores individual psychological experience, whilst retaining a rigorous critique of social forces of oppression. The argument shows how it is possible to theorise the psychological processes and impressions of discriminatory society without pathologising disadvantaged individuals.

Drawing on sociology, social anthropology, psychology and psychoanalysis – as well as clinical material from his own practice – *Towards a Contextual Psychology of Disablism* shapes a view of disabled subjectivity which is embodied, internal and political. Presenting a range of conceptual ideas which describe psychological dynamics and predicaments confronting disabled people in an exclusionary and prejudiced world, this volume is an important new contribution to the literature. It will interest students and researchers of disability studies, including those working within psychology, education, health and social work.

Brian Watermeyer is a clinical psychologist, and a disabled person. During the writing of this book he was a postdoctoral research fellow at Stellenbosch University. He teaches on postgraduate programmes at several South African universities, in disability studies, rehabilitation science, clinical psychology and other health science disciplines.

Routledge Advances in Disability Studies

New titles

Towards a Contextual Psychology of Disablism
Brian Watermeyer

Forthcoming titles

Disability, Hate Crime and Violence
Edited by Alan Roulstone and Hannah Mason-Bish

Intellectual Disability and Social Theory
Philosophical debates on being human
Chrissie Rogers

Towards a Contextual Psychology of Disablism

Brian Watermeyer

Routledge
Taylor & Francis Group
LONDON AND NEW YORK

First published 2013
by Routledge
2 Park Square, Milton Park, Abingdon, Oxon, OX14 4RN

Simultaneously published in the USA and Canada
by Routledge
711 Third Avenue, New York, NY 10017

Routledge is an imprint of the Taylor & Francis Group, an informa business

First issued in paperback 2014

British Library Cataloguing in Publication Data
A catalogue record for this book is available from the British Library

Library of Congress Cataloging-in-Publication Data
Watermeyer, Brian.
Towards a contextual psychology of disablism / Brian Watermeyer.
p. ; cm. -- (Routledge advances in disability studies)
1. People with disabilities--Psychology. 2. Prejudices. I. Title. II. Series:
Routledge advances in disability studies.
[DNLM: 1. Disabled Persons--psychology. 2. Prejudice. 3. Socioeconomic
Factors. BF 727.P57]
BF727.P57W38 2012
155.9′16--dc23
2011052604

ISBN13: 978-0-415-68160-5 (hbk)
ISBN13: 978-1-138-78121-4 (pbk)

Typeset in Baskerville
by Taylor & Francis Books

For Myriam

Contents

Acknowledgements

My precious wife, Rachael, whose constant love, support and pride in my work surprises and blesses me every day.

Prof. Leslie Swartz, my supervisor, teacher and friend, for more than two decades of enormous academic and personal insight, support and wonderful humour.

The members of the psychotherapy group which is part of the subject matter of this book, for what they taught me and for allowing me to document their experience. Especially in memory of A, whose energy and generosity is missed by all.

Chantal Deacon, Tanya Damon, Sonia Fick and Lise Anthonissen, my research and reading assistants, for their hard work, patience, dedication and friendship.

Claire Gregorowski, for her keen grammatical skills, kindness and friendship in the final stages of this work.

Dr. Deryck Sheriffs, my father-in-law, for his careful proof-reading and comments, and for being the immensely accepting and kind person that he is.

Deborah Marks and Valerie Sinason, whose writings and personal communications over several years have vastly enriched my thinking on disability.

The department of psychology at the University of Stellenbosch, for welcoming and supporting me during the period of the book's researching and writing.

The Claude Leon Foundation, for the post-doctoral research funding which was essential in producing this work.

The South African National Research Foundation, for the doctoral research funding which made the original investigation possible.

Introduction

Anyone familiar with disability studies will be aware of its awkward relationship with the question of psychology. Calls to integrate a psychological analysis into the discipline are often not well received, and it consequently carries no coherent model of psychological life in a discriminatory world. This state of affairs is unsustainable for a discipline aiming to mirror the social predicaments of the disabled minority. Many would argue that emancipation must have a human as well as a material face. I agree.

This book is the product of both personal and professional experience. I come to disability studies wearing, as it were, several different hats. First, I identify as a disabled person – I am severely sight impaired. I am also a health professional, having worked as a clinical psychologist for over a decade, with a particular interest in therapeutic work with disabled people. During this period, though, my primary, full-time work has been academic research in disability studies, and disability-related teaching mainly on postgraduate health science courses. These include occupational therapy and physiotherapy, clinical psychology and medicine. I have also taken up various activist roles, such as lobbying for better inclusiveness at my university, taking on media appearances and contributing to the development of disability studies as a discipline in South Africa. All of these identities play a part in the view of disability which I continue to develop. This process has involved an ongoing dialogue between my own life experience, theory, local culture and infrastructure, disability politics and my work as a psychologist.

The usefulness of my multiple roles relates to a metaphor which, to me, describes the fragmented nature of the social phenomenon of disability. I think of disability as a sort of jigsaw puzzle composed of unique pieces, each of which is held by a particular interest group in society. Regrettably though, these stakeholders do not get on. Activists, health professionals, the disabled community and academic researchers very often have relationships which are ambivalent, combative, suspicious or disregarding of one another. For this reason, I aim in my work to make the most of my straddled identities. All the roleplayers just listed have an essential contribution to make in unpacking the disability phenomenon. I use this term to emphasise disability's emotive and multi layered nature. It is of culture, politics, self and body. It creates myths, sustains vendettas and provokes forces of liberation and subordination. It captures the imagination and fills the mind. It is both alien and familiar, palpable and mysterious. Easy agreement over such an issue was never likely. Practitioners, activists, researchers and disabled people themselves all carry a layer of disability reality, as exclusive observers from their vantage point. Disability studies, and scholarship on disability in general, presents an analogous story of disciplinary splits which repeatedly miss opportunities for consolidation and growth. This is not to say that some of the feuding, the critique, has not been well justified; not at all. But it is time now to usher in a new era, one based on co-development and mutual education; one which modifies and improves theory and practice, rather than dismisses it. The work of developing the psychological area in disability studies will, without doubt, require attending to traditional relational splits.

Inconvenient though this may be, it has become clear to me that no single theoretical narrative is able to mirror disability adequately. Different parts of self and society are best described by concepts which do not necessarily interface easily with one another. I have come to accept this compromise, aiming to make the most of what each framework offers in both my personal and academic life. The key shortcoming of the disability studies project thus far is its very limited engagement with the psychological level. This book (along with a few others) is an initial, exploratory response to this lacuna. Liberatory disability politics will miss an essential ingredient of social change unless it accepts the task of conceptualising disabled selfhood, and how this is shaped by ideology. Oppressive ideology informs socialisation, and socialisation shapes the self in ways which serve its purposes. Disability studies has been understandably reluctant to enter this politically prickly area. But if the discipline is to mirror impaired life in a disablist society it has little choice but to explore the psychological realm. Many disability studies scholars choose to rubbish psychology as a discipline, seeing its constructs as too contaminated with pathologisation to entertain. A wholesale rejection would leave disability studies needing to construct its own psychology – an unrealistic challenge to say the least. Constructive engagement is the only option. And I hope, with this book, to begin to demonstrate that it is a workable one.

My own journey has benefited greatly from the politics of the social model, which brings a disdain for psychology as part of its package. The social model device has sparked change in disabled lives around the world, overturning unquestioned logics about how disability inequality happens. So, too, in my own life. I grew up in Cape Town as someone with no sense of entitlement to citizenship rights denied by an inaccessible world. Life as an undergraduate at university was characterised by an instinct to disguise my impairment, as my inability to read in the normal way seemed like a good reason for disqualification as a student. Social model politics partially reconfigured this view in the public realm, but my own experience of impairment remained mysterious. To a large extent, it still does. What does impairment mean … what does it make of one … who, if anyone, is to blame for exclusion … what is it like for others … what feelings are justifiable … what is it reasonable to expect from one's life, oneself, one's career or relationships? These and a host of other questions remain.

It is this personal layer of experience which feminist disability studies has begun to point to over the past few decades, problematising the evasions of materialist disability studies. Like me, these authors found the social model's account of disability helpful, but limiting. Historical materialism's focus on structure leaves it disinterested in individual psychology and development. But it was clear to me that formative aspects of my personal history, as well as the constant realities of material inaccessibility, significantly shaped my experience of my impairment and myself. Somehow, familial relationships, my own sense of self, disablist cultural messaging and structural barriers all needed to find a place in my own disability story.

My teaching and work as a clinical psychologist has been an opportunity to explore and apply psychoanalytic thought in a range of contexts. Its critical, innovative use in making sense of social oppression, group processes and organisational change was prominent in my training, and felt relevant in making sense of my own circumstances. As is well known, psychoanalysis is more often regarded in the social sciences as an oppressive anachronism than a subversive lens of social critique. I was fortunate to be part of a group of colleagues exploring both its problems and its applicability in the developing world context of South Africa – a society defined, above all else, by inequality. This is not a book about psychoanalysis. I draw on a range of disciplines, from medical anthropology to bioethics, social work to literary studies. Instead, it is a work which applies psychoanalytic critique in making sense of social responses to disability at a range of levels. These include the work of institutions, academic formulations, cultural reactions to the impaired body, the nature of disability politics, and much more besides. In so doing, the book uses psychoanalytic thinking to develop ideas on the psychological nature of life in a disablist society. There is no danger here of disability studies being colonised by psychoanalysis. Conversely, my aim is to selectively draw the incisive, and especially *reflexive*, critical power of psychoanalysis into disability studies, which need not fear any loss of identity or purpose. Readers of psychoanalysis will recognise that I have defined terms simply, to be as accessible and specifically relevant as possible.

The problem which has daunted disability studies scholars is how to think about psychological aspects of disability, which tug toward the individual, internal realm, while holding firm to a contextual analysis of structural barriers. This is no small challenge, but psychoanalysis has something to offer. At its heart, psychoanalysis is an attempt to name and describe subtle or unconscious aspects of experiences within and between people. It asks questions about how the self is formed through these transactions, potentially bridging the gap between ideology and the nature of subjectivity. In disabled lives, much of what maintains inequality is unseen and subtle, at times leading to responses or feelings which are difficult to understand. This is because people on all sides of relationships may be caught in a web of hidden meanings about what disability is, what it does and what ought to be done. But this does not mean that psychoanalysis' critical usefulness is restricted to 'soft' or 'close' aspects of relating. It has just as much potential to make sense of policies, assistive devices, social service protocols and architecture as it does of intimate relationships. Its uniqueness lies in the ability to connect these domains, through a curiosity about the unconscious narratives of disability which are held in common. Understanding unconscious meanings of impairment is, in my view, a fundamental part of unpacking the disability puzzle. Psychoanalytic ideas can conceptualise inner experiences in a manner which connects these to the relational world – the world of the family, of media and culture, of material deprivation and of institutions and politics. Disability is about unequal relationships. Surely it is relationships which require study. It is important to clarify that a critical psychoanalytic view is concerned with disability meanings held by all, disabled and nondisabled alike. It does not centre on the nature of disabled subjectivity, but is interested in this as part of a pervasive field of meanings which shapes all social disability phenomena. The psychological meanings of disability for all are under scrutiny.

This book is no more than an initial pebble dropped into the largely undisturbed waters of this area; undisturbed, at least, by the discipline of disability studies. As such, it is an imperfect and incomplete account. Its main purpose is to argue that conceptualising the psychological nature, impact and perpetuation of disablism is essential. The ideas presented here are based on a combination of clinical data, my own experience and a psychoanalytically oriented synthesis of theoretical material. I make no claims that what I have to say is generalisable to a wider context. My aims are far more modest, and primarily to do with stimulating thought, reflection and the creation of a freer, more curious discipline. What the material does demonstrate is how subjective life with impairment in a disablist world exists against the currents of a range of silencing forces, both internal and external. If the experiences described in this book are not resonant, I hope the reader will respond by reflecting on what is, and contributing their account. In this way, my wish is that a growing store of conceptual ideas will accumulate, empowering disabled individuals through naming the often shadowy aspects of inner and relational life which maintain inequality.

In the early phase of both disability studies and the disability movement as a whole, a relatively depersonalised and simplified view was warranted, even needed. Such ambiguous phenomena as functional limitation, pain, fatigue and emotional struggle would have offset the traction of a social oppression view. Instead, the binaries of the social model were adopted, and certainly have served a purpose. But in so doing, a tract of human complexity had to be silenced. Both the discipline and the movement are now challenged to move toward a more mature, nuanced phase, making space for the contested features of disability just named. Again, the challenge is substantial. The experience of impairment, embodiment and emotional life are extremely difficult to represent, and the problem of articulating these with the political world remains. The core task of this book is to begin to find usable ways of thinking integratively about these disparate layers. After taking stock of the depth of the problem through examining critiques of materialist disability studies, I invite the reader to struggle with me in the place to which these lead. Psychoanalysis can help here, as a framework unusually comfortable with acknowledging what we do not know, or cannot precisely define. Being impaired in a disablist culture embodies a psychological predicament composed of historical, relational, cultural, political and material aspects. It is both immediate and teleological, internal and relational, symbolic and manifest.

Psychoanalysis has provided conceptual tools helpful in piecing together my own experience of these circumstances. Each area covered in this book is included because it illuminates something of the predicament of disablism, holding meanings which are simultaneously personal, political and theoretical. What ties all of these aspects together is lifelong disablist socialisation, comprising both psychological and material levels. Conceptualising its cultural elements, the psychological quandaries it creates and the impressions it may leave is the central concern. Interwoven with this exploration is a range of recurring themes which I explore, demonstrate and argue for. I highlight these here, as many represent a significant break from mainstream disability studies, as well as social model discourse more broadly. Many will be surprising, some awkward. New, risk-taking engagement is the challenge and the experiment of this book. Here follows a short description of each theme.

Disability's emotive nature

We all have feelings about disability, which tend to be strong, diverse and at least partly hidden. Cultural and political forces leave us extremely uneasy with most of these feelings, save a small set which satisfy the requirements of political or altruistic correctness. But beneath the surface the simple truth is that all, disabled and nondisabled alike, struggle with the cultural phenomenon of disability. This should not surprise us, and is no cause for shame. As humans, difference is something we find hard. And disability combines profound perceived difference with an immense history of segregation. Anxiety, fear, ambivalence, pity, helplessness and a host of other emotional responses to the visibly impaired body, or its imagined experience, are normal. This is important because emotional responses to disability exist and impact measurably on relationships whether we acknowledge their presence or not. In fact, the more we disallow and disregard our feelings, the more likely these are to shape relationships in unconscious ways. Political correctness, cultural mores and the social modelist resistance to all things psychological have meant that an authentic conversation about how we all *feel* about disability is yet to begin. May it begin here. Friends, family members, health professionals, disabled people, charity workers, activists and citizens; if we all struggle with disability, let us start exploring how, and what this brand of struggle leads to in our work and relationships. Real relating must be based on taking ownership of fears and fantasies about difference. We need to overcome a shared shame, and with trust, humility and humour begin a new, robust engagement with one another. This is a new conversation that the binaries of social model politics cannot hold, and as such, it may at first seem a little frightening. But the critique of society which the disability phenomenon invites carries the immense promise that it does precisely because of its confounding of our comfortable categories. All sorts of relationships to do with disability are powerfully mediated by unconscious, emotional currents. Until we begin the honest conversation of which I speak, we will not have the opportunity to understand, disconfirm or separate from our fantasies about difference, thereby maintaining a futile drama of opposing constructs, rather than actual relationship. Disability is, before and beyond everything we see in material society, a profoundly emotive issue.

Disability is hard to think about

Psychoanalytic ideas about the developing self describe our need to feel *thought about* by others – by parents and carers, in adult relationships, or even by the state. This is an experience of someone being open to what our world is like, allowing us to feel cared for, and growing our ability to treat ourselves with compassion. Because we find disability emotionally evocative and difficult, it is literally hard to think clearly about disabled life. This is not because of its actual nature, but because of our fantasies about it. Because disability speaks to disquieting parts of our inner lives, all find it hard to relate in an open way, undisrupted by pre-existing ideas or apprehensions. Consequently, social responses to impairment are substantially shaped by fantasy rather than actual contact, creating the experience of a misattuned, unresponsive environment in disabled lives. Part of what is created by this world of fantasy is the real-life experience of marginal, excluded and materially deprived positions in society. If we were less threatened by unconscious evocations, and able to think more clearly about this appalling reality, we would by now have achieved more to change it. Instead of being thought about by society, disabled people tend to be controlled, managed, treated, measured, and otherwise 'dealt with' in distancing, material ways. Emotional evocations underpin the difficulty of thinking about disabled life, hence the need for their exploration. With this book I try to model an effort at making awkward feelings more sayable and complexity more admissible. As an example, I discuss a store of psychoanalytic disability research which is regarded by many – at times justifiably – as oppressive and offensive. My purpose (in part) is to deliberately model an engagement with realities which are often hidden, and always complicated. The critique of this decontextualised work I give is, I believe, rigorous enough. But what I reject is an attitude of totalising splits between players in the disability arena who are right and good, and those who are bad and wrong. This splitting is both a key determinant of disablist oppression, and a powerful obstacle to our developing better understandings of its layers. It is a problem faced by theorists and activists, as well as 'oppressors'.

Integration

A good portion of the material in this book is not new to disability studies. But what I attempt here is a fresh synthesis which sees these ideas, along with some additional ones, in an innovative, aligning light. This is done through applying a psychoanalytic lens across the board, comparing lines of theory and narrative which previously seemed at odds, or are products of feuding disciplines. Returning to the jigsaw puzzle analogy, anyone familiar with disability research will understand the often destructive camp formations which divide disability studies from a range of health professions, rehabilitation science, medical sociology and other disciplines. The dismissal of entire research traditions is not uncommon. It is hard to find real initiatives towards open-minded disciplinary integration from within disability studies. As mentioned above, my inclusion of a critical discussion of previously slated psychoanalytic work is one response to this. A further rationale for examining this work is the need to base new theoretical developments on an honest assessment of what has gone before. Much of what I term the 'traditional' legacy of psychoanalytic work on disability implies that people with impairments are psychologically damaged, while paying little attention to discriminatory structures. But notwithstanding its very real ideological problems, a simple rejection of this work is wasteful and unnecessary. We cannot afford to lose fragments of insight because these occur against an ideologically flawed backdrop. Again, this does not mean foregoing or relaxing critique; not in the slightest. But it does mean resisting disciplinary splits. Further, there is value in closely examining politically problematic theory, as we stand to learn much by unpacking its social origins. The psychoanalytic legacy on disability, for example, brings insights about research pitfalls to be avoided, common misunderstandings about disability and how these arise, as well as precious fragments of knowledge to build upon. It is not by accident that these theorists missed a key layer of the disability phenomenon. The split thinking at work here is not qualitatively different from that which confounds current, 'critical' attempts at theorising disability.

Complexity and pragmatism

Disability studies research, especially that informed by the social model approach, has taken an overtly partisan, emancipatory position. While justified, this has at times impoverished conceptualisation. There is a fine balance to be struck between allowing for political impact, not underestimating complexity and taking care not to forego methodological rigour. The assumption has been that an honest, thorough attempt to mirror disabled subjectivity – including psychological aspects – is at odds with an emancipatory approach. We need to take a more courageous position. Complexity may complicate politics, but it allows the disabled constituency to see their experience mirrored more accurately in conceptualisation. The integrative approach I take is one which does not demand, or even expect, minute conceptual correlations. The key criterion is to do with what is helpful and illuminating – what explains subjective experience in a manner which tells us where we are, and helps us think about where we need to go. As alluded to above, psychoanalytic ideas in this book are explained in ways which may, technically, be not altogether complete or strictly accurate. The intention is to make these ideas accessible and, more importantly, practicable in signposting the obscure terrain of unconscious disability symbolism, relational dynamics and internal experience.

Empathy

If, as this book proposes, we all share disquieting unconscious associations to disability, it makes sense that we all do our best to proceed from a position of empathy.

This is a non-judgmental empathy for the disability-related conflicts of others, as well as for our own. Splits, feuds, misunderstandings and vilifications surrounding disability are ever-present; in academic life, service provision, the world of charity, political activism and elsewhere. These arguments are regularly to do with important issues, and some positions are without doubt more humanitarian, critical and defensible than others. But a culture of outrage sometimes obscures what we have in common, which is a struggle with difference. Health professionals often do not understand the predicaments of disabled people, and may be apprehensive about exploring these. Disability activists seldom, if ever, carefully consider the quandaries, attacks and traumas faced daily by health practitioners. Nondisabled citizens who have grown up in segregated societies have had little or no chance to get used to bodies and lifestyles different from their own. None of these difficulties and disjunctures should surprise us. But what is problematic is the heatedness of engagements which make no space for real communication, and hence for mutual adjustment.

If our first port of call is righteous outrage, we foreclose a conversation about hidden struggles with identity, which then remain unaddressed. Somehow we need to create a safer, more generous terrain of engagement, where stereotypes (of all) are left behind, differing predicaments may be heard, and real talking and listening may begin. In the first place, this form of engagement between the disability sector and organizations of health professionals is a fundamental need. There is stereotyping on all sides, missing the opportunity for optimising limited resources.

Trauma

One reason why we struggle to engage constructively around disability is because it is associated with trauma, both real and imagined. This may be the trauma of deprivation and exclusion, of acute experiences of accident or illness, of observers' fantasies about life with impairment, of the shame engendered by prejudice, and so forth. This is not to stereotype disabled lives as traumatic; some are and some are not, and reasons for trauma vary from contextual to relational and embodied factors. But be it in reality or fantasy, our association of disability and trauma is ubiquitous. What defines trauma is an experience or image which is beyond our frame of reference, feels impossible to make sense of, and therefore perforates our defences. Known or imagined, trauma is difficult to think and talk about. The powerful, prejudiced cultural significations of disability and dangerous silence regarding shared feelings about bodily difference combine in keeping disability trauma obscured. It appears as a spectre which is largely mediated by imagination, rather than the words of people living with prejudice, exclusion and impairment. The reality of lived trauma as well as shared apprehensions about imagined trauma are key aspects of the disability story which disability studies has hardly touched upon. To begin, trauma has a wholly understandable influence on the culture of disability politics. Equally, it must be influential in the practice of health professionals who are often poorly supported and under-prepared for the human realities of both acute and ongoing trauma. Family life around disability may involve trauma, for reasons which defy easy categorization. Understanding these and other relationships around impairment must include an examination of the impact of trauma.

Building relationships

What many threads in the above discussion point towards is the need for all disability stakeholders to commit to building relationships. At many points in this book I criticize a pervasive brand of separatist disability politics, which feeds more on the identification of oppressors and in-group idealisation than thoughtful engagement with the issues and roleplayers involved. Slogans and active resistance have an important place in the disability movement, but can become a defensive end in themselves. Dynamics of adversity and inequality are always collusory, and organisations preoccupied with the nature of their oppressors tend to be very poor at self-reflection. Justly or not, it falls to the disability movement to reflect on the problems of its combative politics, the unfairness of some of its pronouncements and the need to find ways to trust in a new era of relationship. The same need for reflexivity applies to health professionals, but until now this was the only group seen as requiring change.

Political correctness

This is, in part, a book about the limits of politics. If not applied with ongoing reflexivity, the drive of political resistance can ultimately narrow the worlds of those it aims to liberate. Political correctness, often in the form of terminology, is a good example. Of course derogatory terms should be disallowed. But in an attempt to create a respectful arena of engagement, politically correct terms often create orthodoxies which constrict thought, serving more as devices of social closure than meaning-making tools. The problem is not the terms themselves, but how these are used for the purpose of identifying who 'out there' is *really* wrong. The hopeful fantasy of a single, grand narrative which makes sense of disability is again evident here, visible in the clarity with which heroes and villains are divided. It is very seductive to believe that if we just use the right terms and follow the correct protocols that everything will fall into place. This is a dangerous mistake, which misses the essence of what drives disablist oppression – that is, the world of the irrational. Narrow, orthodox politics works directly against both group-based and individual reflection among disabled and nondisabled people alike. Ironically, the most important conversations we can have, in my view, are ones which are brave enough to forego political correctness; that is, real, authentic engagements with the contradictory meanings all carry about disability. The generosity of engagement mentioned above is needed to allow our mistaken ideas about one another to come to light, even if this involves the dropping of a few political clangers. This is not colluding with prejudice, but engaging in a way which models openness, and the recognition of a long, shared history of separation. The permission to begin relating in a real way is a first step to mutual awareness, co-education and collaboration.

Universality of human struggle

At the root of this work is the idea that 'disability struggle' is not unique to disabled people, or qualitatively different from other human suffering. We can, however, show in measurable ways how the disabled population is systematically subjected to experiences of deprivation, shunning, control and a range of other assaults on identity which are less likely to befall nondisabled people. But disability experience is human experience. Subtly visible in disablist culture is an assumption of qualitative difference between disabled and nondisabled subjectivity. This is a dangerous myth, which functions as a defence against painful thoughts about 'how I would feel' if subject to the social circumstances of impaired life. The suffering of disabled people is, in fact, perilously nearby, by virtue of the universal frailty of the body and the reality of societies shot through with inequality of every sort. No-one is safe, leading to the need to shore up an illusory differentness. The more we are able to hear disabled subjectivity, the more we will see the contribution this can make to our common understanding of the human condition. Psychological fantasies and bodily realities of frailty are in all, and all are finally subject to the ideological and medical controls of the body we see impacting so powerfully on disabled lives. A recognition of this commonality, where this is achievable, will change the way disability is constructed and responded to.

I turn now to a short signposting of the chapters to come. In Chapter 1, we begin by reflecting on the cultural phenomenon of bodily symbolism – the resilient logic that the nature of the soul, or the self, is 'written on the body'. Culture, as we know, carries strongly held ideas about the psychological nature of disability. Adding the material layer of social responses to impairment, I then sketch the worldwide development challenges facing the disabled community. This is to provide a basic orientation to the international arena of disability politics, against which debates about the psychological level take place. In some sense, these sections embody a problem statement, with the balance of the book examining theoretical responses to it.

Chapter 2 is the first of five primarily theoretical chapters, which structure the main body of the argument. In this chapter, I lay the groundwork by describing and critiquing politicised responses to disablist oppression. The social model's opposition to medicalisation, its own theoretical shortcomings and the difficult question of embodiment are considered in turn. We explore what social modelist disability politics disallows, ushering the reader into the uncertain space beyond its theoretical reach. At issue are a range of difficult compromises, centring on the political need for simplicity, and the human reality of complexity. The experiences of both body and self require attention, bringing conceptual and political challenges. But tackling these arenas also carries the promise of a richer, more real representation of disabled life.

In Chapter 3 I introduce psychoanalysis, with a view to exploring what it may offer to the conceptual problems at hand. As psychoanalysis' ability or appetite for social critique is contested, we begin with an honest assessment of this debate. The many criticisms levelled at psychoanalytic thought here lead logically to the next section, which is a review of the largely problematic history of the discipline's work in the area of disability. This is essential as a point of departure for developing updated psychoanalytic ideas on disability. A new, critical psychoanalytic approach to disablism is then outlined, highlighting the unconscious mediation of discriminatory culture. This examines how unconscious forces shape social responses to impairment at a host of levels, providing important micro-mechanisms of socialisation. Particular psychological defences triggered by the unconscious evocations of disability are described, along with how these distort social perceptions and obscure the nature of disabled life. Four related concepts – stigma, liminality, monstrosity and abjection – are then explored, and tied in to the psychoanalytic framework. At every stage the intention is to even-handedly assess research material and conceptual ideas, with the psychoanalytic lens showing up important, unifying commonalities as well as problems.

The theoretical groundwork of Chapter 3 paves the way for a conceptual discussion of a range of aspects of socialisation in a disablist world, which will span forthcoming chapters. In Chapter 4, I examine debates regarding disability and quality of life in the field of applied bioethics, enquiring about their unconscious narratives. Contested issues such as prenatal testing, assisted suicide, and the cultural viewing of some lives as 'not worth living' are explored, along with a psychoanalytic critique of prominent standpoints. The final three sections of the chapter examine the disability movement's identifying of a purported 'eugenic threat', the distrubing emergence of evidence surrounding disability hate crime, and experiential aspects of the disabled figure's encounter with medicine. What comes into relief is a picture of the psychological predicaments and ideological meanings which compose the lifelong socialisation of disabled people, as well as an argument for psychological perspectives on every aspect of the disability arena.

The theme of socialisation is greatly extended in Chapter 5, which traces concentric layers of culture as these are impressed on the disabled self. The first three sections deal with narcissistic, capitalist culture; artistic and literary representations of disability; and the discourse of charity. In each case the ways in which the disabled figure is constructed as other, as subject or as commodity are investigated, building a picture of the psychological dilemmas which result. Narrowing the focus on cultural shaping of the disabled self, I move then to the emotive and difficult area of the family. Thorny debates to do with constructions of families with congenitally impaired members, the advent of 'normalising' surgeries and unconscious narratives of parenting in disability are addressed here. Social and political forces which make it hard to think clearly about disability in families are a central issue for discussion. Combining all of these aspects of socialisation in a disablist world, the discussion then moves to the difficulties with establishing a solid, shared disabled group identity. Attempts at creating solidarity among a diverse disabled population meet obstacles, which are seldom considered from a psychological point of view. The nature of selfhood, clearly, has much to do with the public identifications one chooses to make.

In Chapter 6 we explore concepts of psychological oppression, along with ideas about change. In the first section, moves from within social model-oriented disability studies to incorporate 'psycho-emotional' aspects of disability are critically examined and contrasted with the philosophical foundations of this book. Thereafter, we take stock of the under-theorised but very important idea of internalised oppression, relating disablism to aspects of psychoanalytic work on racism. Next is the Winnicottian notion of mirroring which, I argue, is central to understanding disablist socialisation. The final two sections pose questions about psychological change; first, against a development studies backdrop, and second, in the vexed association of disability with psychotherapy. I do not provide conceptual solutions to these difficult problems, but critically examine obstacles to constructive debate, outline possible theoretical resources to draw on and offer suggestions to a disability movement which tends to neglect the psychological experience of its constituency.

Chapter 7 is the first of three chapters which are in part informed by my own clinical material. These experiential accounts were gathered in psychoanalytically oriented group psychotherapy with severely physically impaired adults. Theoretical material is interspersed with clinical quotations, which are intended to enliven and humanise the ideas being discussed. This section of chapters represents some initial conceptual suggestions which flow from questions posed by the theoretical foundations outlined before.

Chapter 7 begins by describing how the unconscious evocations of impairment systematically distort relationships, and hence socialisation. We consider the implications of inhabiting a body that evokes discomfort in others. One consequence is a socially engendered silencing of the voice of disabled experience. Thereafter, I suggest an approach to the difficult issue of combining personal, intra-psychic narratives of trauma with a broad, contextual analysis of disability.

In Chapter 8, the pivotal issue of the distortion of personal and psychic boundaries in disabled lives is examined in some depth. The stereotype of disabled people demanding the status of 'exceptions' to normal social responsibilities appears in Freudian theory as well as popular culture. I examine this theoretical proposition, its possible social origins, and critical responses to it. Various relational dynamics which leave disabled people's experience unseen are then described. At times these may worsen material predicaments which carry their own hardships. The defences of a world at pains to distance disabled experience show up repeatedly, in forms such as the need to apply 'solutions', blaming and avoidance. Disabled people socialised in this way may be drawn into colluding with subtle dynamics of inequality. Along with ascriptions of inferiority, though, comes a demand from the social world to achieve higher levels of 'independence', fostering conflict around needs for assistance. The modern self relies heavily on the subjective experience of control, which is a psychological resource often denied to disabled people in an inaccessible world. All of these aspects of social mirroring, both material and symbolic, carry personal meanings which shape selfhood.

Punitive levels of self-discipline and drive in some disabled people are one consequence.

In Chapter 9, the emotive issue of loss and its cultural association with disability is examined. The social model's understandable aim to disprove stereotypes of loss and tragedy have, I argue, contributed to some disabled people becoming alienated from the universal human reality of loss. Finding one's personal narrative, one's truth, is extremely difficult against the hum of a world relentlessly preoccupied with defining and redefining conceptions of disabled life. At times, disabled people may experience a 'loss of self', through living in opposition to ascribed characteristics, rather than in terms of authentically held ones.

Chapter 10 provides concluding reflections, including a return to some of the themes described in this introduction. The lasting impression is of disability as a dynamic process, definable only in dialectical terms. As a human phenomenon, its experience is by nature unique, but the predicaments it creates, at both material and relational levels, can be collectively conceptualised. Paying attention to this challenge will contribute to a more mature, far-sighted and inclusive political movement. Examination of the psychological level is an essential part of the struggle for disability equity.

Brian Watermeyer
Cape Town
November 2011

1 Cultural othering and material deprivation

> If we had a keen vision and feeling of all ordinary human life, it would be like hearing the grass grow and the squirrel's heart beat, and we should die of that roar which lies on the other side of silence.
>
> (*Middlemarch* – George Eliot, 1871, p. 207)

Introduction

The history of disability as a societal phenomenon is probably as old as humankind itself, incorporating a myriad of cultural responses to the 'marked body'. A central argument of this book is that the tendency of bodily difference to evoke visceral, partly hidden emotional responses is an important mediator of the social forces which have driven disabled people to the margins of society. The modern era has witnessed an immense institutional and cultural othering of the disabled minority, leading to a host of systematic exclusions from social participation. Biomedical diagnosis, bureaucratic categorisation and prejudice maintain exclusion of disabled people from the economy, as well as the mainstream production of culture. Around the globe, the hallmarks of the social predicaments of disabled people are poverty, mass unemployment, shunning and discrimination. Inequality is woven deeply into the structure and function of societies designed and developed with the needs of only the nondisabled majority in mind.

Over the course of the twentieth century, the rise of biomedical health care in Western nations saw academic and institutional responses to disability becoming dominated by medicine. But critics of modern health care pointed to its lack of attention to social factors which mediate the way illness or disability is experienced. Biomedicine's tendency was to view disability as a problem of dysfunctional or diseased bodies, neglecting the reality of discrimination. This meant that the social and economic marginality of disabled people tended to be ascribed to individual, impairment-related factors, rather than contextual ones. What became perjoratively termed the *medical model* effectively placed responsibility for the poverty and exclusion of disabled people at their own door, as an unfortunate, but inevitable outcome of functional defects. In response, disabled academics and activists began to galvanise political resistance, shaping the disabled community into a civil rights movement lobbying for change.

The crux of their position was that it was discrimination and systemic disadvantage, not bodily frailty, which was at the heart of the marginal, deprived status of disabled people. Under the banner of this new *social model* approach, marginality became understood as a product of oppression. In addition, it was argued that discriminatory societies selectively ascribed the 'disabled' identity to some citizens, as a means of absolving the state from responsibility for fulfilling citizenship rights. The architects of this new model were academics from disciplines such as sociology and social policy, who mainly subscribed to an historical materialist model of society. This paradigm views access to participation in the economy as primary in shaping social inequality, tending to regard cultural or psychological factors as less important. Along the way, the discipline of disability studies was born, with strong foundations (especially in the United Kingdom) in a partisan, emancipatory approach to disability research. Social modelists vehemently rejected the diagnostic and rehabilitative methods of medicine, seeing these as instruments of social control rather than upliftment. But the social model-dominated disability movement was to bring its own silences. These were based on materialism's strategic eliding of unique, personal aspects of disability experience, as well as the domain of the psychological.

To the political vanguard of the social model, psychology had been at the forefront of pathologisation, characterising disabled people as inherently damaged rather than victims of social injustice. Exploring psychological aspects of disability, in this view, would divert attention from the real, material issue of barriers to participation. Consequently, the cycle of victim-blaming would be perpetuated. But as disability studies has developed, mainly feminist scholars have objected to the materialist orthodoxy of the social model. These writers argue that a focus on the public domain of structural barriers sidelines the equally politically important worlds of the personal, the bodily and the psychological. The social model was unable to make provision for disabled subjects who were diverse and embodied, with personal and psychological histories upon which social suffering had left impressions. George Eliot's roar of human experience which lay beyond the silence required by the materialist view would present significant political dilemmas. The social model's need for this sterile disabled figure was clear, but it left much of the real-life experience of the disabled population un-theorised and uninterrogated.

Historically, it is true that most psychological theory on disability has taken an individual, pathology-oriented position, ignoring social realities almost completely. But this does not mean that a critical, contextual psychology of disability is impossible to create. To begin, a new model would aim to use psychological concepts to illuminate the intra-psychic and interpersonal mechanisms of prejudice, as well as tracing the psychological predicaments of the self in a disablist social milieu. Lifelong processes of socialisation, in which disablist culture impresses itself on impaired individuals, would be a central focus of study.

This book is an initial, exploratory response to the theoretical challenge sketched above. At centre stage is the question of whether we can create a psychological model of life in disablist society which mirrors individual intra-psychic reality, while making sure to retain an analysis of structural forces of inequality. Beyond this, dynamic psychological factors must be at work in both the origin and perpetuation of prejudice. These elements must be conceptualised if we are to understand their workings and begin to imagine change. I believe that the discipline of psychoanalysis has much to offer disability studies in addressing these difficult challenges. Like other branches of psychology, psychoanalysis' traditional theorising of disability has lacked any real contextual analysis – to most disability studies scholars its appearance here probably seems incongruous. Seldom recognised, though, is the power of psychoanalysis as a framework for social critique, aiming to unpack the unconscious narratives of inequality. Psychoanalysis is curious about the formation of the self and, in its more critical incarnations, how selfhood and ideology are connected by socialisation. The issue of the social mirroring disabled people are subject to applies directly here, posing questions about how disablist culture shapes the self. Further, psychoanalysis has much to say about the psychological nature of unequal intergroup relations, the scapegoating of minorities and the unconscious forces at work in political movements. From a critical psychoanalytic perspective, disabled people are used as containers for the projection of the disavowed existential conflicts of a control-oriented, self-centred modern world. There can be little question that disablist inequality has an influential unconscious narrative. We need psychoanalytic ideas to conceptualise this. As corollary, 'oppression' is not a visible, unidirectional force emanating from the dominant group. Instead, it is a dynamic social process, often involving the internalisation of disablist culture by those who are subordinated. In this model, change will require an understanding by all of their participation.

This work begins to develop psychoanalytically informed concepts which connect psychological experience to semiotic and material aspects of disablist culture. What is required is a psychological account of the trauma of socially situated disability, which carefully connects subjective struggle to the distorted social formations which surround the disabled body. In contributing to this project, this book uses the psychoanalytic lens to create a new, interpretive synthesis of a broad range of theoretical ideas on disability.

After thoroughly examining the epistemological crossroads at which disability studies finds itself, I use psychoanalytic ideas to explore socialisation in a disablist world. Besides the re-interpretation and evaluation of existing ideas, I draw on my own experience of psychoanalytically oriented group psychotherapy with severely physically impaired adults. The aim is to describe the often subtle psychological predicaments of life in a disablist culture, bringing dynamics of inequality into relief. The difficult, conceptually awkward reality is that disabled people have inner lives, histories and unique impairments. Somehow we must make a place for the subjective world of disablism; emancipation must surely depend on our ability to describe the lived effects of ideology. The poorly theorised state of problems such as internalised oppression constitutes both a critique and a limitation of disability studies and the disability movement. In addition, the interest in unconscious aspects of the disability phenomenon applies as much to the nature of disability theory and politics as to the underpinnings of oppressive social structures. Psychoanalysis can throw much light on the reasons why the terrain of disability is as contested as it is, incorporating heated disciplinary disputes as well as political conflict.

In the balance of this chapter we consider the cultural phenomenon of bodily symbolism; that is, the resilient logic that the nature of the soul, or the self, is 'written on the body'. On examining these meanings, there can be little question that disability has a trajectory of psychological experience which is rooted in culture and socialisation. After this I present a brief orientation to the worldwide development challenges facing the disabled community, orienting the reader to the global arena of disability inequality and politics. These short sections begin to sketch a world of distorted cultural and material responses to the impaired body. The balance of the book explores theoretical and political reactions to these problems, the lack of a psychological strand and possible new conceptual directions.

Written on the body[1]

Across world culture there exists a long history of explaining behaviour, and indeed self, through the nature of bodies. Somatic characteristics are by their nature compelling and material, instinctually drawing attention away from more subtle aspects of personhood, especially in the crucial first moments of contact. The body mesmerises us. It has the potential to indelibly mark out to the observer constraints upon what or whom the soul it carries may be. To the gaze, it is the body which provides a material, 'corporeal anchor' that reflects and that constitutes the psychological realm (Garland-Thomson, 1995, p. 603). Next to gender, the most widely influential bodily signifier is skin colour, which in every context holds a myriad of personal meanings, often expressed as binary oppositions between members of racial groups. Frantz Fanon placed fantasies about blackness at the very core of European civilisation (Fanon, 1952; Frosh, 1989). Further, as Morris (1993) notes, the correlating of physical attributes with undesirable aspects of the psychological self is, to say the least, familiar to the feminist movement. The response of feminism has been to locate such assumptions within a critique of socio-political context. Rosemarie Garland-Thomson (1995) tells of her dismay at a bedtime fairytale she reads to her young daughter, in which the 'good' girl's sexual and personal worth emanate from 'an outer beauty that parallels her inner virtue' (p. 599). Conversely, the 'bad' girl's poverty of morals and character is mirrored and confirmed by her indelicate, unfeminine features. For the 'bad' girl, the already devalued state of being a woman is made more condemning by failure to redeem herself with beauty. Attractiveness, thus, is firmly linked to virtue (Asch and Fine, 1988).

In a world of fervent somatic symbolising, disability is at centre stage. Bodily differences or 'flaws' lend themselves to analogies with deeper moral or civil shortcomings (Mitchell and Snyder, 1997). In Shakespeare's *Richard III*, there is no question that the protagonist's sinister, beastly ways are constituted mutually with his bodily deformity. In fact, he brazenly conspires with the audience, reasoning that since he is not worthy of this world's purer pleasures, villainy and avarice can be his only ambitions. In the horrific unfolding of the play, every twist can be 'traced back to Richard's consciousness of himself as a "deformed, unfinished" man' (Kriegel, 1987, p. 31). Richard is described as having teeth from before his misshapen birth, allowing him to 'gnaw a crust when two hours old' (*Richard III*, II.iv). Clearly identifiable here are ideas of base oral obsession, deprivation and greed, located within Richard from his very birth. His evil, therefore, is not so much a result of his deformity as a co-constituent with it of his overall self.

Modernity's promise of technologies to master the natural world brings hopeful possibilities – which quickly transmutate into obligations – to perfect the body. Bodies successfully made to appear youthful and powerful have 'increasingly become a sign of social worth', and pivotal to the 'notion of the self as a project' (Giddens, 1991 in Turner, 2001, p. 253). The fantasy of a body completely amenable to the perfecting, subduing action of technology singles out those who fail in this task as inferior, negligent or immoral. Davis (1997a) traces the late modern development of scientific measurement and assignation of the bodily identity. This ranges from scores on intelligence tests to fingerprinting. These characteristics supposedly express a coded genetic essence. The allocation of an indelible corporeal character, interspersed with measurements of prowess such as intelligence, laces each individual into an 'identical relationship' with his or her body (p. 15). Ultimately, the body embodies the identity. In this way, one's resultant identity becomes 'as indelible as one's place on the normal curve' (ibid.). Achieving normalcy on that same curve – by virtue of a body that is 'natural and healthy' – becomes a prerequisite for 'a good life … one worth living' (Michalko, 2002, p. 37). As we shall see, for people with 'errant' bodies there is the converse attribution. Namely, that these lives are not worth living.

So prized and praiseworthy are characteristics of vitality, health, vigour and energy in common-sense accounts that questioning their association with virtue may, at first glance, seem incongruous. Habitually, observations of how closely a body approximates the fantasy media ideal are accepted as compliments. Such compliments cleanse and illuminate not only the body, but also its 'inhabitant'. We revel in praise for our stamina, our ability to work long hours, our resilience and energy, our resistance to disease. But a discourse which constructs health not as a chance occurrence, but as an admirable achievement, is heard very differently from within a disabled body. Here, the individual is positioned as not only physically flawed, but also as personally deficient (Wendell, 1997).

In the cases of race and gender, interrogation of societal forces and the action of civil rights campaigns have worked to erode away bodily attributions. The evidence of oppression has grown and (to some extent) overtaken the urge to ascribe poverty, backwardness, immorality or any other form of inadequacy to bodily difference. Disability, though, presents opportunities for symbolisation which are legion, provocative and fantastic, rendering fantasies about the disabled self correspondingly florid. If the shape of the disabled body is infinitely diverse, infinitely contorted, so must be the shape of the disabled soul. Fantasies of limitless bodily dysmorphology feed, and feed upon, ideas regarding the frighteningly diverse states and shapes of the human character.

Through an examination of the history of the American freak show, Garland-Thomson (1997b, p. 59) shows how a distorted body may be so saturated with symbolism as to become 'pure text', obliterating humanity. Such 'enfreakment' (ibid.) is at one extreme of a continuum on which varying admixtures of body and self are able to be heard. But what her image demonstrates is the pervasive squeezing away of the self by bodies that are all-too-readily appropriated as text. The hegemonic position of the body as a text of identity is evident in universal drives to repair, correct and enhance its nature. When we improve our bodies, we improve ourselves. Paradoxically, this position both frees and entraps. We are seduced by the modernist possibility of change, while endorsing a meaning system which affixes our selfhood to an ultimately fragile and failing body. We have the illusion of control, at the cost of subjection.

The textual message emblazoned on the disabled body is, first and foremost, one of suffering and abjection. Throughout history, writes Henri-Jacques Stiker, disability and suffering have remained inseparable (Stiker, 1982). As liberal societies organise life and identity around axioms such as free agency, mastery, progress and individual will, the image of the disabled person destabilises the very foundations of convention, appearing as the absolute counterpoint to the 'good life' (Garland-Thomson, 1997b). In popular media in the United States, Hevey characterises the image of the impaired body as the 'site and symbol of all alienation ... the contorted body is the final process and statement of a painful mind' (Hevey, 1992, p. 73). So dominant are cultural associations to bodily frailty, according to Susan Sontag, that it is not possible to 'take up one's residence in the kingdom of the ill unprejudiced by the lurid metaphors with which it has been landscaped' (Sontag, 1991, p. 3).

Linguistic traces of the association of impairment with misery appear in a range of popular discourses. For example, allocation of individuals to the categories of 'fortunate' and 'unfortunate' occurs around a fulcrum of the body. In the midst of life crises or losses, the mantra that one is, in fact, 'fortunate' to have 'my health' is almost proverbial. Bodily impairment, consequently, is seen as prohibiting temporality or change in how one's sense of self is viewed. One simply is 'an unfortunate'. The unspoken nature of disabled experience occupies the pinnacle of a shadowy, yet consensual, hierarchy of suffering. If the self is written on the body; the wretched self is written on the impaired body.

One aim of this book is to present a new synthesis of ideas on why and how disablist inequality is so prevalent. But before tracing a course through the varying explanations offered by theoretical ideas, it makes sense to begin with an outline of the socio-political circumstances under which disabled people live. My discussion now moves to a short review of what is known about the structural disadvantages faced by the world's disabled population.

Disability: the international development context

Although substantial gaps in data exist, it is incontrovertible that a vast majority of the world's disabled population live in conditions of extreme disadvantage. Charlton calls this reality 'a human rights tragedy of epic proportions', which embodies 'a fundamental critique of the existing world system' (Charlton, 1998,

p. ix). Poverty, indignity, exclusion and the routine contravention of basic human rights are the touchstones of the social predicaments of the world's disabled population.

Disablist oppression is part of the structure of societies designed in ignorance of the needs and lifestyles of people with impairments. Exclusion manifests in visible and invisible, deliberate and inadvertent, active and passive aspects of everyday cultural, economic and political life. Rather than being the work of a bigoted minority, disablist exclusion recruits all as participants. Providing only for the needs of the nondisabled is a shared legacy.

Defining disability is a notoriously complex, contested task. Consequently, widely divergent definitions have provided global prevalence data sets which are 'inherently problematic' (Coleridge, 1993, p. 104). Combining this bewildering store of data has inevitably involved compromises, leading initially to an international prevalence estimated at 10 per cent of the population. This quickly became prominent in the discourse of disabled lobby groups worldwide. The 10 per cent figure was convenient as a hold-all descriptor for slogans, but was soon shown up as a coarse over-simplification. The estimate fostered the incorrect assumption that approximately one tenth of any population will be disabled, not allowing for the substantial variation in prevalence across contexts. This led to errors in estimates of resource provision. The largest and most sophisticated international data sets currently available are those reflected in the *World Report on Disability* (WRD), launched in mid-2011 by the World Health Organisation (WHO, 2011).

The report draws on two sources, the WHO World Health Survey of 2002–4, gathering together data from 59 countries, and the WHO Global Burden of Disease study of 2004. Confirming familiar difficulties, these data sets are not directly comparable, due to applying different instruments for measuring disability. The *WRD* confirms the broad variation in national prevalence, showing higher rates in developed than developing nations. According to the World Health Survey data, the average incidence of disability in the adult population (18 years and above) across all 59 countries was 15.6 per cent. This prevalence refers to adults described as experiencing 'significant functioning difficulties in their everyday lives' (p. 27). Prevalence rates for adults with 'very significant difficulties' were estimated at 2.2 per cent (ibid.). If these figures are interpreted to cover adults of 15 years and older, this translates into an international population of 720 million disabled people with functional difficulties, and a further 100 million with severe functional difficulties (ibid.). In reviewing the report, Shakespeare and Officer (2011) speak of 'the world's one billion children and adults with disabilities' (p. 1491). Global prevalence is set to escalate for many decades to come, due to population ageing, deterioration in the natural environment and the ongoing incidence of violence (Albrecht and Verbrugge, 2000 in Braddock and Parish, 2001).

It may surprise us that the statistical prevalence of disability in the developed world is considerably higher than that of the developing world, though the majority of the disabled population reside in developing contexts (Barnes and Mercer, 2005a). The greater prevalence of disability in wealthier countries is attributed to three major causes. First, in developed contexts the greater life expectancy and consequently larger population of aged persons leads to higher incidence of age-related impairment. The second cause relates to higher availability of health and other support services in wealthier states, producing higher survival rates in both congenital and adventitious impairment. As an adjunct, individuals are more likely to identify themselves as disabled if services are in place. Last, a range of less conspicuous impairments are probably under-identified in developing contexts. Conditions such as dyslexia may go unnoticed, or not be seen as carrying sufficient functional limitation to justify recording as an impairment (Coleridge, 1993; Barnes and Mercer, 2005a; WHO, 2011).

In both wealthy and under-developed nations, however, disabled persons remain among the poorest of the poor (Coleridge, 1993; Schriner, 2001; Barnes et al., 2002a). Schriner (2001) assures us that it does not 'overstate the case' to declare that disabled people are 'almost universally on the bottom rung of the socio-economic ladder' (p. 645). Through the course of the 1990s, international rates of unemployment among the disabled population changed little, despite the fact that anti-discrimination legislation was introduced in several countries during the decade (Oliver, 2001). Within even the world's most developed nations, rates of unemployment among disabled persons are frequently of the order of 80 per cent and beyond, with average personal income falling in the lowest decile (Braddock and Parish, 2001). Taking the United States as an example, by 2002 72 per cent of the disabled population remained out of work, with the poverty rate among working-age disabled adults topping three times that of their nondisabled compatriots (Davis, 2002). One third of disabled children in the United States live in poverty (ibid.). It is safe to assume that the economic circumstances of disabled communities in less affluent parts of the world are, for the most part, that much more dire.

Economic disadvantage is often interwoven with lack of access to resources needed for participation in social life. For example, gaining and retaining employment is impossible for a mobility impaired person in the absence of appropriate, accessible transportation. Mutua (2001, p. 105) relates how, in Kenya, many physically disabled individuals survive in a 'uniquely paradoxical state of being … present, yet completely invisible', as a result of being shut off from societal participation by the lack of usable transportation. The WHO estimated in 2001 that around 1 per cent of disabled people in the developing world have any form of access to rehabilitation or other institutional disability-related services (Barnes and Mercer, 2005a). Disabled children, especially girls, are regularly denied formal schooling in developing nation contexts (UNESCO, 1995; UN ESCAP, 2003; both in Barnes and Mercer, 2005a). In Flood's (2005) approximation, 2 per cent of disabled children in the developing world receive a meaningful education.

The absence or under-resourcing of disability-related social services in the developing world contrasts dramatically with palliative, preventive and rehabilitative care in wealthier countries (Barnes and Mercer, 2005a). But it should be kept in mind that such services are typically insulated from the broader social exclusions suffered by most disabled persons (Hagrass, 2005). In rich and poor countries alike, disabled citizens face 'formidable barriers to housing, transportation and freedom of movement, as well as exclusion or segregation in education and public accommodations' (Hahn, 2002, p. 165). Reviewing the development of accessible transportation in the European Union over the previous decade, Lawson and Matthews (2005) conclude that only moderate progress towards acknowledging the problem has been made, with reparative actions described as tentative and grossly insufficient. Where attempts at providing key resources such as housing, education, transport and public accommodations have been made by developed world administrations, disabled people have typically been positioned in life-worlds characterised by 'a more pervasive form of segregation … than the most rigid policies of apartheid enacted by racist governments' (Hahn, 1997, p. 174; see also Drake, 2001).

The voracious capital imperatives of a rapidly globalising economy, characterised by deregulation of employment, international trade and the global labour market, seem set to further compound the economic exclusions of disabled workers (Kelly, 2001; Holden and Beresford, 2002). Priestley (2005) poses important questions regarding the complex, often conflictual interchange between European Union disability policy and the particular national interests of member states. This highlights the defining influence of capital. Unfettered market forces have historically provided for a strong link between disability and poverty, which, according to many critics, is likely to deepen internationally. Holden and Beresford (2002) observe that the accelerating market imperatives of a global economy are unlikely to position issues such as the reform of disabling physical and administrative structures as a pressing priority. Events continue to validate this. The global financial crisis of 2008 and the subsequent recession have done much to reinforce these circumstances.

This backdrop challenges disability scholars to re-orient analyses to take account of the new, integrated global economy, including a critique of the influence of multinational corporations and financial institutions (such as the International Monetary Fund and the World Bank) on forces shaping management of labour (Sheldon, 2005). Globalised capital appears most ominous for poorer nations, but a lack of research, as well as poor infrastructure and service provision, mean that little is known about the life-situations of the majority of developing-world disabled people (Charlton, 1998; Barnes and Mercer, 2005a). Filling this knowledge void, myths and stereotypes regarding the 'backward' or 'traditional' treatment of disabled people in these contexts abound. Such myths include the belief that people in non-Western countries 'hide, abuse, and even kill' their disabled family members (Ingstad, 2001, p. 774). There is no denying that cases of abuse and hate crime occur. How incidents become representative reflects bias. As Ingstad puts it: 'we do not take single cases of child abuse to be typical examples of child care in industrialised countries' (Ingstad, 2001, p. 775). Beyond the lack of evidence to support such stereotypes, there is a danger of providing an excuse for governments who wish to obscure the reality of premature deaths resulting from poverty and a lack of health care (ibid.).

Although disability prevalence in developing nations is believed to be significantly lower than in wealthier countries, some researchers believe that as much as one half of such impairment would be prevented by better administration. In particular, effective policies to fight poverty and malnutrition, improvements in sanitation and the quality of drinking water and reforms in labour conditions are key influences on prevalence (Charlton, 1998; Barnes and Mercer, 2005a). The exclusion of disabled people from the world of work in many poorer countries, argue Harber and Davies (1997), is policed by the institutional gatekeeping of education. Being excluded from the educational system in early life is the experience of a large majority of disabled children at the economic periphery. This deprivation is used to legitimate lifelong inequalities, through the attributing of low occupational status to failure in educational achievement (Harber and Davies, 1997 in Barton and Armstrong, 2001).

Within international policy frameworks, interest in disability as an axis of inequality began emerging in the 1970s, beginning with the United Nations' *Declaration of the Rights of Mentally Retarded Persons* (1971) and *Declaration of the Rights of Disabled Persons* (1975) (Barnes and Mercer, 2005a). This was followed by 1981 being proclaimed the *International Year of Disabled Persons*, and the 10-year period from 1983 to 1992 the *Decade for Disabled Persons*. However, many critics view the impact of these seemingly substantial developments as limited by the predominance of an individual, medical and decontextualising view of disability (ibid.). The United Nations' *Standard Rules on the Equalisation of Opportunities for Persons with Disabilities* (1993) were formulated to provide an international benchmarking of standards for disability-related legislation, policy and programme implementation, although carrying no legally enforceable obligations (Braddock and Parish, 2001).

Meanwhile, the WHO attempted to develop a conceptual framework for research and policy development in disability, initially launched in 1980 as the *International Classification of Impairment, Disability and Handicap* (ICIDH) (WHO, 1980), and revised in 2000 as the ICIDH-2 (WHO, 1999) (later renamed the *International Classification of Functioning, Disability and Health*, or ICF). While the revised version represented a substantial attempt to move away from a traditional biomedical view of disability, the framework still sustained a heavy critique from disability studies quarters (Pfeiffer, 2000; Thomas, 2002). In essence, the WHO's approach has been seen by many disability scholars as prioritising the prevention of impairment, rather than foregrounding lived contextual realities such as discrimination and systematic exclusion (Marks, 1999a). In addition they argue that the schema's inherent logic ultimately ascribes disadvantage to intra-individual, impairment-based factors (Lunt and Thornton, 1994; Fougeyrollas and Beauregard, 2001; Thomas, 2002), although this is disputed by some (e.g. Bury, 2000; Shakespeare, 2006). Pfeiffer (2000, p. 1080) goes so far as to brand the ICIDH-2 a 'threat to the disability movement worldwide', due to its lack of a critical, constructionist approach to such issues as normalcy. With a mischievous tone, Miles (2001) pokes fun at attempts at developing an all-encompassing disability vocabulary. To Miles, such 'heroic linguistic labours' as those undertaken around the ICIDH and ICIDH-2 to establish internationally consistent terminology, are simply futile (2001; see also Altman, 2001; Fujiura and Rutkowski-Kmitta, 2001).

Over recent years, many have welcomed the emergence of the UN Convention on the Rights of Persons with Disabilities (CRPD) (UN, 2006) and the *World Report on Disability* (WHO, 2011; co-sponsored by the WHO and the World Bank). The CRPD was adopted by the UN General Assembly in 2006 and came into force in 2008. For many, it represents a landmark in international disability development policy. It is the first binding global treaty seeking to protect the human rights of the disabled population, requiring signatory states to provide equal access to services and prohibiting both direct and indirect forms of discrimination. There can be little doubt that the adoption of the convention is an important achievement, but questions regarding its enforcement and measurable effects will only be answered in time (Stein and Lord, 2010). The WRD, in turn, is a first step in developing analyses needed for successful implementation of the stipulations of the Convention. Bickenbach (2011) regards the WRD as ushering in a new, more critical and integrated era of international disability research. The emphasis is on evidence-based policy and the widest possible sourcing of data from the global disabled population (ibid.). The tone of this new initiative is one of attempting to get beyond traditional, unhelpful splits such as those between research and activism or medical and contextual models of disability. Shakespeare and Officer (2011) wholeheartedly support this approach, seeing the report as a 'tremendous opportunity to raise the profile of disability and rehabilitation across the world' (p. 1491). We await critical reviews of the WRD from other disability studies scholars.

One strategy aimed at countering the economic exclusion of disabled persons is anti-discrimination legislation. Leading an international trend towards this approach was the United States, where the Americans with Disabilities Act (ADA) was promulgated in 1990. Many believed the advent of this legislation would bring about a 'watershed moment' for global disability rights (Braddock and Parish, 2001, p. 50). As a point of departure, the new law affirmed that it was socio-political factors such as discrimination and the history of segregation which underpinned disability inequality in modern society, rather than intra-personal characteristics such as impairment (ibid.). Accordingly, the Act recognised discrimination against disabled individuals in the domains of employment, public services, public accommodations and telecommunications as unlawful (ibid.). This obliged employers to undertake reasonable adjustments to physical environments and practices in order to facilitate equitable inclusion. During the course of the 1990s several other nations followed suit, either adopting similar legislation or amending constitutions to prohibit disability-based discrimination; these included Great Britain, Australia, Germany, Austria, Brazil, South Africa, Malawi, Uganda and the Philippines (ibid.).

With hopes pinned on this legal experiment spearheaded in the USA, the disability movement was to be sadly disillusioned. In what Lennard J. Davis has described as 'a judicial backlash', well over 90 per cent of cases of discrimination brought by disabled citizens in terms of the ADA have been denied relief in US courts (Davis, 2002, p. 148; Colker, 2005). Judges in these cases have adopted a narrow and conservative reading of constitutional stipulations. They reached judgments overwhelmingly unfavourable to disabled plaintiffs (Hahn, 2001). This pattern, Harlan Hahn argues, is founded upon nondisabled lawyers and judges approaching disability civil rights issues from a 'functional limitations' rather than a 'minority group' paradigm, and hence abrogating 'their historic role of defending disadvantaged minorities and seeking to fulfil the promise of equality' (Hahn, 2001, p. 62). Hahn, along with a substantial proportion of disability studies scholars, has now forsaken the hope that significant progress towards collective disability equity can be achieved through the splintered, and often toothless, strategy of litigation (ibid.). Bickenbach and colleagues conclude ruefully that disabled people 'cannot expect emancipation by appealing to one of the many social institutions that oppress them' (Bickenbach et al., 1999, p. 1180).

An episode that was to become a milestone in the early galvanising of the global disability rights movement took shape at a world conference of Rehabilitation International (RI) in Winnipeg, Canada, in 1980. A dispute regarding adequate participation of disabled people in policy decisions led to the 250 disabled delegates deciding to boycott proceedings (Barnes and Mercer, 2005a; Flood, 2005). This sparked a drive for collaboration between the disability sectors of many countries, creating a new organisation called Disabled People International (DPI) which was composed of and run by disabled people (Barnes and Mercer, 2005a). The first international congress of DPI was held in Singapore in 1981, despatching a vehement message to the world that it was henceforth unacceptable for disability issues to be discussed without an equitable participation of disabled people (Flood, 2005). Worldwide, there is minimal adherence to this principle (Hahn, 2002; Hurst, 2005).

In terms of sheer numbers, the disability lobby is destined to swell considerably over the coming decades. The world's population is ageing due to shifts in patterns of reproduction, advances in medical technology and access to safer resources which increase longevity. How the disabled individual is constructed carries many incongruities, of which the following is a striking one. Age-related impairment somehow escapes the devalued disabled identity. According to Pope and Tarlov (1991), the average individual who reaches the age of 75 will experience limitation due to impairment for 13 of those years (Pope and Tarlov, 1991 in Marks, 1999a, p. 136).

It seems that the fact of ageing being our universal fate has led to the cultural fashioning of an artificial gulf between the 'real' disabled, and honorary 'normals' who are merely 'old'. We will examine this in more detail later. But for present purposes, the WHO predicts that by 2020 the planet will house more than 690 million people over the age of 65, in comparison with the estimated 380 million of 2002 (Davis, 2002). This massive inflation in the elderly population will radically change epidemiological patterns and health care needs (ibid.). Of key interest is the extent to which global ageing impacts on governments as well as citizens in mobilising change towards societies which are more accessible to people with impairments. If used strategically, the ageing of the world's population has potential to reposition disablement as a universal variable, rather than a characteristic of otherness.

In this opening chapter I have sketched the cultural idea of the body mirroring the self, as well as briefly outlined the development challenges which the world faces regarding its disabled population. From here we begin an examination of ways of making sense of both issues – cultural othering and material deprivation.

Note

1 After I decided on this descriptive phrase, I became aware that it is also the title of a novel by Jeanette Winterson (1992).

2 Theorising disability

The body, ideology and society

> For centuries, people with disabilities have been … isolated, incarcerated, observed, written about, operated on, instructed, implanted, regulated, treated, institutionalised and controlled to a degree probably unequal to that experienced by any other minority group.
>
> (Davis, 1997b, p. 1)

Introduction

Lennard Davis' strongly worded description of disability-based oppression would probably seem surprising, even incongruous to most people around the world. While we are accustomed to the idea of race and gender as axes of injustice and discrimination, common-sense thought has not yet come to associate the words 'disabled' and 'oppressed' (Watermeyer and Swartz, 2006). Instead, disability is viewed as a personal misfortune, with social consequences which – while regretted by all – are seen as inevitable, 'natural' effects of biological reality. Olkin (1999) neatly demonstrates how un-primed for exploring disability-based oppression we are. She asks us to think of the restaurants we have visited which are not accessible to wheelchair users. If one frequents restaurants, these are plentiful. We freely patronise these establishments which bar access to mobility impaired people; yet how would we feel about eating in restaurants which refused to serve Jewish or black people? To most thoughtful people, this would feel deeply 'unpalatable'. But with respect to disability, we calmly support social institutions drenched in discrimination and exclusion, in terms of practices, assumptions, built environments, delivery of services and every other aspect one could name.

Until recently, this unawareness was mirrored in academic discourse. Indeed, Abberley (1998, p. 80) remarks that 'the most common response of modern social theory to the disabled person's enquiry "what about me?" *is silence*' (my emphasis). Theoretical approaches to disability examined in this chapter thus appear against a behavioural sciences backdrop which has largely ignored disablist oppression. One intriguing demonstration of this is the reluctance of feminism to relate the cultural origins of gender inequality to the predicaments of disabled women (e.g. Garland-Thomson, 1997a; 1997b; McLaughlin, 2003). This is remarkable, since the body has – naturally – been the central arena for political contestation in feminist discourse (Wendell, 1997). Prominent nondisabled feminist scholars ignored disabled women's oppression, instead constructing this group as 'childlike, helpless and victimised' (Thomas, 1999a, p. 66). Disabled women found themselves ostracised from feminist ranks, as the movement sought to promote 'more powerful, competent and appealing female icons' (ibid.).

The attributions we make for the deprivation suffered by social groups tell a tale about our prejudices. In the case of disability, an absence of critical inquiry has allowed culturally condensed assumptions about the cause of inequality to remain invisible and unquestioned. In other words, our socialised understandings of what disability is and does have simply not been brought to light, let alone critically scrutinised. Until we problematise it, hegemonic racism parades as 'common sense'; disability prejudice remains in this realm of self-evident, unremarkable 'truth'. Typically, colloquial accounts reflect an 'individual model', which sees the marginality of disabled people as unfortunate, but ideologically neutral.

To help us examine ways of thinking about disability, Priestley (1998) provides a matrix for theoretical models, which incorporates two key dichotomies. These distinguish individual from social approaches, and materialist from idealist positions. Models applying an individual unit of analysis may be concerned with medical aspects, or management of identity and social roles at the individual level. That is, such accounts may have a materialist or idealist focus – prioritising physical or psychological features of bodily impairment respectively. Correspondingly, socially oriented models may be preoccupied with structural aspects of society or cultural representations of disability (ibid.). Paradigmatic roots of these orientations reflect an enduring debate in sociology between materialist (often Marxist) analyses, emphasising the influence of the economy upon culture, and idealistic standpoints rooted in the work of Max Weber, which argue the converse. But what is noteworthy for our purposes is that Priestley's taxonomy allows, at best, for an awkward space for accounts of disability which aim to relate the social and the psychological. It seems that analyses focused on the psychological realm can, in his view, only be 'individualistic'. Priestley's (1998) position is representative, underscoring how limited disability studies has remained in the quest to bridge ideology – the societal realm of beliefs and practices – with individual subjectivity. To be sure, an examination of the history of psychological accounts of disability seems to support the thesis that an intra-psychic focus cannot, by its nature, lead to critical, contextual and hence politically useful theory. This book aims to call this assumption into question. Instead of eschewing the psychological, the aim is to direct attention towards the development of bi-directional conceptual links between disablist culture and individual subjectivity, operationalised through the mechanisms of lifelong socialisation.

The question confronting us is whether it is possible to think about the psychological experience of disability while retaining a contextual, politically relevant analysis of discrimination. Are we able to overcome the reasons why these strains of disability theory have historically been mutually exclusive? But before we can explore the possibility of a synthesis, it is essential to map the theoretical and political landscape by examining the broad, opposing views of what disability is about. In the balance of this chapter we consider the so-called 'medical' and 'social' models of disability and the tensions and interactions these have generated.

The 'medical model'

Over the past century, the rise of Western biomedicine embedded a philosophy of health and illness centred on the scientific investigation and treatment of the body. Within this dominant paradigm, an epistemological hierarchy positions biological realities as the most important mode of attribution in making sense of human experience (e.g. Kleinman, 1987). What this means is that the core business of Western medical professionals has been the identifying and correcting of structural and functional 'defects' of the body; and that human struggle is viewed primarily as a consequence of such defects. But a host of critics take issue with the orientation's lack of provision for the 'social, psychological and behavioural dimensions of illness' (Engel, 1977, p. 130). Medical anthropologists have spearheaded this critique, bemoaning biomedicine's disregard for the socio-political contexts in which illness is experienced (Kleinman, 1986; 1987; Swartz, 1999).

Within the discipline of disability studies, the so-called medical model of disability – rooted in biomedicine – has been specifically slated for paying no attention to contextual factors which disadvantage disabled people (e.g. Oliver, 1986; Barnes, 1990; Abberley, 1996; Barnes et al., 2002a; 2002b; Barnes and Mercer, 2005a). These writers are critical of the biomedical approach as applied to all populations, but argue that its bodily focus places disabled people in especially invidious circumstances. At issue is the reality of the disabled population as a socially and economically marginal group; the gaze of biomedicine tends to attribute this marginality to bodily shortcomings rather than societal injustice. Abberley encapsulates the point elegantly: the 'medical model', he writes, 'functions to link together the experiences of an individual in a logic which attributes disadvantage to nature' (Abberley, 1996, p. 62). In examining 'defective' bodies, rather than how societies treat disabled people, social factors implicated in keeping disabled people at the margins remain unaddressed. The resultant, default view is that it is the intra-individual reality of impairment – 'nature' – that is at the root of disadvantaged status. In this way, the unwillingness of societies to correct avoidable exclusions remains papered over with wordless justifications.

Logically, it shouldn't surprise us that health professionals trained in biomedicine rather than social critique are drawn to bodily factors in making sense of individual lives. Very little in the training or occupational environments of such professionals is likely to direct attention towards social or ideological factors shaping disabled experience. But the effect can be a sustained depoliticising of the struggles of disabled individuals, who may themselves be subsumed into a generalised view of disability as bad luck rather than social oppression. Consequently, accountability for human rights contraventions is not tracked back to the ills of the social order. Instead, the 'damaged' body is excised from its world of power relations and capital exchange, disguising the reality of social suffering (Kleinman et al.,

1997). Implicated too, is the 'moral zeal' with which biomedicine pursues cure, with the drive to repair disseminating a culture of 'normalisation' which places those with irredeemable bodily differences in a questionable moral light (Marks, 1999a, p. 75; Hughes, 2002a). In this sense, disabled people may be subject to a more stringent version of the disciplinary regulation of bodies exercised upon all by modern health care (Foucault, 1976). Evidence of the moral imperative to 'healthy normalcy' is all around us; public health campaign messaging, for example, routinely depicts disabled people as the negative outcomes of unhealthy or irresponsible lifestyles (Lollar, 2001). Another influential political feature is the clinical encounter between disabled 'patients' and health professionals, which has traditionally been distinctly unequal, characterised by 'experts' defining and delivering services to 'passive recipients' (French, 1994a, p. 103).

While it seems clear that the disabled community has historically had good reason to problematise the approach of medical professionals, this position has at times become an extreme, destructive stereotype. A fashion for the zealous, simplistic vilification of health professionals en masse has emerged as an unfortunate side-effect of disability studies' critique of Western medicine. Misleadingly, the term 'medical model' appears to refer to medicine as a whole, and it has thus come to be experienced as a slur directed at all medical practitioners (Shakespeare, 2006). More confusing still, since the concept itself embodies a critique, no-one chooses to publicly espouse the 'medical model' (ibid.). To address such contradictions, some writers prefer the broader designation of 'individual' models of disability, of which medicalisation is one significant element (e.g. Oliver, 1996).

My own view is that the term 'medical model' is useful to denote a particular clinical stance which may, to a greater or lesser degree, be present in health care practice. It is thus not medicine per se, but rather a mode of performing medicine. The essence of this stance is an embedded curriculum of signs, overt communications and assumptions which identify bodily impairment as the central signifier and causal variable which shapes the social destinies of disabled people. Bodily difference is at centre stage, flanked by meanings such as loss, damage, dependency and a mandatory, even moral striving for normalcy – for cure. As noted, such ideas are not at all universally held by health professionals, nor restricted to them. On the contrary, medicalising views of disability are deeply entrenched in culture and socialisation on the broadest scale, assuming the imperceptible, hegemonic status of 'common sense'. As alluded to, practitioner and patient alike may therefore accept medicalising assumptions without question.

All who have grown up in a racialised society internalise differential conditioned responses to race groups, based on signs and meanings accumulated through the formative years. Critically examining the medical model sheds light on an analogous set of meanings we have accumulated regarding bodily difference. Careful reflection is required in order to bring 'natural truths' into relief as, in fact, culturally specific assumptions. Such self-exploration can reveal potent ideas about what impairment does, and why exactly it is that disabled people need our empathy. The prominent idea is that disabled people suffer shame, helplessness and deprivation arising from the brokenness of the body; not from social exclusion. Consequently, what is needed is care and cure, not political representation or social reform. The problem of disability, in short, is one of damaged bodies, not damaging societies. This somatic logic is what one would be likely to find among average citizens on a suburban street, where the words 'disability' and 'oppression' remain un-linked.

All around us – and dwelling within – is a raft of assumptions about what shapes and embodies disabled lives. Medical preoccupations, with associations of loss, compassion, shame and misfortune combine patient, practitioner and public culture in a consensus which sees the disabled person as a tragic unfortunate. Disability activism has put much effort into loudly opposing this image. I turn now to a discussion of the international disability movement's counterpoint to the medicalising view.

The 'social model'

An alternative, critical social model of disability emerged among disabled social science scholars in Great Britain during the 1970s. This group vehemently argued that it is the inattention of social systems to the participation-needs of impaired individuals which relegates disabled people to the margins (Oliver, 1986; 1990; Abberley, 1987; 1996; Barnes, 1990; Swain et al., 1993). According to the new, radical view, the exclusion of disabled people from participation at all levels of society is an avoidable social accomplishment – an ideological artefact, rather than one based on bodily dysfunction.

Launching a searing critique of dominant, prejudiced beliefs about disability, these authors demanded that discriminatory societies come under interrogation. At the centre of their approach was a conceptual distinction between the notions of *disability* and *impairment*. In the new schema, impairment was defined as a narrow, medical account of difference or dysfunction of the body. Separating off this diagnostic, somatic layer prepared the way for a new, subversive definition of disability, designed to bring oppressive ideology into relief. The wording below is a useful example of how social modelists came to construct disability:

> Disability: The loss or limitation of opportunities that prevents people who have impairments from taking part in the normal life of the community on an equal level with others due to physical and social barriers.
>
> (Finkelstein and French, 1993, p. 27)

This conceptualisation inverted the prevailing logic on disability, situating society itself as the 'patient' to be investigated. The new ailments under scrutiny were a complex, layered array of barriers to participation of impaired persons based in every level of social life – tangible, cultural, legal, institutional and so forth. So would begin a long and intricate process of unpacking society's distorted and discriminatory responses to the impaired body – a daunting task. From the stubbornness of prejudiced myths to the sweeping narrative of socially engineered segregation; from rehabilitation, normalisation and control to the demeaning exploitation of the freak show; from educational and occupational exclusion to the alienation engendered by a physical environment racked with unnecessary barriers; these things and much else became the subject matter of the social modelist cross-examination. In contrast to the scientific crispness of medical attributions, the social model's searching questions aimed to uncover complex layers of oppression woven into the very fabric of society's organisation. A model of disability with oppression at its epicentre had come into view, in which being disabled meant being subject to 'a complex system of social restrictions' inflicted by a 'highly discriminatory society' (Abberley, 1996, p. 61).

Social model theorists drew attention to how so-called 'normal' modes of living are structured by cultural and material worlds which only incorporate the needs of nondisabled people (Abberley, 1996). Medically sanctioned ideas of normalcy and aberrance emanating from this arrangement serve, in turn, to justify ongoing deprivation and ostracisation suffered by the disabled community (Braddock and Parish, 2001). Fiercely attacking biomedicine's individualising account of disability, social modelists branded the medical approach a personal tragedy theory (Oliver, 1986), underscoring how modern medicine's somatic fixation reduced collective injustice to chance personal misfortune. The depoliticising sleight of hand which construed disability struggle as natural, immutable and not subject to the structural mechanics of society was rejected in the strongest terms (Barnes et al., 2002a).

To writers such as Mike Oliver (e.g. 1990; 1996), the medicalising view of disability represented one victim-blaming ideological device among many others, all obscuring the structural origins of economic and political disadvantage. Other examples include the use of deficit theory to explain poor scholastic performance, character weakness as a cause for poverty and sickness as an explanation for criminal behaviour – the pattern is one of individuals being condemned, while social critique is circumvented (Ryan, 1971; Oliver, 1986). The onus for dealing with 'deficit' in all of these situations is placed squarely on the individual. Thus it is that despite the design apartheid of Western cities, mobility impaired persons are required to confront and 'deal with' built environments riddled with impossible obstructions (Imrie, 1996). Although not without its shortcomings, the social model continues to serve a valuable purpose in facilitating recognition of the everyday contravention of citizenship rights (Thomas, 1999a). The model proved capable of shifting disabled individuals from domesticating, static positions of self-deprecation to the just anger which grows out of recognition of discrimination. The social model message was a timely clarion call to political action.

At its extreme, the model construed disability as a completely material, social accomplishment, with no implications independent of history and context. The inference here is that a fully accessible society is feasible, in which impairment may be present without disability. As one moves away from this original, squarely materialist version of the social model – described by Priestley (1998, p. 80) as a 'social creationist' view – the orientation begins to intersect with a more social constructionist interpretation. In the social constructionist philosophical paradigm (Berger and Luckmann, 1966; Gergen, 1985) reality is viewed as intersubjectively socially constructed, redefining disability as an illusory cultural artefact. The two orientations are on a shared continuum, with the Marxian historical materialist geneology of the social model prioritising structural disadvantage, and constructionism foregrounding cultural representations.

A constructionist view of social oppression typically focuses on how positive identities are shored up through othering – a strategy involving the devaluing of an out-group (e.g. Tajfel and Turner, 1979). Othering rests on a view of the social world as composed of binary oppositions – so it is that there can be no such thing as 'madness' without the idea of 'unmadness', no 'reason' without 'unreason', and so forth (Oliver, 1990, p. 47; Foucault, 1995). The notion of disability, resting as it does on the ascribing of deviance, therefore only becomes feasible through the creation of the able-bodied or nondisabled identity (Oliver, 1990). Despite – or perhaps because of – the staunch materialist leanings of early social model theorists, a lacuna which calls for psychological concepts is already noticeable here; that is, an inability to explain the psychic need to disown unwanted parts of self through othering. Cixous and Clement (1975, p. 71) view the need for affirmation of identity through the denigrating of a social 'counterpoint' as so intrinsic to human emotional functioning that 'if there were no other, one would invent it'. A key aim of this book is to lay foundations for a merger of social and individual analyses of the disability phenomenon as, in my view, overlooking psychological aspects has greatly limited the usefulness of the social model. Quite simply, this deficit has meant that the model's ability to mirror and validate disabled life in a discriminatory world has, at best, been partial. Much more will be said about this later, after continuing our brief orientation to the emergence of disability politics.

The historical materialist view of social model thinkers such as Finkelstein (1980) – focused as it is on participation in the economy – traces the marginality of disabled people to early industrialisation in Europe. New, differentiated demands for labour mobilised the bureaucratic categorising of people according to labour power, over time creating the binary classes of 'disabled' and 'nondisabled'. This was the beginning of a sustained operation of identifying, measuring and separating out those with compromised capacities to participate in production (ibid.). Over time, these divisions solidified into segregation, the rise of institutionalisation and the entrenchment of disability as a key axis of structural discrimination (Barnes, 1990). The social circumstances of disabled people during mediaeval, pre-industrial times are an issue of some dispute. Accounts range from an idealised picture of an integrated, diverse society not yet contaminated by the distortions of capital markets (e.g. Finkelstein, 1980), to one of disabled lives marked by unmitigated hardship, ostracisation, deprivation and death (e.g. Winzer, 1997; Borsay, 2002).

In the Foucauldian discourse analysis tradition, Stiker (1982) adds to the picture by associating the horrors of 'the war to end all wars' with the rise of biomedical rehabilitation, and its normalising strivings. The colossal devastation during World War 1 of the material and cultural stuff of which society is composed was mirrored, macabrely, by the multitudes of 'distorted' bodies to be re-assimilated into its ranks. A need to believe in quasi-magical repair for this desolation found form in prosthetics, and generalised to a view of individuals – and society at large – as machines amenable to reconstruction (ibid.). But the goal of such restoration took shape as an unreal, idealised fantasy of what came before the apocalypse – a perfect, harmonious society populated by pristine, functional bodies. The normalising gaze of rehabilitative medicine had begun to impress itself on the impaired body (Foucault, 1979). Stiker (1982) carefully distinguishes between 'cure' – defined narrowly in relation to health – and the ideological forces of uniformity and control characteristic of 'normalisation'. Correspondingly, most social model proponents, although critical of medicine's purported imperative to normalise the body, emphasise that accessible and appropriate health services are a basic human right.

Although both founded broadly on social model principles, the political strategies of the UK and US disability rights lobbies assumed differing courses in the late twentieth century. In the USA, the diversity of the population and the rise of the civil rights movement in the 1960s pointed towards a strategy relying on litigation and the promise of anti-discrimination laws (Hahn, 2001). The Americans with Disabilities Act (ADA) of 1990 was the culmination – albeit a deeply disappointing one to most – of this policy. Many now view the American strategy – known as the minority model approach – as a blunder which fragmented the disability issue into the legal ramifications of individual cases, missing the opportunity for a mass challenge to the status quo (ibid.). Conversely, the Marxian class politics roots of the British social model movement defined disability struggle collectively, in terms of the denial of access to the means of production (ibid.). This attack on inequality relied heavily on group solidarity, arguably fostering the enforcement of orthodoxies – that is, beliefs about the 'real' nature and origins of disability. The UK and US approaches have faced formidable obstacles to social change, not least of which is the fact of disability in the developed world as a multi-billion dollar industry, incorporating an elaborate web of professional, organisational and cultural interests (Albrecht and Bury, 2001).

One arena of social modelist orthodoxy is the ever-present and, at times, acrimonious debate surrounding politically correct terminology. An example is the quarrel regarding *people first* language – advocated by US minority model adherents, and heatedly rejected by UK social modelists (Albrecht et al., 2001). People first language is of the form 'people with disabilities' rather than 'disabled people'; it is intended to stress disablement as one attribute among others, not something intrinsic. Into the bargain, the usage seems to fit well with an American capitalist emphasis on the individual, and the litigation-based counter-oppression strategy of the US disability movement (ibid.). To social modelists, the favoured term 'disabled people' connotes the anti-medicalising idea of 'people disabled *by* society'. People first language, on the contrary, is seen as naively accommodating prevailing ideas of disability as individual defect, rather than exogenous ideological force.

Our introduction to psychoanalytic thought must wait until the next chapter, but this issue provides a helpful opportunity for the first of a few previews. In movements forged around suffering, injustice and social change, disputes over politically correct language are ubiquitous. Sinason (1992) argues that the endless flux in permissible language stems from the need to quell intolerable parts of unconscious life stimulated by provocative ideas such as impairment. For her, the clamour around appropriate terms for sexual orientation, mental illness, race, disability and the like reflects an insatiable craving for euphemisms able to thwart the painful reality of human difference. The wish to deny difference, though always only gratified temporarily, maintains the need for new ideals, and new villains. The world of learning disability (or intellectual impairment/mental retardation/mental handicap) is a case in point.

For the architects of the social model, re-authoring disability as a collective predicament meant adopting a certain 'strategic essentialism' (Garland-Thomson, 1997a, p. 283). Perhaps inevitably, the need to create some sense of homogeneity led to the masking of a mosaic of diverse experience; in fact, a reluctance to engage with the multiplicity of impairment later became an important criticism of the social model. Interestingly, this difficulty was presaged many years before by Irving Zola, an early disability studies scholar. Zola (1988), seemingly cautious about politically expedient over-simplifications, viewed disability as a continuum, rather than a categorical absolute (Altman, 2001). In the following three sections, I will discuss the social model's lack of nuance and flexibility, along with related criticisms.

Criticising the social model

It should not surprise us that a movement dedicated to political action and based on an historical materialist view of society falls short in mirroring disabled personhood. Nuanced, finely toned representations of social reality do not fit well with galvanising revolutions. Instead, the anger of oppressed peoples is harnessed through the cutting of binary distinctions between villains and victims. In psychoanalytic terms what we see here are the defensive simplifications of *splitting* (in the Kleinian object relations tradition), drawing all into reverberating, inflexible distinctions between self and other (Klein, 1946) – much more on this topic later.

Critics of the early social model took issue with a host of its authors' assumptions. As noted above, the strategic essentialism approach meant that the rubric disabled people must connote commonality – a shared predicament of oppression (Oliver, 1990). This enforced sameness provoked steady objections from feminist disability scholars (e.g. Morris, 1989; Wendell, 1996; Thomas, 1999a). At issue was the variable impact of other, superimposed identities on the circumstances of disabled people. As early feminist theory was critiqued for being rooted in white, middle-class Western assumptions, social model pioneers were accused of reducing the experiences of a diverse disabled population to the common denominators of their own lives; that is, the circumstances of middle-class, white, male, Western wheelchair users (Marks, 1999a, p. 87). A model forged amid such a group, the argument went, could not adequately illuminate the struggles of disabled members of ethnic or sexual minorities (Begum et al., 1994; Shakespeare et al., 1996), or of people with different impairments, such as those of a sensory, psychiatric or intellectual nature (Crow, 1992; Morris, 1992; French, 1993a). Instead of an amalgam of contextual and impairment factors, the social model was solely focused on material 'barriers to inclusion' – at that, barriers prominent only to a subset of impaired people.

The need for a counter-narrative to the biomedical view had created a model unable to accommodate unique aspects of individual experience. The reality of diversity, in this climate, appeared as a contaminant to the force, clarity and unity of the social model movement. Exploring difference came to be seen as akin to self-sabotage, opening the way for a regressive confirmation of precisely those medicalising, individualising views that the social model aimed to dismantle. As we shall see, the personal was to be prohibited. Recognition that the social model prism can only shed light on a segment of disabled life led some authors to allege – or concede – that it is more a political device than a theory. Thomas (1999a, p. 26) understands the model as an essential conceptual point of departure, but one which 'poses rather than answers important theoretical questions about disability'. At the heart of the model is the disability versus impairment binary, which presumes that culture has no corporeal substrate, and that a pristine, presocial body exists independent of social construction.

As noted, the social model's failings should not prevent us from giving the viewpoint its due. Overturning acquired wisdom, the approach unearthed a store of suffering and dispossession which before had likely translated into self-blame, or been written off as deviance. Without the model this sea change would not have occurred. But the consequent, emergent psychosocial debris is too complex, too tangled between society and soma to be dealt with in dichotomies. Shakespeare (2006, p. 12), in an at times scorching appraisal of the British social model 'establishment', describes the approach's key insight as 'important and unarguable', but having sedimented into a misleading orthodoxy. The essence of this 'dogma' is that disability is '*everything* to do with social barriers, and *nothing* to do with individual impairment' (ibid., my emphasis). By contrast, a number of disabled authors describe their experience as ambiguous and shaded – not entirely impairment based or entirely socially produced. As example, Sally French (1993a) – herself closely associated with the social model perspective – emphasises how her life has been shaped by discrimination based on her sight impairment. But she also points out how a layer of her difficulties lies 'in between' her body and society – not reducible to impairment, but also not amenable to social intervention. For instance, her inability to recognise faces, though dealt with in repeated clarifications with others, continues to create misunderstandings which disrupt easy relating. She warns against the illusion of a disability-free Utopia, where complete equality is achieved by removing all barriers.

One field in which this illusion may arise is that of assistive technology. As a partially sighted university student, French (1993a) had required assistance from librarians in identifying and sourcing literature – traditional, paper-based library systems are very much sight-oriented. Later, and with a little fanfare, her university installed a computer data-base system which used voice synthesis technology, for use by sight impaired students. Enthusiastically endorsing the principle of disability as an eradicable social artefact, university authorities declared that sight impaired students now had full and equal access to library research. In the experience of French and others this was quite untrue. In a familiar paradox, assistive technology never fully meets the diverse needs of the impaired population; what does occur, though, is that feelings of entitlement to personal assistance are diminished (ibid.). Of course, this does not question the human rights obligation to provide assistive technology in promoting equal access – on the contrary. But the idea of a barrier-free society which provides fully for a very diverse impaired population is, as French (1993a) warned, a dangerous myth.

The modus operandi of social model politics has been to foist every fragment of disability struggle onto structural exclusion. And of course, the disadvantaged, even dehumanising circumstances under which a vast population of disabled people live worldwide lends good reason to this approach. The dogged focus on social barriers is an irate reaction to a world that seems entranced by the 'failings' of the body; a world in which the belief that inherent defects will always mean inequality routinely justifies a failure to address avoidable barriers. The common logic at work here is that 'we can't change society to suit everybody … everybody's needs are just too different', or 'it will cost too much'. The reality of an inevitable, residual layer of 'impairment effects' (Thomas, 1999a) is regularly used as a rationalisation for doing nothing at all to promote equity in the lives of the most marginal.

The social model's problem with integration of diverse, individual impairment factors with structural barriers to participation is no small matter. Shakespeare (2006) reasons that since the disability–impairment distinction is elemental to the social model, and its logic is unsustainable, the model should be abandoned. In his view, a British ivory tower of social model orthodoxy has impoverished disability studies, isolating contributors seen as not subscribing strictly enough to its politics. Potentially important work has, on the basis of politically incorrect terminology or adherence to the maligned ICIDH and ICIDH-2 (Bury, 2000), been relegated to the research junk-heap labelled 'medical model'. Very relevant here is the fact that the US disability studies tradition is substantially more wide-ranging than its UK counterpart, with roots in the liberal arts and humanities, in addition to the social sciences (Hughes, 2009). Less constricted by social model prescriptions, American researchers have thus been more responsive to recent shifts towards postmodernism, cultural studies and embodiment (ibid.). Nevertheless, American writers as eminent as Lennard J. Davis, Harlan Hahn and Susan Wendell are among those who have seen their work denounced for its purported lack of political clout (Shakespeare, 2006).

The labour politics roots of the social model, for Shakespeare (2006, p. 27), show up in the 'hard, combative and ideological' methods of its campaigners, who view a progressive respect for human rights and inclusiveness as impossible in the absence of their approach. The picture, at times, tends towards a fundamentalism which refuses critique and, according to Lee (2002, p. 148), promotes an immature politics which 'inhibits the development of realistic strategies' which may promote individual inclusion. The model's disdain for the personal precludes what Lee (2002) calls a 'politics of individual actions and interventions' (ibid.). Rather than vilifying medical intervention in disabled lives, such a politics would make nuanced theoretical provision for it, allowing conceptually for unique aspects of disabled experience. Lee (2002) underscores the point by drawing an analogy between the social model and leftist intellectual accounts of poverty. While it is certainly accurate to see poverty as a problem generated by systemic capitalism rather than individual failings, to suggest that we may only eradicate it through a wholesale conquering of capital represents a 'phenomenally simplistic politics' (ibid., p. 148). Oppression, here, is seen as a unidirectional force exercised on faceless individuals who are altogether subjectified by crushing ideology – a system of villains, victims and malevolent hegemonies to be overthrown. By contrast, Lee (2002) is correct in asserting that it is 'naïve' to presume that individual behaviour in no way contributes to the perpetuation of poverty. In the disability arena this recognition places us on the threshold of what is, to social model thinking, the unspeakable terrain of complicity. The response of social model writers to this theoretical moment has been the spurning of all things psychological. As already noted, it is only fair to recognise that the history of psychological accounts of disability shows that fears about oppressive, pathologising individualism are not at all unfounded; but it is now time to brave more nuanced, uncertain waters.

If political movements choose to rely on oversimplified binaries for the good of their cause, the identities of oppressed and oppressor become increasingly reified. Social constructionist thinkers on disability assume an opposite course, attacking oppression through disrupting the category of 'disabled person' itself. But adherents of a narrow social model approach have instead endorsed the disabled–nondisabled dichotomy, and hence invested in developing a positive disabled identity (e.g. Swain and French, 2000; 2008). The strategy here is to reclaim and re-validate the disabled identity, rather than question its logic. With Shakespeare (2006), I believe that progressive disability politics need not rely on such separatism – a strongly contextual position can also provide for theoretical and individual variation. Disability studies is not alone in these challenges; on the contrary, this debate reflects a watershed moment in radical politics on the broadest scale (Paterson and Hughes, 1999). This is a time of 'turmoil and reorientation', where 'the Marxist certainties of the past have given way to post-Marxism and post-modernity, to a context in which politics spills into culture, if not amorphousness' (ibid., p. 600).

The need to rely on separatist, polemical rhetoric emanates not only from recognition of the social predicaments of disabled people, but also from the evocativeness of disability itself. No matter what one's position on the social–medical debate, disability as a construct is deeply imbued with associations of suffering and trauma; as such, it is perennially emotive, divisive. Valerie Sinason's (1992) comments above on the emotional motives for political correctness correspond closely here. Because of this provocativeness, disability dwells, for all, in a realm of thought shaped by the defence of splitting (e.g. Bion, 1970). Put simply, because of its meanings disability is difficult to think about; in the face of these meanings, we find refuge in dichotomy. This observation does not at all question the material suffering caused by the negligence or cruelty of disablist societies, or devalue the motives of those who strive for change. The point is this. To get inside the disability phenomenon we must theorise the mutually constitutive interaction of both social and psychic variables. These are played out in our political positions and actions, our awareness and unawareness. The social model movement, like other revolutionary formations, is incomplete without an account of the personal and psychological, but simultaneously unable to accommodate one.

Prohibiting the personal

> Our anger is not about having a chip on the shoulder, our grief is not a failure to come to terms with our disability. Our dissatisfaction with our lives is not a personality defect but a sane response to the oppression which we experience.
>
> (Morris, 1992, p. 163)

Jenny Morris reflects above on the moment in feminist discourse in which the subjective struggle of women – of rage, grief and confusion – ceased to be viewed as an endogenous product of biology. Thus began the exploration of women's experience as a phenomenology of gender domination, not the outpouring of individual or biological temperament. The growing awareness of the social model's inability to conceptualise the psychological carries strong parallels. This is about disabled people realising that their experience is worthy of contemplation, and that the roots and consequences of oppression are to be found in both inner and outer worlds (Thomas, 2001; Hughes, 2002a). Emotional turmoil, here, may show up as a sane response to 'mad' circumstances, rather than evidence of madness (Griffin, 1982 in Morris, 1992). Like the psycho-political predicaments of women, disabled life-worlds are littered with cultural mechanisms which promote the turning inward of anger or distress, reducing social oppression to personal shortcoming. The backdrop of exclusion in a host of domains, especially education and employment, structures a limitless supply of subject matter for self-pathologisation. Further, continued subscription to a Cartesian separation of body from society relegates personal experiences of impairment to a shadowy inner world. In this realm, these may interact with the residues of degrading socialisation, which make sense of struggle through self-blame.

In the gender realm, to split public and private worlds means to collude with the pernicious idea that such matters as familial roles, sexuality and domestic violence are not, in fact, 'political' concerns (Thomas, 1999a). The social model's material and public focus brings about equivalent oversights, through what has been called 'contextual essentialism' (Söder, 1989 in Shakespeare, 2006, p. 56). It is inaccurate to accuse social model authors of completely ignoring the psychological realities of disablism, but it is undeniable that the model allows for the most awkward of spaces to examine these issues. Responding to the critique of Morris and others, some social model authors have argued that emotional struggle should, in fact, be regarded as a most direct and painful manifestation of oppression (Abberley, 1993; Finkelstein and French, 1993; Oliver, 1995). Still, these same writers discourage exploration of the psychological level (e.g. Finkelstein, 1996), holding firm to the idea that 'exclusion from the world of work is the most important factor in what happens to disabled people' (Oliver, 2001, p. 149).

In steering clear of an embodied and psychological construct of personhood, the social model seems clumsily out of step with contemporary shifts in social theory. Noted psychoanalytic social theorist Stephen Frosh remarks that 'something unexpected' has taken place across social science disciplines, where the political has truly become personal – in fact, 'some might say it has become so personal as to no longer be political' (Frosh, 1991, p. 1). Increasing notice is being paid to how ideology coalesces at the intra-psychic level, investigating the self as a product and agent of social power. Contemplating his own political development, Hoggett (1992, p. 3) comments with surprise at how prior paradigms unabashedly ignored the individual. He writes: 'the mysteries of life and death, of feeling and passion, of dreaming and imagination, of love and terror – it was as if these things didn't exist'. In this Marxist world, one only qualified as 'politically committed' through aligning oneself to a 'shallow view of life' (ibid.). For Hoggett and others, a materialist orientation which denies the materiality of the body – its flux, advance and decay – just made no sense. In addition, neuroscience's emerging picture of the psyche as an entity with 'its own laws of structuration and process' (ibid.; Pinker, 2003) was set to further upset the Marxist picture of humans as 'some kind of putty on which social forces work' (Hoggett, 1992, p. 6). Axel Honneth (1995) is similarly critical of traditional social theory's fixation with material interest, with its consequent disregard for how moral feelings shape the social order. Significantly, he stresses that even though a collective interest may correspond with a social conflict, the conflict is not necessarily reducible to that interest. Social struggles, to Honneth (1995) have a 'moral grammar' – that is, a narrative of meanings and motivations which may coincide with material interests, but have their own basis in psychology, identity and culture. Very recently the beginnings of a recognition from within disability studies that the psyche is itself a cultural, ideological artefact have emerged (Goodley, 2011a; 2011b). Goodley (2011a), however, takes care to limit his analysis to the 'valued other' – that is, the psychological lives of nondisabled people under exposure to disability imagery. And as we shall see, his point of departure has been one starkly dismissive of psychology as a discipline. Nevertheless, this work seems to echo my own call for an exploration, within disability studies, of the relationship between ideology and selfhood.

For our purposes, one implication is that the social standing (the esteem, the identity) of disabled people must be included as part of a mutually constitutive dialectic which, along with material realities, shapes social destiny. Borsay (2002) applies this logic in disputing the social modelist understanding of the emergence of disablism during the development of modern Western economies. As described earlier, this view sees the rise of industrialisation, with its centralisation of economic and political power, as primary in forcing disabled people to the margins (Barnes, 1990). Borsay (2002) argues that this account is not only historically flawed, but also conceptually inadequate, since it tells us nothing about cultural factors. A convincing historical picture must hold 'materialism and culturalism – or structure and agency – in tension' (ibid., p. 104).

While thinkers such as Frosh revel in the re-psychologising of the social subject, strong social model adherents are among those who fear that politics will so collapse into the personal as to no longer be political at all. To these scholars, psychological explorations are diversionary, and will inevitably be misappropriated in pathologising disabled people. What Finkelstein, Oliver, Barnes and others seem to be saying is that disabled people cannot afford to make their struggles known, as these will be prejudicially attributed to an 'inherent wretchedness' that accompanies impairment. This will offset the political drive to interrogate exclusion, by confirming disability stereotypes of vulnerability, dependency and damage. Finkelstein (1996, p. 34) describes a concern with personal experience as a 'discredited and sterile approach to understanding and changing the world', arguing that the disability movement has been hijacked by academics bent on replacing the active vision of resistance with 'passive theoretical abstractions'. As we shall see, the debate has remained a vibrant one since these words. But while the social model position has been augmented – particularly in the work of Thomas (1999a; 2001; 2007) – an essential thread of Finkelstein's resistance remains. This book is a direct challenge to this position: in my view, the claim that we may adequately theorise social disability without considering the intra-psychic is at best impoverishing; at worst dangerous.

The distaste which social model theorists feel for phenomenological research finds expression in the fractious relationship between 'mainstream' disability studies and the discipline of medical sociology (Thomas, 2007). This field, also known as the *sociology of health and illness*, explores the experience of chronic illness and disability, focusing on symbolic meanings and the creation of personal narrative (Williams, 2001). Such work is accused of buttressing a medical view through failing to interrogate the context of the disability struggle being depicted (Thomas, 1999a). Theoretical perspectives often used in such investigations combine symbolic interactionism in the tradition of Erving Goffman (1963), and phenomenology, pioneered by Maurice Merleau-Ponty (1962). Critics describe how journeying into the subjective experience of disability renders an ever-deepening, solipsistic and at times quasi-religious account, losing touch with the structures which shape life trajectories (Thomas, 2007). Such narratives capture what Finkelstein (1996) scornfully calls 'inside-out research', which begins with the individual, and becomes so tangled up with the interstices of the internal world that the social is never reached. Instead, the picture is filled with how sufferers 'cope' with chronic illness or disablement, damage to identity and the re-configuring of self-worth; the social origins of subjective states are typically not explored (Thomas, 2002).

In an early response to the political versus personal dispute, Colin Barnes (1998) pointed out that the social model itself grew out of experiential accounts of discrimination – a fact which is typically overlooked. Nevertheless, at this stage, Barnes' influential voice positioned research integrating experiences of impairment, fatigue, pain and depression as inherently unhelpful, as well as a redundant replication of the medical sociological literature. His view (e.g. Barnes et al., 2002a) has broadened slightly to include 'extended' social model work such as that of Thomas (1999a) and Reeve (2002), which we will examine later. But as with Finkelstein (1996) and other members of the social model vanguard, the essence of a steadfast materialist position remains. Barnes is staunchly critical of work which, in his words, 'effectively blurs the crucial distinction between the experience of impairment and the experience of disability' (1998, p. 77). What this position assumes is that somewhere in the tangle of biology, socialisation, perception and subjectivity, a clear distinction between these entities serenely awaits discovery. He then goes on to inform his reader that depression, fatigue and pain are not 'unique' to disabled people, and that large numbers of disabled people will never encounter these experiences. Of course this is true; but of interest is the need to reiterate it here. Understandably, Barnes aims to debunk the cultural connection between impairment, pain and dysfunction, and emotional suffering. But in doing so he risks dissociating disabled people from emotional struggle altogether, shearing off psychology and subjectivity with one expedient, Cartesian stroke. One may accept the critique of medical sociology's partial, skewed account of disability; but to respond to this difficulty with an adversarial, equally partial analysis seems intellectually irresponsible. Thomas (2002) intervenes by proposing that the social model does not deny the functional restrictions and physical experiences of impairment, but that these do not constitute 'disability'. She terms these limitations *impairment effects*, thus 'rehabilitating' the beleaguered disability–impairment distinction. The ideological motivation for this conceptual hopscotch is clear, and admirable. But an insurmountable fault-line in the social model's logic is coming to light.

The quest to develop a multi-layered construct of disability seems to leave one between a rock and a hard place. That is, lost in existential solipsism, or impoverished by an arid, dehumanising materialism. Some authors argue that political vigour can be retained while exploring the 'darker phenomenological waters' of individual narrative (Williams, 2001, p. 139; Turner, 2001). The difficulties with this are substantial – these are the narratives of subjectivities forged within a specific cultural soup of disability meanings. Is it possible to critically examine the origins of subjectivity by studying subjectivity itself? Scholarly and enriching auto-ethnographic contributions to the medical sociology tradition demonstrate – I believe – the problem of creating theoretical strands to connect internal turmoil, bodily difference and the mechanisms of ideology (e.g. Murphy, 1987; Toombs, 1994; Frank, 1995; 1998). Identification with the subject and feelings of pity or empathy tend to eclipse any critique of political context (Mitchell and Snyder, 1997). Importantly though, there remains heated dispute regarding the tension between methodological rigour and an ethical imperative to simply 'hear' and accept individual narrative (Thomas, 2010). Atkinson (1997), for example, is harshly critical of the work of writers such as Frank (e.g. 1995) and Kleinman (e.g. 1988), who view illness narratives as inherently coherent and meaningful, rather than texts to be critically interpreted. Excessively pursuing objectivity and methodological purity, to these authors, means sacrificing something of the subtle, essential value of narrative (Thomas, 2010). Arthur Frank in particular is suspicious of the call to 'neutrality', seeing this as a veiled demand for patients' stories to acquiesce more closely to the authority of the medical gaze (Frank, 2000). In general, it seems fair to say that the emotional hyper-arousal around cultural meanings of disability does tend to obscure material deprivation – personal tragedy captures the imagination much more readily than discrimination. It is a tragedy typically incorporating a paradox of enmeshed sentimentality and potent othering; a powerfully prejudiced construct. But to bury the tragic imago[1] is simultaneously to conceal real disability experience, including the painful impressions made on subjectivity by disablism. This stance tends to disregard oppression operating in personal domains such as self-identity, interpersonal relationships, sexuality and family (Thomas, 1999a). Thomas goes on to say that materialism's eliding of these concerns leaves critical disability theory vulnerable to 'psychologists and others' who would 'not hesitate' to apply an individualising model in filling these theoretical breaches (ibid., p. 74). While her point is clear, the depiction of psychologists – of whom I am one – demonstrates a startling degree of discomfort with imagining a critical, ideologically situated psychology of disability. She is not at all alone in her impressions of the discipline – disability studies has predominantly viewed psychology as a 'pathologising, voyeuristic, individualising, impairment-obsessed discipline that has contributed to the exclusion of people with impairments' (Goodley and Lawthom, 2005, p. 136). As an antidote to this 'scourge', these authors present community psychology and participatory action research, setting this field up in opposition to a homogeneous, oppressive monolith. Clinical psychology, here, is seen as inherently – immutably – disinterested in political engagement. In a direct rebuttal, Forshaw (2007) describes this position as 'outdated'; I would add short-sighted. The disability-related problems of applied psychology, as with all health disciplines, must be addressed through building relationships of mutual openness, resisting the splits which have so often led to the abandoning – rather than transformation – of valuable resources.

Frosh (1989) is very clear that the curse of racism is perpetuated as much in the individual psyche as at the level of collective interest. A psychological model of racism, thus, is not a substitute for a socio-political analysis, but an essential complement to it. Psyches forged in fields of ideological meaning and competing interest imbibe significations which become tangled with subjective life, confusing and hybridising agency with ideology, volition with power. This psychic precipitate of social process appears in all, shaping the unconscious lives of oppressor and oppressed alike. Frantz Fanon (1952), similarly, viewed racism as 'a story that takes place in darkness' – an internal darkness – thus requiring that 'the sun that is carried within me must shine into the smallest crannies' (p. 29). In other words, if oppression is to be overcome, all actors within a social system must look inward.

The crux of Frosh and Fanon's view is that racism – prejudice – is in part embedded in irrational layers of ourselves; these are places where appeals to reason carry little sway. Returning to disability, Clegg (2006) reports findings on the meanings which learning disabled clients attach to 'rational' social service policies. As per their social model origins, these protocols deal only with environments and behaviour, not personal experience. But searching questions reveal that service users attach personal meanings to material conditions. For example, it was found that learning disabled boys using respite care often imagine that they have done something wrong, as their siblings are not required to stay away from home. Similarly, people who had been physically restrained often understood this as an arbitrary decision, with implications for how safe and wanted they felt in their residential setting. As we shall see, Valerie Sinason's (1992) ground-breaking work on the social suffering of learning disabled people demonstrates the impact of such meanings. Sinason (1992) showed the immense influence of trauma – the trauma of consciously or unconsciously recognising that one is not wanted – on both the emotional and cognitive functioning of her learning disabled subjects. Meanwhile, a study by Morris (1989) appeared to confound social modelist expectations about the core concerns of disabled people. In her interviews with women with spinal injuries, Morris (1989) found that their most common difficulty with health care professionals was a lack of consideration of emotional aspects of disability. It is becoming clear that the world of disability has human reach which extends way beyond the material and rational, beyond tangible barriers, to the recesses where these are mirrored in psychic life.

From a development studies perspective, Coleridge (1993) rejects the view that material interventions such as legislation can change 'human nature' with respect to the treatment of disabled people. He refers, of course, to legal mechanisms such as the USA's Americans with Disabilities Act (1990), Great Britain's Disability Discrimination Act (1995),[2] and many similar policies. To maintain a strongly materialist view, Coleridge contends, is to declare both education and development redundant. There is an accusation levelled at the social model here, inferring that materialist positions militate against resources being allocated to the development of human capital. While provision of basic needs such as food, shelter and health care is essential, Coleridge (1993) takes issue with viewing 'development' as limited to this. He writes:

> The problem lies in the fact that such needs are passive: if these needs are met, so this approach asserts, then 'development' has happened. But there are other needs which are just as basic: the need to be creative, to make choices, to exercise judgment, to love others, to have friendships, to contribute something of oneself to the world, to have social function and purpose. These are active needs; if they are not met, the result is the impoverishment of the human spirit, because without them life itself has no meaning.
>
> (Coleridge, 1993, p. 213)

Disabled lives carry every aspect of human complexity; of relationship, uncertainty, self-regard, loss and hope. Accordingly, a model aiming to validate disabled life must provide conceptually for each level of personhood. One important layer of disability which social model dualism has consigned to the margins is that of the body; of impairment. The embodiment of self has traditionally been as much an anathema to the materialist figure as has the psychological domain.

The vanishing – and reappearing – body

Viewing material barriers as the nub of disability steered the social model movement towards a somatic impasse. Although the model was conceived to oppose the traditional medical view, the disability–impairment binary at its centre inadvertently endorsed medicine's mandate for managing the body. By asserting, perhaps impetuously, that disability is purely contextual, social modelists relinquished impairment to the purely biological (Thomas, 1999a; Hughes, 2002a). In so doing, the social model aligned itself with Cartesian medicine's view of the body as 'a domain of corporeality untouched by culture' (Hughes, 2002a, p. 67), correspondingly projecting disability as a disembodied phenomenon. In other words, impairment was construed as a reality unmediated by its cultural milieu (Marks, 1999a), reaffirming biomedicine's abstraction of the body as a 'faulty machine' (Hughes and Paterson, 1997, p. 329). The irony of this convergence is remarkable. Social model politics had informed a collusion with biomedicine's decontextualised view of bodily experience – the view so problematised by medical anthropology. Its disregard for post-structuralism's attack on enlightenment dualisms allowed for the embracing of irreducible polarities such as body and society, medicine and politics, therapy and emancipation, pain and oppression and, of course, impairment and disability (ibid.). The urge to dissociate from the vagaries of 'sentimental autobiography' had, crucially, generated an insurmountable obstacle to the creation of a sociology of impairment (Hughes, 2002a). Susan Bordo (1993) provides a dramatic contrast to the social model's 'biologism', seeing the body as everything but a stable, acultural constant. Instead culture is always, a priori, inscribed through the living of our bodies. There is no 'natural' body – instead, in Michalko's (2002) words, 'natural' is 'the script of culture writ large on the body' (p. 58).

While disability studies was abandoning the corporeal, the body was set to become a central site of engagement in other arenas of social struggle (Hughes and Paterson, 1997). Hancock and co-workers describe the scene as follows:

> Meanwhile the body was making itself ever-present in social and political life, be it in the shape of a battered woman, a terminated foetus, a victim of torture or televised war, a proud celebration of womanhood, disability, colour or homosexuality, an organ in transit for transplantation, a human-machine stepping on the moon, a sample of DNA under the microscope, a man who was a woman or vice versa, a body transformed by diet, exercise or the surgeon's knife, a homeless person camped on the streets of the world's richest nation, a mass grave, another world record smashed.
>
> (Hancock et al., 2000 cited in Hughes, 2002a, p. 66)

But for disabled people relying on the social model account, the living, breathing body had vanished; in its place a 'timeless ontological foundation' (Hughes and Paterson, 1997, p. 327). In their landmark critique of materialist disability studies, Hughes and Paterson seem near amazed as they describe the social model's construction of the impaired body as a 'dysfunctional, anatomical, corporeal mass obdurate in its resistance to signification and phenomenologically dead, without intentionality or agency' (ibid.). Social modelists intent on furthering the cause continue to show little appetite for the conceptual intricacies of aligning body, mind and society. But this neglect can leave the lived reality of impairment in limbo, between the control and invalidation of biologism, and the unwelcoming disdain of a repressive populism.

Some authors have defended the social model by pointing out that analyses of impairment have appeared within their framework. But rather than investigating impairment per se, this work is concerned primarily with its social origins (e.g. Abberley, 1987; 1996; Oliver, 1996). Abberley (1996) asserts correctly that forms of impairment occur within historical and political contexts which influence prevalence, and support exacerbation and amelioration. Unsafe working conditions, the efficiency of health systems, access to vaccines, levels of public safety – these and many other factors shape the incidence and consequences of impairment (ibid.). Though undoubtedly important, such an analysis falls very short of examining impairment as a complex, embodied process comprising both societal and personal aspects. Instead, Abberley (1987) introduces us to the social underpinnings of impairment, but then abruptly sets aside the resultant phenomena as a consensual, unproblematic reality (Paterson and Hughes, 1999). For Paterson and Hughes (1999, p. 598), the social model's evasions eliminate the possibility of disabled people building an 'emancipatory politics of identity', based upon the delineation and mutual validation of interwoven threads of cultural and corporeal existence – that is, the 'sociology of impairment' referred to earlier.

As we have seen, social constructionism and the postmodern tradition offer an alternative strategy for making sense of what disability is. Because these viewpoints provide only for versions of reality, it is not only disability, but also impairment which is up for grabs as a socially constructed artefact. In body as in identity, the secure ground of intrinsic characteristics is left far behind, replaced by a subject composed of continually shifting and negotiated repertoires. Constructionist disability theorists aim to wrest control of 'disability meanings' from positivist accounts, characterised as holding a 'western conception of objective, individualistic, ahistoric knowledge' (Gergen, 1985, p. 272). This is a valuable counterpoint to medical essentialism, but the liability of the constructionist view lies in the caveat that all such alternative accounts are equally illusory. By consequence, a strictly constructionist view of disability allows the body to be momentarily rescued from biologism, restoring it as a frame for discursive struggle. But it is then immediately engulfed by the imperative of deconstruction, sanitizing it of all non-contingent meaning (Price and Shildrick, 1998; Turner, 2001). As we have seen, the social model accedes to biologism by abstention, allowing no scope for the unique 'living' of the disabled body. But the constructionist position fails to balance the equation, replacing a barren biological essentialism with an equally depersonalising 'discursive essentialism' (Hughes and Paterson, 1997, p. 333; Hacking, 1999). Instead of breathing life into the body, deconstruction dissolves it into nothing more than its constituent cultural signifiers.

Rosemarie Garland-Thomson (1997a) takes a pragmatic position which draws on both constructionist and essentialist conceptions of the body. First she suggests we employ a 'strategic constructionist' argument in order to launch a 'denaturalising' assault on the view of disability as bodily incapacity, replacing this with a contextual account focused on the interaction between bodily difference and a misattuned cultural world (ibid., p. 283). Here, delineation of the 'disabled' identity is unclear; an illusory product of ascribed characteristics. Although also attacking disability as a social accomplishment, the social model's compatibility with this position is limited by its reliance on binaries.

Second, Garland-Thomson argues that this constructionist view be amalgamated with a 'strategic essentialism', in order to affirm the historical 'reality' of the disabled body. Embodied differences, such as living with a wheelchair, or without sight, can thus be claimed and elaborated by those who 'live' them (ibid., p. 283). Here, notwithstanding its investment in 'disabled' as a minority identity, the social model's position again seems awkward, due to its non-engagement with the experience of impairment. Garland-Thomson explains her compromise position as follows:

> Thus, a strategic constructionism destigmatises the disabled body, locates difference relationally, denaturalises normalcy, and challenges appearance hierarchies. A strategic essentialism, by contrast, validates experience and consciousness, imagines community, authorises history, and facilitates self naming.
>
> (Garland-Thomson, 1997a, p. 283)

The Foucauldian discourse analytic tradition forms a central thrust of social constructionist work on disease and disability (Foucault, 1976; 1995; Stiker, 1982). Although these accounts provide piercing social critique, especially around the notion of normalisation, little attention is given to subjective life or individual agency (Whyte, 1995; Turner, 2001). In fact, on everyday lived experience discourse analysis is altogether silent. Further, while the strategic essentialism suggested by Garland-Thomson (1997a) admits the body as palpable, the biomedical realm which is its natural home is also unsuited to exploring subjective embodiment. Garland-Thomson (1997a, p. 282) develops her position by positing a 'universalising disability discourse', which draws on feminism in asserting the body as a 'cultural text which is interpreted, inscribed with meaning, [and] indeed, made within social relations of power'. The critique here is essential in destigmatising 'damaged' identities, but it also tends to obscure the lived effects of identifiable difference, destabilising the identity categories which make oppressed experience collectively meaningful (ibid.). We are oppressed by identity categories (gender, race, disability), but also require their reifications to legitimate our experience, as well as for critical social analysis. Deconstructing identity can free individuals from a 'narrative of essential inadequacy', but simultaneously sacrifices 'the particularity of … embodied experience' (ibid.). The presumed difference of bodies is at the heart of medicalisation, but it is the specific nature of this embodiment that must be recognised as an essential part of the lived reality of oppression, as well as of identity itself (Turner, 2001). Deconstructing labels will, to some extent, disrupt the politics of material inequality. But reducing the body to a phantasm of representations risks invalidating the experience of those living with a subordinated identity. At present, it would appear that the disability movement simply cannot afford to discard the 'disabled' category. Interestingly though, a sector of the deaf community has adopted this tactic, promoting their identity as a cultural and linguistic minority, and disidentifying with the disability movement (e.g. Corker, 1994). This position not only assails 'disability' as an arbitrary socio-linguistic product, but 'impairment' as well. The politicised position that deafness is not an impairment now underpins intense debate surrounding cochlea implant surgery for young children, which would effectively redirect their cultural and linguistic identity development (Kermit, 2009; Sparrow, 2010). But in sum, doubts about the extreme relativism and poor explanatory capacity of radical constructionism seem well founded (Thomas, 1999a; 2002). Perhaps more significant, though, is the groundswell of feminist writers in disability studies mentioned earlier, who call for a common-sense return to the lived reality of bodies.

With this visceral, matter-of-fact tone, Crow (1996, p. 208) describes how social model thinking has marginalised her experience of impairment, through constructing it as 'irrelevant, neutral and sometimes positive, but never, ever as the quandary it really is'. To her, 'glossing over' impairment means masking the contradictions and complexity, the confusion and ambivalence which are part of the physicality of social life in an impaired body. If pain, for example, is subjectively meaningful it must therefore also be culturally meaningful (Paterson and Hughes, 1999). This socially mediated view of pain sees it not as 'physical sensation with overlays of meaning' but as 'permeated with meaning – permeated with culture' (Jackson, 1994, p. 211). The 'naturalisation' of what is, in fact, a cultural process could only be seen as an impediment to political conscientisation (Michalko, 2002). The myth of the 'natural' body thus leaves Crow (1996) abandoned in her 'quandary'. But for Hughes and Paterson (1997) the alarms run still deeper – surely, in their analysis, a biomedical view which has had free reign over impairment would produce bodies and subjective states in line with its categories. In other words, 'a particular genus of body with its appropriate signs, symptoms, behaviour and normative expectations' (p. 333). Some may argue that the social model is implicated through a passive collusion with biomedicine's colonising of subjectivity. The challenge for disabled people such as Crow, therefore, is not simply to express the experience of impairment, but first and foremost to find it among the silence and control of both biomedical and political socialisation.

Thomas (1999a) adds her voice to the 'grounding' of impairment experience, commenting that the everyday reality of impairment remains irreducible to both medical and deconstructionist abstractions. 'Surely', she writes, 'it is obvious that some restrictions of activity are caused by limited physical, sensory or intellectual functioning?' (ibid., p. 38). Far from devaluing impaired life, this position invites an exploration of the diverse ways in which it may be lived and imagined (Wasserman, 2001). Wendell (1997), with a candour probably disarming to materialists and constructionists alike, states that many impairments tax energy and stamina, limiting functioning in areas beyond those directly disrupted by the impairment. Similarly, Vehmas and Mäkelä (2009) seem bewildered at 'mainstream' disability studies' reluctance to recognise impairments as 'biological facts' (p. 45) with real-life implications. Again, the peculiar ambivalences of the social model are shown up here, seeming to sanction biomedical diagnosis (as in the original definitions of impairment), yet eschewing the idea of bodies which hurt or falter. More bluntly, Shakespeare (2006) underlines his identity as social model dissident by stating that 'people are disabled by society and by their bodies' – and, that it is 'inescapable that some forms of impairments are more limiting than others' (p. 56). His 'critical realist' position makes space for 'bodies which sometimes hurt, regardless of what we may think or say' (p. 54). It is important to point out that arrival at this seemingly self-evident conclusion can belie the very real, complex political concerns which made the journey such a meandering one. This conceptual location – where impairment may be re-admitted – is altogether different from the biomedical point of departure at which physicality informs social status. The social model must somehow realign its dualistic nature to provide for a body which is 'part of the domain of history, culture and meaning' (Hughes and Paterson, 1997, p. 326). Opinion is divided on whether it is sufficiently robust to survive such seismic changes.

Thomas' (1999a, p. 125; 2002) defence of the social model rests on her addition of a 'materialist ontology of impairment and impairment effects', which is 'neither biologically reductionist nor culturally determinist'. Unlike Shakespeare (2006), she sees it as feasible to apply these constructs alongside the essence of the social model, in an 'extended' social-relational approach. As noted earlier, her concept of 'impairment effects' is defined as 'restrictions of activity which are associated with being impaired but which are not disabilities in the social-relational sense' (Thomas, 1999a, p. 43). These 'effects' are 'profoundly bio-social; that is, shaped by the interaction of biological and social factors', and 'bound up with processes of socio-cultural naming' (ibid.). With these important adjustments in place, she sees the social model as relevant and flexible enough to retain. What seems unclear though, is how the model's key binary – the disability–impairment distinction – can continue to have meaning under this new dispensation; we will revisit questions surrounding Thomas' theoretical contributions later. The position of Hughes and Paterson (1997) on social modelist disembodiment is, compared to Thomas', wholly unforgiving. To these writers disability and impairment cannot in any way be construed as discrete, but part of 'a complex interpenetration of oppression and affliction' (ibid., pp. 335–36). Seeing the body as the very 'stuff of human affliction and affectivity', and the subject and object of oppression, directs us towards a phenomenological sociology of the body (ibid.). Here, the lived body incorporates selfhood as intrinsic to its functioning, its viscera and sensation. The body incarnates the individual's point of view on the world; it is, like the notion of the self, not possessed, but lived (Toombs, 1994). In this new landscape, the body reappears, filling up the sterile spaces of positivism with desire, sensation, flux and caprice. The view of embodiment emerging seems beyond symbiosis. Instead, the mutually constituting currents of cultural and somatic processes show as unitary phenomenology, as self.

This position is, I believe, quite compatible with the critical realist view recommended by Shakespeare (2006). Williams (1999, p. 806) draws attention to how critical realism provides for 'mind-independent generative mechanisms', where the body and (cultural) experience of the body are indissoluble. In its 'living', the body is not so much 'written upon' as 'written'; it has an ontological depth untouched by constructionist epistemological claims' (ibid.). In dramatic contrast to both materialist and constructionist propositions, 'humanity', therefore, 'is never a gift from society' (Archer, 1995, p. 285; Williams, 1999).

For the purpose of this book, a very important aspect of the critical realist position is the idea that layers of experience, of embodied selfhood, lie beyond consciousness. Though probably uncomfortable to both materialists and post-structuralists, this feature provides for the model's 'critical' and 'emancipatory' attributes (Williams, 1999) – for the possible uncovering of oppressive, internalised layers of embodiment. 'Emancipation' here, is something 'far more concrete and tangible than the shift to alternative discursive registers' (Williams, 1999, p. 810). Instead, awareness is directed towards 'structural internalisations' (ibid.) – the business of an emancipatory interrogation of self.

So the social process of making, becoming and being a body incorporates the making and living of the self (Turner, 2001). The significance for theorising disability is clear – embodiment and enselfment are interwoven projects (ibid.). Disability, then, is not a function of oppressive societies or impaired bodies, but an emergent phenomenon flowing from the interplay of structural constraints, physiology and culture. Williams (1999, p. 813) summarises this consolidated view of disability as follows: 'a dynamic, dialectically unfolding process between body and society, located within a temporal frame of reference (both historical and biographical)'.

The body is allowed to live, although we remain wary of the snares of biologism. A phenomenological approach shows up the continuous life of bodily perception, set against the (critical) reality of cultural signification and societal structures; the impaired body is a lived cultural phenomenon. From here, a space for theorising the socially situated, embodied nature of disabled selfhood begins to open. It is a space beckoning us towards psychoanalysis.

Notes

1 An unconscious, prototypical figure which is invested with emotional materials of varying valency. The disabled imago, for example, refers to a culturally constructed tragic figure existing partly as a product of projected unconscious fantasy.

2 Replaced in 2010 by the Equality Act.

3 Psychoanalysis and disability studies

An unlikely alliance

Preamble

To many, the psychoanalytic model may appear a peculiar framework for interrogating disability. The common-sense image of psychoanalysis calls to mind a plush consulting room in an urban, Western setting, with analyst and patient involved in a lengthy and very expensive process of individual psychotherapy – a far cry from the development needs of much of the world's disabled community. We tend to be less aware of psychoanalysis as a lens of social critique, able to make sense of behaviour at the broadest collective level, as well as the individual. The model provides a means for examining the intra-psychic world and making sense of how this realm relates bi-directionally to the 'real world' of politics. But to begin, what do we mean by the term 'psychoanalysis'? Here follows a very brief orientation, to be elaborated upon later.

Towards the end of the nineteenth century Sigmund Freud introduced the world to the radical idea that a sizeable part of the human mind exists outside of awareness. He termed this hidden segment the *unconscious* (Freud, 1912). Broadly speaking, the term psychoanalysis denotes a family of theoretical schools concerned with the investigation of unconscious life. Freud reasoned that, by virtue of having to negotiate difficult aspects of the human condition, we all carry memories, impulses and feelings which are painful or threatening, and thus cannot be tolerated in a pure form in consciousness. More importantly, he asserted that our actions are very significantly influenced by unconscious phenomena – that is, irrational and unknown motivations play a significant role in what we do, say and think. Our ability to manage difficult feelings, and hence to function, is dependent on what Freud termed our *defence mechanisms*. These are strategies the psyche employs to protect our conscious minds. Defences reformulate or 'censor' difficult unconscious feelings which may be pressing the boundaries of consciousness for recognition. But in doing so, the defences also alter our perception of both internal and external reality. Needing to not know about internal parts of our psychological life will, at times, mean needing to deny or distort parts of reality 'out there', such as aspects of the society we live in which remind us of our 'shadow'. In this way internal defences have significant implications for how society is structured, influencing perceptions of important, emotive issues such as oppression, inequality, violence and inter-group conflict. In the case of disability, the question psychoanalysis poses is to do with what the impaired body touches upon in the unconscious minds of members of society. As we will discover, disability awakens discomforting feelings in all of us, potentially triggering defence mechanisms which distort perception and affect the way in which we respond, as societies, to people with impairments (Marks, 1999a; Watermeyer, 2006).

The critical psychoanalytic view of disability just introduced is relatively new; this book is an attempt to develop and apply its ideas. But it is sensible to begin at a more foundational level, by examining arguments regarding whether psychoanalysis does, in fact, have emancipatory political potential. Unhappily, the history of the discipline shows far too little subversive application to social questions. And as alluded to above, many would dispute that psychoanalysis has anything at all to offer to emancipatory politics; foremost among these would be historical materialist thinkers such as the architects of the social model. Here, psychoanalysis may easily be viewed as a symbol of class separation, and the solipsistic indulgences of the bourgeois. But a recurring theme of this book – very relevant here – is an appeal to thoroughly explore what theoretical ideas may illuminate, rather than slating these because of their historically oppressive ideological associations. Let us consider the debate.

Psychoanalysis and social critique: depoliticisation or subversion?

> The political tasks of modern democracy are similar to the psychological tasks of modern therapy and analysis. In both areas, there is a fight between consciousness, liberation and alterity on the one hand and suppression, repression and omnipotent beliefs in final truths on the other.
>
> (Samuels, 1993, p. 4)

While psychoanalysis in its applied, clinical form provides one route to exploring unconscious processes, the implications of analytic knowledge extend beyond the individual. Psychoanalytic insights illuminate the unconscious underpinnings of social structures and intergroup behaviour, exploring how political and psychological realities constitute one another. But as we saw in the previous chapter, to people favouring a materialist view of society the exploration of individual characteristics such as emotion or 'the internal world' is a pointless diversion from the 'real', material issues of socio-political life (Figlio and Richards, 2002).

Such critics accuse psychoanalysis of psychic reductionism – a situation in which social actions such as political radicalism become interpreted as nothing more than the manifestations of unconscious conflicts (Figlio and Richards, 2002). Seeing the origins of struggle as largely internal will distract us from examining material, societal factors implicated in suffering. This view sees psychoanalytic formulations as having a 'dumbing down' function, diminishing feelings of entitlement to engage in political resistance. Psychological wounds inflicted by, say, prejudice may consequently be misunderstood as the results of intra-individual psychological fallibilities. There is little doubt that this criticism has been justified – both idealist (psychological) and materialist thinkers have fallen into the trap of denying the alternative level of analysis. At times we may be drawn to over-psychologised views because of how these turn accountability inward, appealing to our human propensity for self-blame. The result is that culpability is not tracked back to social injustice, missing the opportunity to mobilise change. What is clear, then, is that if a model of intra-psychic functioning is to be relevant, it must interface meaningfully with social realities of history and economics. Instead, some psychoanalytic approaches have viewed society as an individual psyche writ large, circumventing any real integration of historical factors (Hinshelwood and Chiesa, 2002a).

The location of psychoanalytic practitioners and institutions in bourgeois, developed world contexts has only reinforced the discipline's depoliticising image. Added to this, the community of 'traditional' psychoanalytic intellectuals has been described as self-referential, and occupying a rarefied world starkly out of touch with political praxis. This narrow, insular cultural location has limited the discipline's applicability, and left it vulnerable to accusations of prescriptiveness (Samuels, 1993). The problem is this: delineation of how psychological processes such as human development *may* take place quickly becomes transmuted into ideas about how such processes *should* take place, ignoring the slants caused by the cultural embeddedness of all such investigations. The British psychoanalytic establishment has, it seems, done the 'ivory tower' image of the discipline few favours by retaining a highly hierarchical structure, thereby seeming to reproduce rather than subvert social inequalities (Frosh, 2006). The influential *object relations* model[1] within psychoanalysis focuses heavily on intra-psychic and (close) interpersonal explanations for personality development, emphasising the importance of the early years of life. While there is little doubt that such ideas are valuable, an exclusive focus on the familial 'sanctum' can promote a disregard for more collective, socio-political layers of experience (ibid.).

But problematising theoretical emphases or institutions does not equate to the discipline having nothing to contribute. On the contrary, many writers lament the history of psychoanalysis as a series of missed opportunities for powerful ideological critique (e.g. Wolfenstein, 1990; Samuels, 1993; Gordon, 1995; Hinshelwood and Chiesa, 2002a; Frosh, 2006). Gordon (1995, p. 287) charges that psychoanalytic intellectuals hide behind the anonymity required by clinical practice as an 'excuse for doing nothing' in the public domain. Feminism's recognition that politics is not only lived in the public realm, but also in the personal, led to the vision of a psychoanalytic 'politics of everyday life'; the hoped-for fruits of this enterprise have been scant (Figlio and Richards, 2002, p. 192). In its place, the discipline has positioned itself in a primarily palliative clinical role – offering a 'band-aid' to society in lieu of advocacy (Gordon, 1995, p. 285). While this may well be true, psychoanalysis is by no means alone in battling to combine examination of personal, internal reality with the political; it is no easy task. The idealist–materialist split means that either approach misses half of what is important, often defensively discounting the alternative layer. We see evidence of this same split in common-sense understandings of our own lives. Think of how we may explain our own and others' experiences of distress as being *all* due to society's injustices, or *all* the fault of the individual. These views, respectively, show up a struggle with acknowledging the darker conflicts of the internal world, or the painful realities of social oppression.

As noted above, psychoanalysis' focus on the family and early life in shaping subjectivity has clear value. What is, thus far, disappointing is the discipline's failure to create conceptual threads which expand this model outward to the group-political sphere, as some theorists in human development have attempted to do (e.g. Bronfenbrenner, 1977). Importantly, it should be borne in mind that in theorising the ephemeral, unseen layers of the internal world, models and concepts are difficult to validate empirically; one is, after all, attempting to map subjectivity itself. Under scientific scrutiny, therefore, much psychoanalytic theory may appear more like doctrine than fact (Frosh, 2006). But as we shall see, it is on this ethereal plane that underpinnings and effects of oppression are imprinted, and, in part, maintained. No matter how slippery internal phenomena may seem, these must be part of our conceptualisation. Slavoj Zizek (2008) is clear that psychoanalysis presents the only theoretical modality able to trace the hidden contours of power in societies shot through with the divisiveness of modernity. So what is it that psychoanalysis has to offer?

Psychoanalysis brings a certain constructive suspiciousness to our study of society. In the words of Paul Hoggett (1992, p. 3), the objective of the discipline is assisting us to 'lie to ourselves a little less than we do'. Human motivations are complex, and carry valencies which – contrary to Marxist principles – are not reducible to how many removes one is from the means of production. Psychoanalysis is well acquainted with the ambiguous nature of human subjectivity, and not at all reliant on the hoped-for stability of a two-dimensional material world. Although in the minority, a radical political strand in psychoanalysis has a long history, beginning with Freud's *Civilisation and its Discontents* (1930), continuing through the so-called Frankfurt school, and taken up by a range of later feminist theorists. In the wake of World War II, Wilhelm Reich (1945; 1946) used psychoanalytic ideas to make sense of the catastrophic, irrational social phenomenon of the age – the rise of fascism. For Reich, the role of psychoanalytic critique in politics was clear. He spoke of:

> … the area in historical materialism where psychoanalysis has to fulfil a scientific function, which social economy is not in a position to accomplish: the comprehension of the structure and dynamics of ideology, not of its historical basis.
>
> (Reich, 1946, p. 28)

Reich's aims – as those of this book – were to explore how the 'facts' of political economy interact in a mutually constituting dynamic with individual subjectivity. As observed, this is shifting and slippery conceptual territory, but unlike positivism, a strength of psychoanalysis is its capacity to tolerate 'limits, gaps, vulnerability, and a lack of knowledge' (Cooper and Treacher, 1995, p. 3). In historical materialist accounts of social inequality the identity of the 'villains' is generally all too clear, protecting us from the painful reality that social relations are dynamic and collusory; that both victims and perpetrators shape the ongoing social tangle which is oppression. The role of unconscious aspects in mediating these relationships is key – and to the discipline of psychoanalysis the inevitable ambiguity of such phenomena is familiar, even comfortable terrain. Psychoanalysis does not offer solutions to these problems. It does, however, provide a means for understanding the effects, and hence the reproduction, of relations of power at the psychological level. If critically – that is, *subversively* – applied, the paradigm can unlock psychic realities which overturn stereotypes and confound simplistic, reified views of the division of social power. Unlike materialism, psychoanalysis carries the capacity to free from within, through bringing to light the human effects of ideology. The aims of this book are modest: simply to demonstrate the necessity of such an investigation, and suggest some tools with which to begin. A key debate regarding the use of psychoanalysis in interrogating society traces back to the mid-twentieth century altercation between the Frankfurt school (including theorists such as Marcuse and Adorno), and the Revisionist psychoanalysts (in particular, Fromm, Horney and Sullivan) (Frosh, 2006). The disagreement hinged on the Revisionist idea that it is possible to separate out universal human needs from the nature of the social order; their opponents strongly rejected this claim (ibid.). The view that human needs are intrinsic and identifiable implied that psychoanalysis could inform a set of humanistic ideals to shape a utopian society. The belief here is that if optimal circumstances are created, social ills will dissolve away. This idea that humanity is innately good, that ills come from 'the outside' and that an ideal, harmonious society is within reach is very tempting. Would elaborating the prerequisites for such a society not be a noble task for psychoanalysis? Let us consider some implications.

Within the Revisionist stance, if psychoanalysis is to engage with social change it must accept the existence of a 'non-social subject'; a pre-social human self which, although developing in the social world, is not *fundamentally* conceived by it. To some extent Freud's early contributions imply this position, through not allowing enough for the integration of social history. Later, the work of Melanie Klein – as we shall see – made far more provision for relating the nature of the individual psyche to society. The Revisionist position's opposition to this increasingly socio-cultural emphasis carries some worrying inferences. It constructs a pristine self, regarded as the only 'real', and hence healthy self; the sort of self that will respond positively to nourishing treatment. The key issue is that this self is viewed as beyond the reach of deconstruction; questions regarding its shaping through ideology are obviated (ibid.). Wolfenstein (1990), along with the Frankfurt scholars, regards the idea of such a self as a dangerous fantasy. If psychoanalysis assumes the authority to define the nature of this essential self it becomes (all the more) the gatekeeper of normalcy, specifying what people *need*, based upon a presocial theory of what people *are*.

For the Frankfurt school every layer of psychological life is, by definition, profoundly social. In their view the Revisionist account would lead to a situation specific psychoanalytic humanism, privileging psychic functioning which fulfils its normative expectations. Here we might recall Rod Michalko's (2002) ominous, cautionary words from the previous chapter regarding how 'nature' is 'the script of culture writ large on the body' (Michalko, 2002, p. 58; Bordo, 1993). To accept the Revisionist position, in my view, is to miss out on the crux of what psychoanalysis has to offer; that is, a radical framework which interrogates normative expectations and the privileging of sacred cows. In the disability world the humanistic psychoanalysis of the Revisionists might inform a 'rehabilitationist psychology', which identifies who the disabled subject *is*, and consequently what she or he needs in order to function or integrate. This would leave no place for investigation of the nature or ideological roots of disabled subjectivity. The history of psychological theorising on disability shares with such an approach a problematic assumption of inherent attributes which require interventions. If disablist prejudice does indeed have deep psychological roots, and is often ideologically hidden as hegemony, an unwavering critique will be required to uncover its mechanisms. In other words, theoretical space must be made for ideology.

In the decades since Freud the emergence of Kleinian object relations theory (Klein, 1946; 1948; 1952; 1957) provided new concepts to connect the intra-psychic world with the social. The helpfulness of Melanie Klein's ideas in this regard is surprising, considering that she showed little interest in understanding socio-political processes. Ideas such as projection and projective identification (both examined later) have become central in psychoanalytic investigations of society (Richards, 1989). In Klein's model, bi-directional, reverberating connections exist between an inner world of conflicting *objects*, and a real world of political battles. Actions on either terrain may be motivated by, and have consequences for, the other. Intra- and inter-group dynamics may thus be understood as deeply entwined with the internal conflicts of ongoing object relations (Hinshelwood and Chiesa, 2002a). It is a misappropriation of Kleinian theory to portray these ideas as a reductionist pathologisation of individual political action. Freud's key to psychoanalytic critique lay in the multi-determined nature of thought and behaviour; that is, its roots in both rational, material and unconscious, personal realms. To examine personal psychic investments in unfolding societal history does not mean blaming the 'recalcitrant' victims of social ills.

Let us return to defence mechanisms – this time with a Kleinian slant. Klein introduced what she termed the *psychotic defences*. In her model, infancy was a time of immense anxiety for all of us, based on the combination of utter physical dependency and the lack of intellectual resources with which to distance ourselves from our feelings. This combination is a very powerful one: an internal world full of unprocessed emotion, reliance on caregivers for one's very survival and none of the refuge from anxiety provided by sophisticated cognition – by memory. Memories are extremely useful to us as containers for anxiety, allowing us to recall a similar distressing situation to the current one, and how it 'turned out all right'. Without such resources the infant lives in a state of being repeatedly psychologically overwhelmed by emotion, with only the most rudimentary means to make sense of it. These rudiments are the *psychotic defences* – so termed because of their association, in Kleinian thought, with psychotic illness. To Klein, psychosis was an adult state in which the mind remained dominated by infantile ways of making sense of the world – that is, by means of very crude, distorting defences. But the psychotic defences are not restricted to babies and mentally ill persons; not at all. Instead, Klein described how all carry a psychotic layer; a stratum of the psyche which is expressed when aspects of our worlds speak very directly to our most vulnerable parts. When this happens, we revert to the crude sense-making of babyhood, as the intensity of our fears echoes that early vulnerability. To put it simply, when we are afraid and our psychic equilibrium is under threat, it becomes difficult to think. At these times even the healthiest mind becomes prone to viewing aspects of the world in a 'crazy' way. A range of primitive defences will be examined later, but for now let us return to the idea of *splitting* introduced in the previous chapter. Splitting is a psychotic defence with which we make sense of a bewildering, at times frightening world by dividing what we see into polarities – what we may term 'black and white thinking'. In this frame of mind it is clear to us what is good and what evil, who are victims and who perpetrators, what is entirely true and absolutely false. In each case we unconsciously choose to ignore complexity and opt to categorise, rendering a denuded world populated with idealised good figures and persecuting malevolent ones. The hated figures are seen as wholly negative because disavowed parts of ourselves have become split off – that is, disowned – and then projected onto a devalued other. The dichotomous reifications of racism are an initial example to ponder.

It is no coincidence that racist stereotypes about black people – for example, to do with immorality or low intelligence – reflect vulnerable points hidden within the psychology of the dominant group. Here, insecurities and fears regarding our 'real' nature have triggered a defence which insulates us from a devalued 'other'. In Kleinian theorising on social process, base defences against primitive anxieties are centrally implicated in social ills such as racial hatred or disablist prejudice, rigidifying divides and adherence to the status quo (Bion, 1961; 1967; 1970; Young, 1994). In other words, for internal reasons we may need to construe social reality in a particular way. When the psyche is under threat and psychotic mechanisms are activated, thought becomes narrowed, creativity stifled and we assume a concrete position of defensive hostility rather than openness and engagement. A consequence is that if society is to change it will require exploration of the 'common anxieties and unconscious collusions underlying the social defences determining fantasy social relationships' (Jaques, 1955 in Young, 1994, p. 88).

For the purposes of this book this simply means that all need to explore, understand and take ownership of their complex feelings about disability – no matter which political, professional or embodied vantage point one begins from. In Klein's conceptualisation, social actions are driven by an internal world of fantasy, and thus heavily shaped by emotion rather than rationality. To put this another way, we relate to what we imagine, not what is; and importantly, our imaginings are unconsciously, psychologically self-invested. Racism, for example, is everything but rational; to understand it we must explore the emotional payoffs of the reality it constructs. The investment is always to do with protecting ourselves from some painful knowledge, often to do with our own identity. If we take on Hoggett's (1992) injunction to lie to ourselves less, it means accepting ownership of fears about ourselves expressed in the scapegoating of minorities. An important consideration is that defensive constructions of the world germinate as shared aspects of group behaviour. One way in which identity and group allegiance is often conveyed is in how out-groups are thought of. Here, internal and institutional (that is, group-based) defences inform and reinforce one another. In Klein's words the group's reality is repeatedly introjected (taken in) by the individual, and his or her internal views are repeatedly projected into the group, creating the self-fulfilling expectation that these are shared by all. In the intergroup arena the illusion of homogeneity (in 'what we believe' or 'what they are') and real homogeneity are, in effect, interchangeable.

The ideas above may seem abstract and difficult to grasp, but will become more animate later as we apply them to disability. But before trying to construct a new *psychoanalysis of disablism*, it is important to cast a critical eye back on the discipline's prior work on disability. I term this early work 'traditional' in order to differentiate it from the critical, contextualised psychoanalytic model of disablism at the heart of this book. Much of this research is highly problematic in its construction of disability, and has been roundly slated by disability studies. While the critique is warranted, I nevertheless believe there are valuable lessons for our discussion in this examination. These include pitfalls to be avoided and hidden pieces of understanding, most of which will be explored later. But there is another lesson here. Against the backdrop of a psychologically sterile disability studies, this emotive, politically problematic material presents a challenge to all to suspend totalising ideological judgments, and to consolidate the precious fragments of insight to be found amidst an outmoded approach. Somehow we need to grow in our ability to hold politics and theory in tension; remaining critical, but avoiding the obliteration of either by its counterpart.

Psychoanalysis and disability: a brief history

Historically psychoanalysis has paid very little attention to theorising disability. This is surprising. One would imagine that cultural and personal aspects of bodily difference would be important to a discipline concerned with human subjectivity. There are various ways of reading this silence. Did psychoanalysts see the disabled population as no different from others, and not requiring specific research attention? Or were disabled people regarded as too damaged or too different to be included in the theorising of personality or psychotherapy? Was there an inadvertent, anxious avoidance of work with disabled people? Evidence from the limited literature indicates that psychoanalytic accounts, like most psychological theorising on disability, assume that bodily impairment leads to psychopathology of some form (Lenny, 1993; Oliver, 1993a; Gill, 2001; Wilson, 2003).

As is clear by now, the crux of the social model position is to dispute this, arguing that emotional distress experienced by disabled people – where this occurs – is due to barriers to participation. Reiterating Barnes' (1998) words from the previous chapter, not all disabled persons encounter psychological distress, but as in any population, a proportion will. Social model writers point accusingly at nondisabled mental health researchers from psychoanalysis and elsewhere, whose formulations ignore contextual factors such as discrimination (Oliver, 1993a; Barnes, 1998). The research of Miller and Gwynne (1972) is often held up as the odious epitome of such work. These writers portrayed disabled persons in residential institutions as having psychological problems which were an inevitable outcome of physical 'limitations', an assumption echoed in most psychoanalytic work.

Adrienne Asch and Harilyn Rousso, in their critical review of psychoanalytic research on disability, argue that this work has tended to reinforce prejudices regarding the emotional functioning and potential for productivity and intimacy of disabled people (Asch and Rousso, 1985). Some psychoanalytic theorists have simply labelled disabled people 'unanalysable', based on the assumption that impairment brings severe psychological damage. Other writers have, as in the mistaken logic described above, sought to establish causal links between bodily difference and forms of psychopathology (ibid.); that is, musing upon how body and self mirror and create one another. From this point of departure, attention moves to whether the 'psychological effects of impairment' are 'inevitable, preventable or modifiable' (ibid., p. 4). For example, Thomas and Siller (1999, p. 182) recount that typical reactions to impairment include 'depression, withdrawal, shame, overcompensation and denial', as well as 'considerable sensitivity about the disability' and 'feelings of inferiority' which are managed through a 'generalised hostility' (Siller, 1963; Castelnuovo-Tedesco, 1981; Thomas and Siller, 1999). It is not hard to see why a host of writers across disability studies has slammed such research. While there is no reason to doubt the emotional *states* Thomas and Siller (1999) observe, the problem is that their attributions make virtually no mention of the harmful effects of exclusion and shunning so prevalent in disablist societies. Their identification of unmastered aggression and poor ego maturity as 'symptoms' of disability is echoed by many other contributors (e.g. Burlingham, 1961; Niederland, 1965; Ogden, 1974; Bornstein, 1977; Castelnuovo-Tedesco, 1981). The picture is of an ego battling to manage powerful emotions, and consequently employing primitive, distorting (psychotic) defences. Interestingly, even as these writers point to how the spectre of impairment may trigger such defences in disabled persons themselves, it evidently does not occur to them that it could be equally psychologically provocative for nondisabled persons.

The psychological disturbance most frequently linked to disability in the traditional literature is narcissistic pathology (Harris and Wideman, 1988; Davis, 2002). In simple terms, narcissism is a tendency towards unrealistic self-aggrandisement as a means of protection from inner feelings of damage. Distortions in how the self is viewed are, in turn, reflected in a distorted view of the world. Although, as we shall see, Freud's own utterances on disability are quite ambiguous, Niederland (1965) supports his own position by pointing out that Freud (1914) viewed work with patients with 'organic disease' as a key route to understanding narcissism. In order to explain my main difficulties with this body of research, I will examine Niederland's (1965) work in some detail, in important ways it is representative.

The position of Niederland (1965, p. 518) is that bodily 'defects' function as 'nodal factors' in the development of narcissistic disturbance. It is assumed that a 'damaged' body (from infancy or childhood) will lead to development of a distorted *body ego* – the early representation of the self that emerges as a 'reflection' of physicality. Further ego development will thus be based on unstable, fractured foundations, leading to the emergence of narcissistic defences to protect the self from knowledge of its own damage. The implication of this logic for how we make sense of distress in the lives of disabled people is, to put it mildly, alarming. The 'damage' supposedly underlying such distress is 'pushed' into the impaired body, construing the disabled individual as carrying *inherent psychological difference* emanating from organic factors, affecting perception of self, other and reality. From infancy, it is the 'essentially bodily self-image and cathexis'[2] based on an 'oral-tactile' early concept of body which provides the base for a troubled ego (Niederland, 1965, p. 527). The narcissistic 'symptoms' to emerge later include grandiosity, magical thinking, secretiveness and a florid fantasy life containing themes such as revenge, immortality and birth–rebirth (p. 521). Niederland (1965) restricts his analysis to people impaired since birth or early childhood, but similar effects are posited elsewhere in the psychoanalytic literature for adventitious impairments in adulthood (Castelnuovo-Tedesco, 1981).

The key question here is whether it is viable to argue that the *pre-social* experience of an impaired body may lead to body ego distortion, and hence narcissistic injury. Freud (1923, p. 26) wrote that the ego is 'first and foremost a bodily ego'; the ego is 'a projection' of the surface of the body. This seems to suggest that the nature of the body informs the character of the body ego, and is hence – at least foundationally – formative of the ego itself. At issue is whether culturally condensed assessments of normalcy mediate this 'reflection' of the body as it is precipitated into a body ego. Writers such as Niederland (1965) view this imprinting of injury upon the ego by 'basic physical experiences' as unproblematic (p. 522). But elsewhere Freud implies a far more ideologically situated view of bodily difference. He writes:

> In the aetiology of neuroses organic inferiority and imperfect development play an insignificant part. Neuroses make use of such inferiorities as a pretext, just as they do of every other suitable factor.
>
> (Freud, 1914, p. 99)

Here, Freud (1914) positions bodily difference as secondary to psychic functioning, suggesting that impairments may be used by the psyche as a rationalising 'kernel of truth', allowing material sense to be made of what are, in fact, psychological phenomena. In other words, rather than causing emotional disturbance, impairment may be utilised 'retrospectively' as a hook on which to hang emotional experience. The effect is one of blaming the self – in the form of the body – for emotional struggle. In his account of early development, Winnicott (1965, p. 244) strongly emphasises bodily experience in shaping what he terms 'the imaginative self'. Dwelling within and exploring the 'inside' and 'outside' of the body provides the subject matter, the shape and sensation, of the coalescing self (ibid.; Erskine and Judd, 1994). But importantly, Winnicott's picture does not imply that the impaired body could come to be experienced as damaged without the distorted socialisation invariably associated with bodily difference. The body which the congenitally impaired infant possesses is the only body which he or she has ever experienced; its boundaries and shape, its motility and sensation – these are not experiences set against some pre-existing ideal, but primary apprehensions of a unitary physicality. Highlighting this contradiction, Asch and Rousso (1985) summarise their critique of psychoanalytic work on disability as follows:

> Our major criticism … is that by asking what impact a physical disability has on adult psychopathology, many authors overlook the impact of parental, familial and societal treatment on the psychological development of their disabled patients.
>
> (Asch and Rousso, 1985, p. 6)

This oversight by psychoanalytic writers is peculiar, as it betrays a disregard for basic tenets of the paradigm. Most psychoanalytic frameworks place early formative relationships – the family – at centre stage in shaping psychic functioning, both adaptive and otherwise. But surprisingly, this principle seems to have been discarded here. We are left wondering: is the hegemony of individualising accounts of disability such that these writers have forgotten the role of parents and others in shaping selfhood? One of Niederland's (1965) research subjects, a woman with a paralysed arm, is portrayed as manifesting grandiosity attributable to her impairment. After recounting this, he then informs his reader of how she was held in traction – flat on her back, and presumably in hospital – for much of her first year of life. Niederland (1965) makes no real mention of the aetiological significance of this experience – that is, the role it may have played in shaping the woman's adult mental state. Instead, he moves quickly to a consideration of her 'revenge fantasies' (p. 521) involving dismemberment, mutilation and the like. As before, while these 'revenge fantasies' may well have been in evidence, the question is revenge *upon whom*, and *for what*? The attribution of fantasies of revenge or grandeur to asocial origins, against the backdrop of striking culturally condensed forces of socialisation, is bewildering. Surely our attention should be directed at the culturally produced meanings of lived bodies, rather than the material, banal, 'presumed' body. Somehow Niederland (1965) sets up impaired bodily experience, even in infancy, against the myth of Susan Bordo's 'natural' body. Taking issue with such a position does not mean diminishing the embodied reality of impairment – very much the contrary. Instead, it underscores the social shaping of meanings which permeate every experience of the body. Niederland, Bornstein, Burlingham and others fail to investigate how their impaired patients have been responded to throughout their developmental years by, in all probability, a fretful and unready social world. Later in the same paper, Niederland (1965) does add a few caveats to the rather bald statements recounted above. He writes:

> While noting these relations between disturbed ego development and early physical defectiveness, I wish to emphasise that I do not regard the latter as the sole pathogenic influence in their clinical picture. I believe, rather, that the defect, in addition to its significance as a concretising and organising experience of pathogenic import from early childhood, adds a 'kernel of truth' quality and multidimensional aspects to the pathological fantasies which are likely to arise during the developmental phases.
>
> (Niederland, 1965, p. 529)

What Niederland seems to suggest here is that the impairment becomes – in Freud's (1914) terms – a 'pretext' into which basic, universal conflicts are projected. This afterthought is helpful, but it is just that – an afterthought. In effect, the overall logic ignores relational factors; these are named, but no effort is applied to imagining the contours or implications of such concerns. Instead, the compelling nature of the impaired body entrenches itself into a monopoly of attributive meaning. Recent investigations in neuroscience have given limited credence to the idea that different forms of embodiment may carry subtle implications for higher order cognition (Scully, 2009). While this may be so, issues both of scale and sequence place the conspicuous realities of cultural responses to the unusual body – *still largely unexplored* – at centre stage as the subject of investigation. A focus on abstract ideas about the possible presocial experience of impaired embodiment is, at best, lopsided in the absence of an examination of palpable realities to do with the socialisation of disabled lives.

A number of psychoanalytic studies have focused on the purported effects of congenital blindness on development. In the mould of Niederland (1965), these workers have typically tried to conceptualise the impact of the 'naked' absence of sight on developing object relations, giving rather unilaterally pessimistic prognoses (e.g. Blank, 1957; Burlingham, 1961; Omwake and Solnit, 1961; Nagera and Colonna, 1965; Bornstein, 1977; Wright, 1991). Burlingham (1961), for example, argues that blind children are constitutionally restricted in learning to manage aggression, through not being able to perceive the consequences of their behaviour. The children she studied feared that their actions had unknown, catastrophic effects, leading to an anxious constriction of agency. With a similar, essentialist tone Bornstein (1977, p. 25) observed that blind children are 'reduced to helplessness and panic' upon repeatedly failing to verify their mother's presence through the 'bitty' modality of hearing. The children in this study showed very poor object constancy[3] at 3 years; this is typically achieved by non-disabled children at about 1 year. Nagera and Colonna (1965) reported how, in contrast to sighted children, blind children remained largely rooted in the early phases of personality development. In their view this was due to problems identifying environmental means of gratification. Because of this difficulty, when such means were found, these were held onto in a state of fixated preoccupation, disrupting progression to more mature functioning. Lastly, Omwake and Solnit (1961) describe therapeutic work with a blind girl. Like Niederland (1965), these authors frame her impairment as the cause of her psychological disturbance, directly after describing the repeated traumas of her early life. Their understanding was that under-stimulation due to impairment prevented her from developing the psychic imagery on which mature defences are based. I have critiqued Kenneth Wright's (1991) influential work in this area elsewhere (Watermeyer, 2002a).

All of these contributions share a fascination with the 'dark world' of blindness, distracting attention from what may be learned from an object relations analysis. What is missing is a close examination of the relational implications of impairment – that is, the largely unconscious, reverberating impact of anxious cultural responses to blindness on early formative relationships. As I shall argue later, impairment's ability to evoke primitive anxieties in the other has the power to disrupt the early developmental milieu, impressing itself on socialisation and selfhood from the earliest moments of life. Providing emotional containment and positive mirroring to an infant is, in any circumstances, a demanding task. The unexpected, unknown nature of infantile impairment can quite understandably heighten normative anxieties about being an adequate parent, especially when parents lack sensitive institutional support. What is required is an empathic exploration of the dynamic emotional circumstances unfolding between parents and infants, avoiding fixation on ever-present fantasies about the abstract, presocial nature of impairment. Research accounts suggest that anxieties evoked by sight impairment in children can disrupt familial socialisation (French, 1993b), and evoke repressive, even bizarre policies in education (Chapman, 1978; Armstrong, 2005; French and Swain, 2006). When we ask searching questions about relational factors we begin to see how the developmental problems described above may be shaped by *disrupted socialisation* which, in turn, emanates from the systemic psychological impact of 'disability meaning'. Significantly, these effects may masquerade all too well as the end-products of naked impairment, particularly if we fail to resist being entranced by impairment and consequently resort to managing our fantasies about difference through splitting.

Let us consider the work of Berger (1967) as a final example. Although developing ideas on chronic illness rather than disability, Berger regards the feeling that one's experience is 'unknowable' as central, attributing this to somatic factors (Berger, 1967 in Erskine, 1994). Now if, as we are beginning to see, the experience of disability or illness is marked with misattunements and empathic failures from an anxious or even hostile world, then feeling unknown, and hence unknowable, is a likely consequence. But here we readily assume that it is not an *experience* of being unknowable which is at work – that is, a relational artifact – but the modernist reality of *being* unknowable. Freud's most important utterances on the issue of disability, in a paper entitled *The Exceptions* (Freud, 1916), show up his own ambiguous position regarding the relative influence of relational and somatic factors on the experience of self. This work is important enough to require special attention, and will be examined in some depth later. In disabled lives then, one imagines that the mistaken attributions described above are subjectively *lived out*, through defences of self-blame; that is, 'I am unknowable', rather than 'I occupy a social world reluctant to know me'. Contradicting this experience, Olkin (1999) cites a raft of findings from clinical settings which disconnects the impaired body from the troubled mind, showing that the nature and severity of impairment does not correlate with psychological morbidity.

The bodily fixation of psychoanalytic writers has, by and large, worked to trace the invisible outline of an illusory 'disabled personality', leaving distorted social relationships uninterrogated. From here, the way is open for such formative experiences to take up a malignant residence in the disabled self, as subjective flaws rather than injustice. Deborah Marks (1999a) has pioneered an alternative, critical psychoanalytic view, aiming to cross-examine cultural influences shaping the lived reality of disability, with an emphasis on the unconscious mediation of oppression.

A critical psychoanalytic view of disability

Critical psychoanalysis takes the viewpoint that both conscious and unconscious processes are 'inextricably intertwined' with the shaping and flux of social structures (Marks, 2002, p. 2; Obholzer and Roberts, 1994). In other words, the landscape of the social order is constituted mutually – in ongoing reverberation – with its intra-psychic concomitants. Society's structures exist for *over-determined* reasons, serving both manifest, logical as well as latent, irrational purposes. Despite its ideological problems, the individual focus of traditional psychoanalysis shows as an unlikely strength here, bringing a wealth of concepts to describe the intricacies of subjective life. The challenge is to weave these intra-psychic aspects into a socio-historical, group-based analysis. If one accepts the interpenetration of social and psychic, it follows that progressive moral changes in society will – as we have seen – necessarily involve painful psychic shifts (Cooper and Treacher, 1995). What this means is that the cultural significations we use to harbour hazardous unconscious materials must be given up, as part of a realignment of defence mechanisms for making sense of the human world. In any form of oppression, unpacking the impulse towards 'civil defence' must involve understanding how this becomes the vehicle for psychic defence (Figlio and Richards, 2002, p. 197). But like myself, these writers warn that interpretation of the unconscious layers of social conflict can muddy the 'automatic rightness' of struggle politics (ibid.). As splits are interrogated and complexity revealed, crude vilifications appear less credible, less useful.

If disablist discrimination was not rooted in unconscious life, simple educational interventions would overcome it. It seems clear that this is not the case (Marks, 1999a, p. 13; Zizek, 1990; 2004; 2008). Rather than a lack of awareness, something far more obstinate is at work; disablist cultural phenomena, to some extent, embody a ransom for psychic stability. It was all too clear to Fanon (1952) that racial equality would never be won through a purely legal case structured in rational, conscious discourse. Instead, the unconscious meanings of skin colour had to be mined. In the critical psychoanalytic view a socially constructed identity such as 'disabled' is formed, reified and internalised in a dynamic, group-oriented manner, shaping identity-meanings and relations of both disabled and nondisabled persons. In a sense, all come to *rely* on the existence of these 'socio-psychic instruments'. Observable disability phenomena such as special schools, rehabilitation units, cultural representations and social service policies come under scrutiny as (*in part*) outpourings of defences which are mobilised by unconscious conflicts evoked by the disabled imago. The global prevalence of disability discrimination, common across all societies, suggests a core of unconscious investments in disablist othering – enacted via social structures. But what are these unconscious disability meanings composed of?

Though not operating within a psychoanalytic frame, Garland-Thomson (1997b) provides an eloquent description of the symbolic burden carried by disabled people. She writes:

> The disabled body stands for the self gone out of control, individualism run rampant: it mocks the notion of the body as compliant instrument of the limitless will and appears in the cultural imagination as ungovernable, recalcitrant, flaunting its difference as if to refute the fantasy of sameness implicit in the notion of equality. Even more troubling, disability suggests that the cultural other lies dormant within the cultural self, threatening abrupt or gradual transformations from 'man' to 'invalid'.
>
> (Garland-Thomson, 1997b, p. 43)

Disabled people are positioned as the symbolic custodians of damage, frailty and defect, their lives consistently constructed as dysfunctional and spoiled (Marks, 1999a). Shakespeare's (1994) emotive axiom 'dustbins for disavowal' captures the image of society's disowning of unwanted 'feelings, processes or characteristics', and the cementing of these to the disabled minority (p. 287). The roots of these unconscious aspects of the human condition lie, I suggest, in our shared experience of growing up.

An object relations view of early psychological development sees *emotional holding* as always imperfect (Winnicott, 1947). Sensitive care and support is essential, but does not save us from the struggles of our existence. The young infant must consequently manage a growing disillusionment – literally, the relinquishing of illusions – as he or she becomes more separate, and begins to negotiate an unknown world. Learning to manage the panic of abandonment is elemental, varying only with the goodness of fit between parent, baby and environment. Later development will bring further challenges: the competitiveness of school, anxieties about intellectual and sexual adequacy, fears about being acceptable and lovable and shame regarding dependency in a world where autonomy is prized. This description is particularly applicable to a Western, capitalist cultural environment, but the difficulty of the changes of human development is universal. Freud's conflict model of mind provides for the repression – the splitting off – of memories and emotions accumulated through the universally bumpy process of maturation. Staying psychologically functional requires that the conscious owning and 'working through' of this store of trauma be selective and limited, so as not to destabilise our ability to manage the ongoing tasks of life. All, therefore, carry unconscious layers of suffering, described by Marks (1999a, p. 176) as 'universal existential anxieties'. Notions and images of disability are convenient, sanctioned vehicles for giving vicarious life to such conflicts. Simultaneously, a lack of realistic representations of disabled life recapitulates a myth of inherent difference, making the disabled figure available as a carrier of struggles seen as having nothing at all to do with the lives of 'normals'. It is telling that psychoanalytic accounts of human fears about normality and acceptability reveal that 'those aspects of disability which generate most anxiety are precisely those areas of human experience which many people struggle with' (Marks, 1999a, p. 170). Cultural depictions of disability offer a semantic landscape brimming with symbolic potential, such as tragic accounts of ostracisation and the irresistible romance of redemption. Marks (1999a) describes this symbolic layer as it plays out in a street interaction with a visibly disabled person:

> As in a child told not to stare, the desire to look, combined with a fear of something dangerous and unthinkable, yet intriguing, create a heady mix of prurience, insecurity and avoidance of the subject.
>
> (Marks, 1999a, p. 11)

In this vignette the onlooker is captivated, yet appalled; drawn by an unconscious desire to find a fragment of herself in the other, but repelled through a defensive fantasy of intrinsic difference. In the stranger before her she sees tragedy, loss, shame, the unknown; each aspect an affront to modernist aspirations. A moment such as this allows little choice; we unconsciously deflect what is raised in us, often seeing the stranger as a personification of our own un-thought wounds. In one author's words, the alternative is to acknowledge that of which disability is a harbinger – 'that life is tragic and we shall all soon be dead' (Hunt, 1998, p. 16). What has taken place is an unconscious transaction, leaving the disabled other as the carrier of an inherent, unequal difference. The absence of such 'differentness' would lay the observer bare to the discomforting, simple reality of disabled people as human subjects who suffer oppression – as I might – and suffer the frailty of the body – as I will. Readmitting disabled people to the shared, human fold also means acknowledging that society is 'shot through with inequity', to which all are vulnerable. In this sense disabled people 'represent a fearsome possibility' (Murphy, 1987, p. 117).

All human relating involves transference (Klein, 1952) – that is, our view of the other is always distorted by projections arising from past relationships. In this sense the disabled identity is an extreme case, where emotional valency is heightened and culture provides a 'disabled imago' to aid projection on an inter-group scale. Because engaging with disability speaks so directly to hidden limitations, cognitions here are especially distorted (Bion, 1957). Primitive conflicts are exposed, prompting a regression to concrete, simplified and self-protective cognitions – the hallmarks of what Klein (1946) termed the *paranoid-schizoid position*. There is no room here for reflection or nuance in interpretation of what we see; instead, our reactions are immediate, unmediated and paranoid. The authoritarian culture and crude, accusatory certainties of political movements on the far right demonstrate this mode of functioning. This violence is analogous to intra-psychic totalitarian parts in all of us, similarly provoked to action by perceived threats to identity. In both cases the threat is *perceived*, as the very nature of the self is built on denial of those self-same characteristics. It is important to note that the resultant split view of the disabled figure may as easily manifest in caring responses based on a stereotyped invalidity, as in hostility or distancing.

Social injustice and attempts at its amelioration are a magnet for the projection of psychological conflict (Richards, 1986). As a result, efforts at social change often carry very personal hopes for healing or relief, even to members of social groups who are materially unaffected (ibid.). In the case of disability's charity discourse, it may be argued that personal investments in struggle inadvertently prop up demeaning representations, confounding change. Institutions aiming to shift the status quo often become entangled in complex and paradoxical unconscious investments, potentially sabotaging precisely those changes initially sought (Fenichel, 1946; Bion, 1962a; Menzies-Lyth, 1988; Foster, 2001).

Gordon (1995) questions whether insight into the intra-psychic correlates of social processes will bring about change, commenting that during the First Gulf War it was no help whatsoever to know that global politics was dominated by projection. Though probably true in this instance, in the case of disability inequality I disagree. Unlike intercontinental warfare, disablism is often woven into intimate, proximal relationships; between professionals and patients, parents and children, carers and cared for – it is on this terrain that disabled subjectivity is forged. In these tightly bound engagements, rich with projection and introjection, insight which fosters the re-owning of disavowed or lost parts of self seems invaluable. For example, supporting parents of congenitally impaired children in understanding the unconscious currents evoked by disability is crucial. This will protect relationships from the confusion and disruption which can so easily take shape. Since disability prejudice is so intermingled with common sense – through the pervasiveness of the medical model – it may be that personal insight is a more essential prerequisite for change here than in other arenas.

Zizek (1990) augments our picture of inter-group division founded on splitting and projection by adding his notion of *enjoyment*. This is an experience of narcissistic gratification rooted in a myth of the sanctity and unique worth of a group identity. Members channel energy towards proving the 'vivacity and plenitude' of group attributes, reinforcing an illusory commonality (p. 52). A pivotal feature is that this involves the structuring of relations towards other groups. In fantasy, 'hazards' to group identity such as an influx of immigrants threaten the security of enjoyment (ibid.). Here, the illusion of a consensual, material 'way of life' comes under threat from the corrosive forces of out-group culture. This nebulous, wishful 'way of life' of Zizek's model precisely describes a group fantasy of 'nondisabled culture'; that which, although undefined, may be spoiled by disability-difference (ibid.). The illusion of distinctiveness referred to above is realised in the materiality of social policies and installations, legitimating the hum of projections which traverse it. While the nondisabled 'way of life' is portrayed as inaccessible – unliveable – to disabled persons, it is 'nonetheless constantly menaced by "them"' (ibid., p. 52). Group myths of enjoyment reinforce internal narcissistic structures. In this way fantasy marshals group power, by making personal consolation contingent on maintaining separateness from those who do not share 'our way of life'. Reflecting on a fantasied 'disabled threat', the historical prominence of demonological beliefs about cause provides clues to the unconscious resonances of this form of otherness (Braddock and Parish, 2001).

The sexuality of learning disabled people brings into view an example of non-disabled life coming under the subjective threat of 'mixing'. Sinason (1992) describes an intense, commonly held feeling of alarm or disgust surrounding the sexual activity of learning disabled people. The threat to majority enjoyment takes shape here as a catastrophic fantasy that the shame seen in learning disabled lives will exponentially reproduce itself, overwhelming civilised existence. The long history of controls enforced on the sexuality of the learning disabled community is testimony to this anxiety. White (2003) provides a corresponding analysis of the history of sex education for blind persons, finding that such 'education' is better described as the fervent enforcing of an especially rigid heteronormativity. One may view such interventions as defensive reactions to fears of encroachment or contamination. In fantasy, disability's unnerving, seemingly infinite diversity readily destabilises cherished aspects of 'normal' life. When such norms are under threat – say, by the integration of visibly disabled children into early learning centres – a need to 'enumerate disconnected fragments' of nondisabled culture may emerge, as queasy fears of 'mixing' surface and social and psychic ranks begin to close (Zizek, 1990, p. 52).

Marks (1999a) orients her exploration of unconscious factors implicated in disablism by posing a number of questions – questions she believes may only be tackled psychoanalytically. She asks:

> What is the origin of the excessive emotional energy (be it sadistic, fearful or kind) evoked by images of disability?
> How do we account for patronising, hostile or avoidant responses of non-disabled people?
> What 'emotional payoff' is achieved by nondisabled persons' involvement in 'altruistic' disability-related work?
> What typically unacknowledged existential anxieties have disability come to symbolise?
> Why are persons with disabilities repeatedly represented in popular media as dangerous, helpless, disordered or infantile?
>
> (Marks, 1999a, p. 22 [paraphrased])

To Marks (1999a), Stephen Frosh's (2006) comment that it is often fantasy that fuels politics, rather than the other way around, is especially true in the case of disability. With different terminology, Murphy (1995, p. 140) concurs, stating that 'stigmatisation is less a by-product of disability than *its substance*' (my emphasis). He continues:

> The greatest impediment to a person's taking full part in his [sic.] society is not his physical flaws, but rather the tissue of myths, fears and misunderstandings that society attaches to them.
>
> (Murphy, 1995, p. 140)

What is threatened by the disabled figure is nothing less than the modernist project itself. Modernism dreams of exorcising the spectre of human frailty through control, separation or eradication (Hughes, 2002b). These controls seek not only to eliminate bodily 'damage', but – perhaps more significantly – carry an imagined extermination of the internal damage which this symbolises. The post-structuralist axiom that difference always resolves into inequality is powerfully played out in this fantasy of 'cleansing' (Garland-Thomson, 1995). Disability unsettles us in the manner of what Freud (1919) termed 'the uncanny' – that which provokes dread because of its perverse intimacy with the familiar. Freud (1919), in fact, makes specific reference to bodily 'deformity' in describing the flavour of this fearful disgust, associating it to images of 'dismembered limbs, a severed head, a hand cut off at the wrist' (p. 244). In the previous chapter we considered Sinason's (1992) critique of politically correct euphemisms that cluster around evocative markers of difference. Arguably though, it is disability which cuts the deepest. Davis (2002) points out a sobering reality. It is familiar to see white people embracing the civil rights cause of blacks; likewise, many straight people have taken up the cause of sexual minorities. But it is a small and exceptional minority of nondisabled persons who identify disability as a social oppression issue and participate in its civil rights agenda. Davis (2002) relates this to the position of the disabled body as harbinger, as prophecy. Observing social inequalities, we are aware that no white persons are at risk of becoming black, and few straight people will alter their sexual orientation. But every 'normal' individual can, and most *will*, become disabled during the life course (ibid.). Disability, therefore, confronts us with Freud's (1919) character of *das Unheimlich* – that which is sinister and discomforting precisely through its closeness to home.

The theoretical orientation being developed in this book combines an object relations-based, critical psychoanalytic position with social constructionism's strength for critiquing culture. The metapsychological foundations of object relations make the discipline more able to include the influence of culture on intrapsychic formations than its purely drive-based forerunners, while a constructionist approach unpacks ideological machinery that shapes subjectivity. In this view, disability meanings and behaviour are strongly unconsciously mediated, yet those unconscious formations are partially – largely – an ideological product. Although it may not at first seem so, critical realism's common-sense return to bodies which are painful or dysfunctional is, I believe, a compatible overlay to this approach. This viewpoint, as my own, draws on a partial application of constructionist critique, and is similarly wary of the binaries of a traditional politicised stance. My critical psychoanalytic view has no need of deconstructing pain or deficit out of existence. It is, however, interested in how fantasies about these experiences (real or not) are played out in unequal societal enactments. In all of this, the question of how disabled selfhood is coalesced is central. In the following sections we examine specific defence mechanisms at play in disabling social relations. In each case, the need to defend the self from disability meanings manifests in distorted social perceptions which, at times, carry oppressive consequences.

Defence mechanisms at work in disablist oppression

The need to subdue unconscious parts of self enlivened by images of impairment harnesses defence mechanisms shaping our responses to the disabled community. As external interventions are applied, these aid in the stilling of internal struggles. Thus it is that many aspects of society's response to the impaired body present, in part, as concretisations of psychic defence. Under the rubric of *social responses to disability* I include elements as diverse as legislation, linguistic conventions, service installations, religious rituals, health care protocols, built environments, education policies and much else. Most, on close consideration, carry a degree of latent, unconscious motivation. This scrutiny often shows the shape of the defence, as this is mirrored in the nature of the social response. In the main, the defences described below act to maintain material and psychological distance between those designated as disabled and nondisabled, preserving the former in the role of available psychic containers.

Splitting

Developing the discussion begun earlier, this is a crude defence which avoids the anxiety-provoking ambiguities of a complex world through endowing people or things with 'all good' or 'all bad' qualities. The template for such sense-making harks back to early life, with the infant struggling to integrate intense, fearful feelings of dependency. For her the world is unknown and frightening, its figures unpredictable. She also does not have the mental faculties to deal with constitutional feelings of aggression, which are consequently experienced as part of the 'dangers' outside. For the infant the primary carer – often the mother – is 'the world'; all fantasies of that world's abundance and danger are experienced as part of her. In order to manage fears of dependency, un-control or cruelty, the baby splits her internal idea of 'mother' (her *maternal object*) into two – what Klein (1946) called the idealised *good breast* and the hated *bad breast.* For the baby, the idea that both good and bad are part of the same carer is far too anxiety-provoking, exposing her to the naked unpredictability of her situation. Instead, she creates a 'good' mother, and attributes all else to an iniquitous 'bad' mother.

In responses to disability, the need to escape feelings of ambiguity is readily to be seen. Disability's associations of inability and brokenness come with an uncertainty about degree. For example, when meeting a sight impaired person, disquieting fantasies about life without sight are deepened by ambiguity regarding the *extent* of impairment.

This may in part reflect a need to gain control through knowing the extent of the imagined danger. Like the anxious infant, the observer here resolves a chaotic world into black and white, rendering the familiar extremes of the 'disabled invalid' and the superhuman disabled person who 'can do anything'. Disabled people in these circumstances have diminished opportunities to be seen as complex, nuanced individuals, instead carrying – perhaps alternately – a wholesale idealised or devalued character. Brokenness perceived in the disabled figure may be flanked, at the edges of consciousness, by a fear of becoming impaired and guilt over 'able-ness', adding to the psychological stakes of the engagement. An important part of the splitting process is between observer and observed – the distancing fantasy of inherent difference, re-creating another as an *other*.

Klein (1960) understood idealisation as a guilty, reparative response to underlying feelings of aggression. If disabled people represent parts of us which we very much need to avoid, it should be no surprise that hostility forms part of our muddle of emotional responses to the disabled body. Hate crime, forced sterilisation and genocide may, under careful examination, show up as extreme forms of these destructive impulses – an overwhelming drive to renounce split-off parts through destroying their symbols. But more subtle, everyday hostility is channelled into the figure of the 'supercrip'. Accounts of heart-warming, plucky resilience in the face of impairment, along with the attribution of unrealistic abilities and ideal traits are familiar in popular culture. Disabled people falling on the opposite side of this split may find themselves holding attributes of a depressed inertia, helpless and inadequate, and deserving of abandonment, punishment or pity. Either formulation leaves little mental space to comprehend the experience and self of the disabled individual, making empathic, authentic relating less possible. One is as unknown by being idealised as by being denigrated. Foster (2001) describes how work with 'vulnerable' populations draws social service workers into split relating. Here, the emotional noise of hostility and guilt interferes with listening, leading to distortions in the helping relationship such as control or infantilisation. It is important to understand that, in my view, our anxiety-ridden feelings and fantasies about disability are not the problem. These are, in all likelihood, relatively universal consequences of fears about difference, and nothing to be ashamed of. What distorts relationships, and at times psychologically scapegoats the disabled figure, is our difficulty with consciously *thinking about* our feeling-associations, in a way which accepts ownership. It is a reliable psychodynamic rule of thumb that we will tend to *act out* that which we cannot consciously own up to; it is the hidden nature of conflict which makes it dangerous, as it continues to seek displaced expression.

To give life to the idealised disabled figure I have elsewhere provided the following example (Watermeyer, 2006, pp. 37–38). In the film *Scent of a Woman* (Universal Studios, 1992), Al Pacino plays an embittered and isolated blind man who, despite his 'limitations', undertakes a range of breathtaking feats including dancing a dramatic tango after merely enquiring about the dimensions of the dance floor, and driving a sports car at breakneck speed under the instructions of a terrified navigator. The 'blind man' is represented here at both extremes of a split concept of what disablement implies. The first portrays Pacino's character as the stereotype of an emotionally damaged, isolated invalid, with a self stunted and distorted by impairment. This image, arguably, reflects fantasies of 'how I would feel without sight' held by the screenplay writer and echoed by societal stereotypes. These ideas form the basis for a unidimensional, broken character. The usefulness of splitting here is the following: in the face of threatening, amorphous imaginings about what life with blindness may be like, the observer attains mastery and control by deciding that the blind person's life is, in fact, the way it is fearfully imagined to be.

Paradoxically, the construction of Pacino's character as able to perform the heroic antics that he does reflects a need, in the observer, to *overcome* the original fantasy of his invalidity and desolation. After the giving over of feelings of damage and incapability stimulated by the blindness imago, these are managed by a form of reversal requiring portrayal of an implausible potency and talent. Remarkably therefore, Pacino's character allows the observer to feel reassured that his life is not the unmitigated tragedy which we fear, and yet simultaneously to have confirmation that it is just that. Distorted constructions such as this prevent us from seeing that disabled lives carry familiar human complexities; strengths and vulnerabilities, hopes and losses, competence and inadequacy. The failure of Hollywood to present disabled characters as normatively complex individuals muddling through life's challenges is most unfortunate, and has been well documented (e.g. Norden, 1994).

Projection

As should be clear, this is the primary explanation for how unwanted parts of self come to be attributed to others. To Marks (1999a, p. 23) the concept is a 'key tool for understanding the psychic mechanisms of prejudice against disabled people'. Klein (1960) presents a picture of the developing child experiencing him or herself as bad, and escaping the ensuing guilt by seeing the 'badness' as a characteristic of others. For the infant, as in authoritarian politics, this attribution reinforces fears of persecution, as the boundaries of the psyche rigidify to hold out the threatening weight of disavowed material. The relationship – again, in infantile or authoritarian psychology – between projection (in effect, prejudice) and paranoia is clear to see. In each case haunting guilt is a feature, arising from hostile feelings or awareness of the victimising sleight of hand of the emotional transaction.

It is quite wrong, however, to view projection as always harmful or pathological – its forms occupy a continuum. At the extreme we see its dangers, but it is also an essential basis for empathy (McWilliams, 1994). As mature compassion, projection is essential if we are to benignly imagine the predicaments of another. 'Maturity', here refers to the pivotal question of taking ownership of one's own fearful parts, rather than projecting these. Relational intuition and attunement would not be possible without a careful measure of projection (ibid.).

But turning to the influence of projection in relationships around disability, let us consider possible unconscious currents in a family with a congenitally disabled sibling. Against the backdrop of anxious unconscious resonances and the physical demands of caring for an impaired child, splits can easily, and understandably, emerge between the 'neediness' or 'vulnerability' of the disabled child and the 'independence' and 'strength' of her siblings (Burke, 2008). Worries in parents about their disabled child's ability to cope with a demanding, unaccepting world make healthy separation harder, positioning siblings differently. Subtle relational dynamics may be internalised by all, leading to frailty or need being seen as the province of the disabled child, with other children growing into identities where needs are less visible, even to the self. Guilt and confusion relating to feeling like one of the 'lucky ones' may deepen the dynamic, through drawing siblings still further away from their own vulnerability. Meanwhile, in broader society insistent media representations of disabled people as damaged unfortunates maintain group-based projection on a mass scale, encouraging the perplexing splits experienced by family members.

In a post-structuralist view of the development of subjectivity, projection (by one name or another) is central, as the illusory self is built upon differentiation from what it is not. To feminist constructionists such as Burman (1996, p. 138), the projected aspects of self have no intrinsic 'realness'; she refers to the fantasy of a prior time of 'unity and completeness' where all had ownership of their own attributes – a time which never existed. I, too, wouldn't endorse the idea of an era of wholeness and unity, but I do allow for a residue of 'reality' in the crossfire of identity fragments. This is the reality of shame-ridden aspects of self, universally present as a result of our experience of infancy and the struggles of development, and lived, in part, through our embodiment. Hegemonic values which see health and vigour as moral virtues, and attach abjection to impairment, provide impetus for alienation from these intrinsic characteristics.

Earlier we saw strong critique levelled at traditional psychoanalytic writing on disability for its disregard of context. But as noted, I feel that scuppering this body of work as a whole would mean the baby being discarded with the bathwater. To take one psychoanalytic contribution vilified by disability studies (Lenny, 1993; Goodley and Lawthom, 2006), let us revisit the work of Thomas and Siller (1999). A closer look shows up surprising worth to an emancipatory, contextual psychoanalytic view of disablism. Siller (1970) found that *fear of rejection* among non-disabled subjects predicted reluctance to associate with disabled people (in Thomas and Siller, 1999). In other words, the ostracisation of disabled people correlates to projected anxieties about acceptability in the broader populace. Other studies cited by these writers (Siller et al., 1967 in Thomas and Siller, 1999) found that expectations carried about disabled persons' emotional response to their impairment corresponded closely to each subject's own psychological struggles. For example, the assumption that disablement would lead to depression or anger embodied a 'direct projection of one's unconscious fears' (Thomas and Siller, 1999, p. 185). Further, such expectations corresponded to fears about specific forms of impairment. They write:

> For example, a woman with intense communication problems expressed greatest fear, if disabled, of being deaf. Paralysis was a particular issue with those showing dependency fears. Cerebral palsy posed a great threat to those

> for whom control is critical, with physical uncontrol objectifying emotional uncontrol.
>
> (Siller et al., 1967 in Thomas and Siller, 1999, p. 185)

What becomes clear is that the system of cultural meanings which shape perceptions of disability interfaces with the 'projection needs' of the community at large. The essence of the psycho-political fix that disabled people find themselves in is, arguably, a specific and amplified version of the predicament of all oppressed minorities – having one's characteristics, one's self, forcefully defined from without. Kriegel (1987), in a critique of representations of 'the cripple' in English literature, concludes that while others cry 'I am what I am', the disabled figure is forced to submit, instead saying 'I am *what you tell me I am*' (p. 33 – my emphasis).

Although not working from a psychoanalytic viewpoint, Hunt (1998) describes, in essence, a majority investment in holding the disabled community as receptacles for projection. He notes a need in the observer for disabled individuals to show evidence of suffering in order to reaffirm the value, the 'specialness', of nondisabled status. If out-group members show no sign of misery this may be awkward for narcissistic self-assurances, which rest on experiences of positive distinctiveness. Zizek's (1990) notion of the precarious status of 'enjoyment' resonates closely. Since we all have bodies in flux, the investment in meanings carried by the disabled imago touches all.

In both racism and disablism psychic parts are projected, then attacked by the selves that disavowed them (Frosh, 1989). But paradoxically, the out-group is also resentfully stereotyped as possessing idealised privileges, or even characteristics, for which it is loathed. In the disability arena this resonates with the familiar, often hateful image of the freeloader who enjoys special privileges and a life of passive, even gluttonous dependency. Mingled in may be a resentful sadness at the 'invalid's' perceived licence for dependency – despised, but unconsciously envied. One fantasy is of disabled people occupying a mythic, nurturant and attuned environment of care – the wished-for safety of the maternal dyad. Sympathy-inducing, infantilising representations evident in disability charity discourse do much to reinforce this picture. By definition we are disquieted by reflections of our vulnerability. Thus it is that our inability to see nuance in the disabled figure correlates with the struggle to consciously experience our own distress. Avoidance of self reduces the other to a monochrome reflection of a fragmented, dingy inner world.

Projective identification

This defence is closely related to projection, but here the recipient is directly emotionally affected by the process (Young, 1994). Whereas 'pure' projection is merely fantasy in the mind of the projector, projective identification involves the recipient being unconsciously co-opted into a collusion, and often an enactment of what is attributed to him or her; a relationship of control or enmeshment has begun. In the case of racism projective identification has been described as 'the internal equivalent of colonial occupation' (Davids, 1996, p. 216). Earlier we considered how 'normals' may need the disabled figure to fulfil expected characteristics. Here, denigrating fantasies move beyond the psychic, into a relational space where the other is actually *created* in a manner which affirms the projection. An examination of the often demeaning social circumstances of disabled persons poses important questions about projective identification. Do modern societies produce disabled persons who are marginal, dependent, uneducated and emotionally damaged in order to maintain a material other who may live out these split-off parts on behalf of the dominant group? In higher education institutions or the workplace, clinical experience shows anecdotal evidence of disabled people who seem – inadvertently – set up to fail; welcomed, yet simultaneously sabotaged by barriers to fulfilling potential.

Elemental to this defence is the recipient becoming *identified* with the projected parts – she experiences these as her own (Segal, 1973; Ogden, 1979). In this sense the creation of a marginal disabled figure occurs not only on the material plane but also – perhaps more importantly – on the psychological. If projected material is to find a home in the other, it must be felt to be familiar, fitting with self and circumstance. In this way what comes in feels continuous with one's own self; medical model mechanisms of self-blame are clear to see here. When projective identification works, the recipient is unaware that anything has occurred, simply taking ownership of the shames of others.

In lives of exclusion and deprivation lived by many disabled people in modern society, questions of responsibility are everywhere – 'Am I to blame?' … 'Or is society to blame?' The split simplicity of this dilemma underscores the anxiety-ridden, concrete thought environment which a culture of othering provides to all concerned. In lives facing massive obstacles to fulfilment, nagging internal mantras direct blame at a self that 'didn't try hard enough', or 'wasn't organised enough', or was 'too needy' or 'too difficult'. These familiar echoes may be read as consequences of projective identification, which blurs internal boundaries between what is 'me' and 'not me', eroding entitlement and, notably, disrupting the creation of a united political minority.

Young (1994, p. 140) emphasises the 'primitiveness' and 'adhesive, binding power' of projective identifications, which cause these connections to be particularly resilient. One upshot is that the defence manifests as a 'profoundly conservative' device, constructing prejudices which are immensely difficult to dislodge, as we remain obsessed by lives offering discharge to our unvoiced psychic fragments (ibid.). This obsession shows not only in passive constructions, but in the need for relating, for exchange, for control. Consequently, the mechanism has deep significance in understanding helping relationships – one need not look far in the disability arena to find individuals and organisations with striking emotional investments in their work. It is not at all my intention to pathologise or denigrate these investments, but simply to suggest that our motivations are complex; both service providers and users stand to benefit from honest reflection on these layered relationships. Along these lines, Dass and Gorman (1985) comment as follows:

> It's as if our vicarious involvement with the trials and tribulations of others engages us in the life process in a way that we seem to need, but also want to be able to control. We want to watch it, but be able to turn it off at will.
>
> (Dass and Gorman, 1985, p. 55)

In helping relationships split-off, shameful parts of self may be unconsciously called forth in the other through modes of treatment which elicit their expression. Dynamics such as these may pervade the lives of visibly impaired people, shaping socialisation in a way which directs individuals towards accepting a marginal place in society. Formative relational experiences such as the limiting of separation by intrusive or anxious caring, controls exerted on life decisions, symbolic and material exclusions and much else may find a home in the disabled individual's internal world. Here, projective identification elicits subjectively natural participation in mutually reinforcing relationships of difference. It is important to bear in mind that both projection and projective identification are seldom, if ever, one-directional. Splitting affects the images of all participants, rendering distorted views of self and other in 'oppressed' and 'oppressor'.

While this initial model is a quite simple, crude one, it begins to show how the cultural idea of 'disability damage' can be chronically re-enacted through relationships steeped in the unconscious whisperings of the disabled imago. Dauntingly, it also shows how difficult real change is. It demands honest, cooperative self-examination by all, in order to identify and dislodge relational schemas imbued with shared, archaic meanings. Of course we must be aware of the danger of pathologising disabled people as co-contributors in oppressive relationships; but it is an equally grave error to ignore the hurtful impact of lifelong distortions in relating which often surround impairment.

Reaction formation

In the case of this mechanism the ego is protected from discomforting feelings about the other by enacting their opposite (Marks, 1999a). Images of disability, always provocative to us, may evoke unconscious feelings or impulses which bring a moral unease, such as aggression or disgust. One way of managing such feelings is through the guilty compensation of 'doing good'. Marks (1999a, p. 22) asks that we carefully consider 'altruistic' disability-related work, and the 'emotional payoff' which it may bring. I have already emphasised that this be done in a thoughtful and non-judgmental manner, rejecting a disability movement split which disparages people in caring roles. A *portion* of the satisfaction or feeling of well-being associated with such work may relate to a safety from darker impulses (towards the other, but also the self) brought on by proximity to the mortal, dependent body. The reparative work of *undoing* (see below) is often interwoven.

The prominence of pity around impairment does provide signposts to our more difficult, unconscious feeling responses; indeed, Freud (1933) explicitly associates altruism with disavowed sadism. This, of course, does not mean that altruistic work is *reducible* to paradoxical unconscious motives – not at all. But if we agree that the atmosphere around disability is thick with unconscious, emotive investments, it shouldn't surprise or shock us that motives for entering caring professions are seldom one-dimensional, and always partially hidden. I happily include myself in this assessment. There can be little doubt that the ideological influence of such relationships – in residential and nursing care, a range of medical professions, state social service institutions, community rehabilitation organisations, charity and religious groups, and a host of others – can hardly be overestimated.

In relations between disabled clients and nondisabled professionals, pivotal issues such as the defining of 'needs' may be strongly coloured by unconscious investments in control, or the fulfilment of a caricatured caring persona. The vast critique directed at health and other social services by disability studies – while excessive and simplistic at times – tells a story of complex relationships characterised by very real inequality and largely unexamined personal motivations. Perennial, charged debates about how disability should be 'managed' reflect both manifest and unconscious struggles for power; personal needs in the practitioner shaping this engagement are seldom examined. Simply put, the question posed to professionals is this: what more subtle, personal needs are filled by your caring role? No-one need be afraid of this exploration, and there is much to gain. There is also solace in the reality that, when it comes to an evocative area such as disability, *none* of us are here entirely by accident. My experience in training health professionals involved in work with disability shows clearly that all have a disability story. A curriculum of disability socialisation plays out in a range of domains, including having an impaired relative, the impressions of religious or charity-based duty, the observing of social distancing and segregation, images of bodily difference in stories or doctrine, the need to relieve real or imagined pain in family members; the list of such emotive meanings is endless. My experience as a trainer and supervisor is that providing an accepting space for reflecting on these stories can bring important, personal threads of a practitioner's relationship with disability to light. On many occasions I have witnessed great relief as someone uncovers what he or she has – on the hidden, personal plane – been *doing*, or *undoing*, in their disability work. Obviously, what all of this points to is the need for an accepting atmosphere of reflexivity between professionals. Much supervision of rehabilitation professionals is of a relatively 'technicist' sort. I cannot emphasise enough the benefits to all of a more open-ended, psychoanalytically curious supervisory space.

Reversal and undoing

These forms of defence are both, in effect, specific cases of reaction formation. In *reversal* difficult feelings threatening the surface of consciousness (such as painful feelings about self-identity or memories of trauma) are managed by switching roles – that is, shifting from the position of subject to that of object (McWilliams, 1994). This describes a situation in which, for example, feeling threatened by traumatic, formative experiences surrounding one's longing for care resolves into the compromise of becoming a carer – perhaps a health professional. Vicarious life is given to the needy self through close proximity to those thought of as helpless, from the safety of a role defined in opposition.

Undoing refers to a pattern of reparative actions, perhaps lifelong, which are rooted in remorse for past mistakes or misdeeds (McWilliams, 1994). These 'sins' may be real or imagined, realistic or exaggerated, but are subjectively felt as somehow definitive of a 'badness' in the self, which must be 'made up for'. McWilliams (1994) describes psychotherapeutic work with an elderly white woman who had dedicated her life to campaigning for racial equality. As a nine year old, she had, with the naïveté of a child, racially insulted a black woman whom she loved deeply. This experience, for her, became the kernel of an iniquity she suspected in herself, around which coalesced a defensive 'characterological altruism' (ibid.). The disability arena is, to say the least, no stranger to highly dedicated workers and campaigners – both disabled and nondisabled. Again, without reducing or pathologising such dedication in either population, clarity about its outcomes will depend on an understanding of its roots. If we do not know why we do what we do, we can understand only a part of the meaningfulness of the goals we seek – goals which, like all of our behaviours, are psychologically over-determined.

Rationalisation

In the case of *rationalisation*, guilt-evoking unconscious impulses or feelings are managed through constructing rational justifications for the actions these inform (Marks, 1999a). All social responses to disability, both institutional and cultural, appear enclosed in an envelope of 'sensible', rational purpose and meaning-making, disguising the additional layer of more subtle, emotional motivations. It is important to be clear here that identifying unconscious motives in, say, the policy of segregated special schooling does not detract from the reality or legitimacy of the conscious, theoretical reasoning. Instead, the intention is to add an awareness of complexity. Developing this example, the following vignette is an illustration (from Watermeyer, 2000):

> Some 100 kilometres outside my home city is a small town which has over several decades developed into a centre for disability social services. These include special schools for visually and hearing impaired children and residential sheltered employment facilities for sensorily, physically and multiply impaired adults. One conscious explanation for locating these services and their consumers in a small rural town surrounds safety – for example, persons with sensory impairments seem far safer in an environment without the heavy traffic of the city. Further, it makes sense to centralise special services and skills required to teach sensorily impaired children. This thinking seems, and is, reasonable. But what other explanations might be reached if we apply a psychoanalytically oriented curiosity? Perhaps at an unconscious level policy-makers were drawn to initiatives which located disabled people out of

> sight, out of the everyday social world. The impaired adult body is often disquieting to us; impaired children probably all the more so, due to our constructions of childhood as innocent, hopeful and full of possibility. Evacuating bodily difference may partly fulfil an unconscious wish that 'damaged' people and, more importantly, the emotional damage of which they are reminders, do not exist. The manifest, overt objectives of disability-related social services fall easily on the ear, supported by beliefs which affirm 'helping' and 'support' as admirable. In fact, we tend to feel uncomfortable, even outraged at the questioning of motives of individuals and organisations dedicated to helping those 'less fortunate than us', with reasoning sometimes traceable to religious doctrine. As a result, unconscious influences on the design of disability social services often remain obscured.
>
> (Watermeyer, 2000, p. 40 [paraphrased])

Unhelpfully, social service organisations working with disability may, as in the example above, feel unassailable to critique. Or critical feedback may be responded to defensively. At times, too, such critique may be of the unfair, vilifying sort associated with some segments of the disability movement. In each case, what is missed is a candid, respectful and cool-headed discussion of the merits and disadvantages of policy, due to a combination of avoidant or controlling unconscious motives, investments in the helping identity and splitting on all sides. If a useful, developmental engagement is to take place it will require a certain empathy from all quarters. Of course, the rage felt by disabled persons whose rights are routinely contravened is appropriate. But if destructive, feuding splits are to fade, all stakeholders must begin by creating accepting space for the complex investments and experience of others. If service providers are to grow in understanding unconscious investments in strategies and identities of care, an empathic, flexible relational environment will be essential. The destructive chronicity of splitting, accusatory relationships with health professionals not only misses the opportunity for improving methods, but also wastes personal capital through a needless alienation of workers with valuable skills.

Medicalisation as a defence

This is not a defence mechanism one would find in a psychoanalytic text. I suggest it here to bring together a range of ways in which medicalising discourse can be used to distance the disquieting voice of disabled experience. These strategies may involve combinations of 'formal' defences; those already described, and others. To begin, health services based on Cartesian principles commence with diagnosis. To some degree, the social experience of impairment is sheared away. The personal tragedy narrative that an uncritical biomedical stance creates can be a refuge from the disturbing reality of social injustice. Instead, inequality is, often wordlessly, framed as inevitable and morally neutral. Paradigmatic, professional, even architectural aspects of biomedicine tend to promote 'looking past' oppression – disciplinary boundaries create somatic silos carrying clinical discourse far from street level. As we have seen, disability provides corporeal hooks – in the form of bodily difference – which are useful in rationalising prejudice. For

Gill (2001) this makes the dilemma of disablist oppression potentially more sticky, more intractable, than that of women or black people. Further, the fact that difficulties such as pain, fatigue or functional limitation are part of life for many disabled people allows these experiences to be misused as blanket foundations for devaluing attitudes (ibid.). These aspects are often generalised or cited in isolation, creating a 'distorted wholesale disparagement of the disability experience' (ibid., p. 365). The collective view that medical factors are pivotal in disabled lives can be understood as a shared introjective identification (Hinshelwood, 1987). In this scenario, individuals have taken in a supportive object – medical discourse – which is collectively, culturally available, but has a personal defensive usefulness. Once taken in, the introject assists in smoothing over the harsh realities of social injustice, as well as possible guilt or helplessness. The resultant censored view of social reality is cyclically re-projected into the cultural arena, solidifying it further into a group-based given, which is again available for re-use.

Introjective identifications may also be forced into recipients against their conscious will, paving the way for demeaning identity ascriptions (Menzies, 1960 in Hinshelwood, 1987). This is a form of subtle psychic coercion, drawing disabled people into submitting to stereotypes. The interweaving of disablist discourse with internal needs to avoid recognising injustice, as well as project unwanted characteristics, limits everyone's ability to imagine a different sort of society. A malignant disabled identity introject may be an ever-present shadow which stalks disabled lives, slowly seeping in, or being 'installed' by institutional socialisation. Kriegel's (1987) description of the disabled individual being forced to submit that 'I am what you tell me I am' feels painfully resonant. In a ground-breaking, astute monograph the anthropologist Robert Scott (1969) demonstrated how the rehabilitation of blind persons by social service organisations in the USA was more accurately described as adult socialisation; that is, an exercise in training the newly impaired in the business of being the society's disabled minority. With disturbing clarity, Scott (1969) showed how clients of rehabilitation organisations were rewarded or negatively sanctioned for modes of 'being disabled' which did or did not fit with official protocols. The script defining the right way to be blind – demeanour, trappings, methods – which carried with it a range of more subtle communications relating to social position, worth, 'reasonable expectations' and the like. For Stiker (1982) the emergence of rehabilitation heralded an age of 'identification' – a drive to make humans identical. In his view, institutions aimed at eradicating alterity bolster a fantasy that it is possible to dissolve 'all that is lacking' from society and create an ideal, homogeneous social whole (pp. 128–32; McRuer, 2006).

Wherever we see the social sequelae of disability, guilt seems always present – in disabled people and others, and at both conscious and unconscious levels. The contradiction of, at times, starkly uneven provision of resources to ostensibly equal citizens distorts relationships with guilt, manifesting in a range of emotional and behavioural forms. The biomedical view offers the observer the opportunity to substitute *disability guilt* with the milder discomfort of *impairment guilt*. The former, I suggest, involves a level of culpability, where the observer is passively implicated in supporting a society which deprives some of its citizens. By contrast, impairment guilt places the issue in the hands of destiny, nature or God, absolving both society and the individual. Dominant discourses of pity and charity fit snugly into this defence, helpfully composing the objects of impairment guilt as chance unfortunates. The onlooker, from here, is left with the opportunity to be both altruistic and powerful in relation to that which earlier brought fault, becoming a bringer of succour rather than affliction.

Troubling fantasies about the abject bodily and psychological experience of disability lead to a range of medicalising defensive manoeuvres in the observer which can distort relating. One strategy is constructing the body as controllable by science or responsible care. Medical discourse can function very well to deny the chance, indiscriminate way in which the body betrays us. The rationalisations at work here are twofold: first, those who suffer the body's frailty do so through their own negligence; and second, those who properly subject themselves to medical authority can be restored to wholeness. Susan Wendell (1997) tells how, after she became severely ill, friends candidly questioned her regarding what she might have 'done wrong' to cause her body to fail. She writes: 'our cultural insistence on controlling the body blames the victims of disability for failing and burdens them with self-doubt and self-blame' (p. 269). Marks (1999a) points to a curative zeal with which health is pursued and delivered, undoing any possibility of illness or disability becoming 'integrated within conceptions of community and humanity' (p. 75). Nutritional fads, exercise regimes, rigidly advocated esoteric practices and other lifestyle imperatives prepare the way for an illusion of somatic and spiritual control, rendering a moral judgment on those audacious or careless enough to flout directives. Sinason (1992, p. 149) comments that, without fail, blame enters the arena of disease, and does so 'with a vengeance'. Fear of illness, disability, madness – all stir an irresistible instinct to blame the victim. Attribution of deviant sexual excess, addiction and delinquency to people living with HIV and AIDS is a powerful example (Sontag, 1997). In a provocative passage psychoanalytic author Tom Main (1989, p. 205) positions medicine and war in parallel, as arenas both saturated with 'issues of life and death, crippledom [sic.] and loss, sadnesses and terrors about external dangers', as well as unconscious fantasies of 'primitive sadism' and 'punishment'. The need to defend the psyche against such threats speaks for itself.

Marks (1999a) and others refer to biomedicine's tendency to ignore bodily experiences it cannot explain as *epistemic invalidation.* Interlaced with the personal, psychic usefulness of a denial of un-control is a professional expediency (Barnes, 1990) which protects medical authority from disruption by wayward experiential data. Medicine here assumes the guise of empirical gatekeeper, barring entry to what Burman (1996, p. 138) calls the 'surplus that will not fit'. Whether this excess is traumatic social aspects of disability or rehabilitative outcomes which do not fit professional goals, the consequent sense of failure or disharmony tends to settle on patients' shortcomings. By contrast, in the words of Colin Barnes (1990, p. 6) 'the "expert" is exonerated from responsibility, professional integrity remains intact, traditional wisdom and values are not questioned, and the existent social order goes unchallenged'.

Exploring this invalidation of the life-world, Frank (1995, p. 80) describes how the medical gaze transforms 'mystery' into 'puzzle'. Biomedicine's curative zeal cannot allow suffering. Suffering is a 'mystery', which can only be faced and tolerated. By contrast, a puzzle admits solution; thus are disabled lives turned into 'challenges', struggles into obstacles with 'solutions', and identities into blemishes requiring disguise or overhaul (ibid.). But experience and identity can only be valued as mysteries which, unlike puzzles, cannot be 'got right' because 'there is no "right" way to get it'; as such, these things are 'a scandal to modernity' (ibid., p. 81).

It is important to remember that medical practitioners, through no fault of their own, very seldom have the benefit of substantive training in psychological aspects of illness or disability. Gliedman and Roth's (1980) observation that psychological expertise tends to be accumulated over decades of trial and error in medical practice, although now dated, still rings true. The curative and relatively depersonalised brand of medicine for which much training is geared can, in practice, reduce medical ethics to issues of life and death, perpetuating the stereotype of practitioners concerned only with controlling the unruly body (Wendell, 1997). This narrow focus means that knowledge about how one may live through illness or disability in interface with society, uncover and communicate one's experience, and manage the uncertainties of pain and functional limitation remains marginal and unsystematised (ibid.). Medicalisation has the potential to pull all towards an arid mode of relating, missing the opportunity for human contact afforded by the exploration of personal experience.

In the rest of this chapter I explore a number of concepts which have something to offer a contextual psychology of disability. While not based in psychoanalysis, I believe that the psychoanalytic lens brings these ideas into a shared relief. To begin, we turn to the medical sociological notion of *stigma*.

Stigma

Erving Goffman's (1963) notion of *stigma*, although controversial, is an ever-present element of most reviews of disability social science. In *Stigma: Notes on the management of spoiled identity* (1963), Goffman painted a stark, at times disturbing picture of distortions in relating surrounding identities such as disability. In his view a major feature of life as a disabled person is the necessity to ward off devaluation provoked by perceived difference. Goffman highlighted strategies to curb denigrating responses, including humour, proof of competence and the disguising of difference. Concealing impairment, if successful, allowed disabled people to pass as 'normals' (Gill, 2001). Conversely, failing to mitigate the current of negative ascriptions meant consignment to the margins; although this outcome was, it seems, subtly anticipated by all. Goffman's (1963) concept is layered, embodying an individual characteristic, an interpersonal process, a social category and an accompanying emotional set (Coleman, 1997) – it rests somewhere between the psychological and the cultural.

Goffman's (1963) work – part of the disdained field of medical sociology – is among that heavily criticised by strong social model authors (Finkelstein, 1980; Oliver, 1990; Thomas, 2007). Their primary, justifiable difficulty is Goffman's (1963) inattention to systemic, material disadvantage. But furthermore, Goffman was accused of representing disabled people as passive victims of prejudice, living with the 'unfortunate but inevitable social consequences of being impaired' (Thomas, 1999a, p. 146). To a materialist analysis, research focused on cultural, relational and symbolic aspects of disability would never offer much. Nonetheless, a re-examination of Goffman's work from a perspective interested in intra-psychic and interpersonal mechanics of discrimination tells a different story. The social modelist view that Goffman's (1963) contribution should be rejected outright because of its perpetuation of stereotypes is, I believe, both over-simplifying and repressive. The desire to foreground images of resourceful and resilient disabled people risks disallowing a candid exploration of the struggles of those whose identities *are*, to much of the social world, a source of shame or disgust. Finkelstein and others seem to view an examination of stigma as generalised slander, rather than an attempt to describe a most painful aspect of oppression. The 'stereotypes' described by Goffman exist – unfortunately – as very real sources of shame and suffering in marginal lives. Ideological concerns and empirical realities are, as so often in the social model tradition, at odds. But it need not be so. One view is that Goffman's (1963) descriptions can be read as implicitly problematising what he sees. Perhaps it is the *silencing* rather than exposing of denigrating treatment which demeans. It is fair to say that Goffman's (1963) account is very inadequate in socio-political critique, but probably no less incomplete than a correspondingly bald materialist view. Goffman (1963) is clearly no essentialist; stigma is a phenomenon of historically situated cultural relations. He is describing 'what is', not 'what is inevitable'. A more reasonable criticism is that Goffman underestimates the resourcefulness of individuals negotiating stigma, describing desperate attempts at survival rather than calculated coping (Frank, 1988). My own view is that the key phenomenon under scrutiny is the hum of distorted relating which emanates from the ideals of modernist culture – be it resourcefully managed or not. With different terminology, Goffman (1963) points to projection and projective identification, highlighting the predicament of life in the face of ongoing, psychologically embedded othering.

Perhaps most objectionable to social modelist critics are Goffman's (1963) intimations about how stigmatised people may be drawn into endorsing a demeaning view of self (Frank, 1988; Watson, 1998). Surprisingly, the view that an individual suffering stigmatisation may – even for a moment – weaken in the face of assaults on identity is seen as prejudiced. Psychoanalysis' space for human ambivalence is an important counterpoint here to the concreteness of materialism. Indeed, if we apply an analytic lens to the materialist view we might see it (in part) as a wholesale, retaliatory re-projection of internal suspicions of damage. As Hoggett (1992) implied earlier, an extreme materialist position demands the disavowal of humanness itself. The idea that prejudiced meanings can rain in upon an individual for a lifetime without in any way shaping his or her view of self – conscious or unconscious – is perplexing, to say the least. Far from dooming people to 'eternal stigmatisation in their own eyes as well as those of society' (Ablon, 1981 in Frank, 1988, p. 96), Goffman was forging the beginnings of a model of oppression which incorporated the relational, and hence the psychological. Gill

(2001, p. 356) takes issue with Goffman's (1963) lack of attention to 'deviants' who choose to reject the struggle for acceptance by 'normal' society. This, too, is a fair objection, but Gill (2001) may not recognise that the constant current of disablist projections is sustained by all, no matter one's political stance, and thus remains a relevant subject for scrutiny. Besides this, if Goffman (1963) expresses a subtle pessimism for the possibility of a 'solidarity of deviants' based on the affirming of marginal identities, it is not entirely facetious to see his view as foreshadowing recent critiques of identity politics (e.g. Fraser, 2000). Gill (2001), on the other hand, takes issue with Goffman's view that 'deviant' persons who choose to reject mainstream culture in favour of forming alliances with other similarly stigmatised individuals risk inadvertently validating difference and reinforcing marginality. This position is politically inconvenient, but what Goffman has tried to do is describe the double-bind of stigma, and hence of disability. His opinion – that attempts at some form of 'affirmation model' (Swain and French, 2000; 2008) of marginal identities will tend to become snarled in the very categories it seeks to overturn – has been shown in recent debates to have substance.

Liminality

The anthropologist Victor Turner coined this term to describe the situation of members of society who have no clear status, because a prior identity has been expunged and re-allocation has not yet occurred (Turner, 1969). Famously, Turner described such people as 'betwixt and between', occupying a state of suspended animation outside the protocols governing social life, and often in the midst of rites of passage. Fellow anthropologist Robert Murphy, in his auto-ethnographic disability monograph *The body silent* (1987) regarded the concept as strikingly apt to the social predicaments of disabled people, writing that:

> The long-term physically impaired are neither sick nor well, neither dead nor fully alive, neither out of society nor wholly in it. They are human beings but their bodies are warped or malfunctioning, leaving their full humanity in doubt. They are not ill, for illness is transitional to either death or recovery. … They are neither fish nor fowl; they exist in partial isolation from society as undefined, ambiguous people.
>
> (Murphy, 1987, p. 131)

Turner likened social liminality to other ambiguous states of existence, including death, being in the womb and being invisible (Murphy, 1987). The ambiguity was often part of an unfinished cultural transition, but also mirrored a deeper instability to do with one's fundamental nature (Golden and Scheer, 1995). Murphy et al. (1988) argue that disability rehabilitation echoes ritual transitions marking passage from one identity to another in 'traditional' societies. Newly impaired individuals are withdrawn from society to undergo training in modes of living to fit their new ascribed status. Scott's (1969) critique of rehabilitation as 'adult socialisation' resonates perfectly. Rehabilitation here functions less as a palliative than a strategy for restoring society's taxonomy. But to Murphy the disabled individual's transition is never fully over; instead she is caught between liminal isolation and an unviable social emergence (Gill, 2001). Such individuals are 'sociologically dead', and thus present a chronic threat to the validity of the social order (Gill, 2001, p. 358). This nuisance is managed by a sort of sequestering, which only allows for the social participation of disabled people within narrow, ritualised bounds – that is, the 'disabled role'. In Murphy's words this signals relegation to 'the twilight zones of social indefinition' (Murphy et al., 1988, p. 237).

The idea of disabled people as 'out of place' also resonates with Mary Douglas' (1966) anthropological model of society's management of contaminants – anomalous presences which disrupt the cultural categories that make social life meaningful. In *Purity and danger* (1966) Douglas elaborated the cultural symbol of 'dirt' – discordant elements defying society's schemas of control and predictability (Garland-Thomson, 1995). For Douglas (1966, p. 35) 'dirt' cannot exist in an isolated, acultural space; its menace only appears as opposition to a stipulated relational order. Disability, here, presents as a menace to invisible hallmarks of normalcy. What requires our attention, therefore, is Honneth's (1995) 'moral grammar' of modes of exclusion, rooted in cultural mores which carry the mythic essences of our beloved 'enjoyment' (Zizek, 1990). The awkward, specific and complex needs of disabled people seem to embody the disquieting essence of anomaly; that which is ill-fitting, unworkable and haunted by a shadowy threat of systemic failure. The failure of the system is at the heart of Douglas' construct of the unthinkable, harnessing restorative ritual which squeezes the disjuncture back into the individual. In this way, the legitimacy of the system relies on the chronic liminality of the misfit, keeping taboo and contagion at bay.

Douglas (1966) outlined five strategies societies employ to deal with polluting anomaly, which seem to mirror aspects of the disability world rather accurately. First, ambiguous phenomena are assigned to single categories, often in binary sets (Garland-Thomson, 1997b). The disabled–nondisabled dichotomy, with its refuge from anxious uncertainty about degree, is a clear example. In the second strategy the delinquent element is simply eradicated, as in the extermination, sterilisation or abortion of disabled bodies. Third, avoidance of the phenomenon is arranged, calling to mind the global ideology of segregation and institutionalisation (Garland-Thomson, 1997b). In the fourth instance the troublesome element is distanced and controlled through labelling, often with institutional legitimation. Last, ambiguous elements may be incorporated into ritual, to 'enrich meaning or to call attention to other levels of existence' (Douglas, 1966, p. 40). This last strategy is the only one with positive, socially transformative potential. For our purposes, it highlights the contribution an exploration of disability stands to make to our understanding of how societies work, as well as deepening conceptualisations of the human condition in the broadest sense. But alas, more likely is the appropriation of the disabled figure as metaphor in literature or art, with conservative implications. Murphy (1987) adds to this picture of the subduing of anomaly by pointing to Claude Lévi Strauss' assertion that the most fundamental binary in the human world is that between nature and culture. In this 'grand dualism', bodily impairment signifies the intrusion of nature, which 'undercuts one's status as a bearer of culture' (p. 132). Combining Goffman (1963) and Douglas (1966), one may suggest that human stigmata present in the modern world as 'social dirt' (Garland-Thomson, 1997b, p. 33). Clear resonances with a psychoanalytic view are evident here, assisting in naming and describing intra-psychic correlates of society's shared repression.

One startling demonstration of the constructed nature of 'disability dirt' shows up in the naming of elderly people with impairments. In a peculiar incongruity, child- or adulthood impairment squarely implies aberrance, while in old age it is viewed as a 'generational norm' (Priestley, 2006, p. 86). Cultural permission for functional limitation 'rehabilitates' impaired people who are, then, not considered disabled but simply old. Conversely, the ascription of a negatively valued disabled identity is again shown up as a cultural whim. Somehow, culture contrives to simply look past the 'dirt' of impairments of later life, since to not do so would be to open the door to a weighty, undigestible portion of the universal reality of bodily frailty.

Monstrosity and abjection

The Latin word *monstra*, from which the English 'monster' is derived, means 'sign', and also forms the root of the verb 'demonstrate' – to *show* (Garland-Thomson, 1997b). This etymology expresses how bodily differences, especially birth malformations, have been regarded as omens throughout antiquity. Through the nineteenth and early twentieth centuries the freak show enjoyed its heyday, giving 'normals' the opportunity for the cultural and psychological othering afforded by the spectacle of extravagant bodily difference (Bogdan, 1988). Amid the thrills of P. T. Barnum's travelling shows citizens of the early United States got to grapple with dilemmas of classification, and in so doing to hone the skills of creating self through othering – the skills of nation-building (ibid., p. 246). Fiedler (1978) provides a rich history of the cultural phenomenon of 'freaks', exploring the role of bodily disparities in the development of subjectivity. Through religious doctrine malformed bodies came to carry the projected weight of God's wrath poured out on a wicked humanity. Indeed, as in the 'Monster of Ravenna' (b. 1512), specific aspects of malformation were interpreted as divine messages decrying human evils (ibid., p. 25). Clinical experience shows traces of this idea of divine communication in the emotional struggles of parents after the unexpected birth of a congenitally impaired infant. In Fiedler's (1978) view our psychological need to differentiate ourselves by means of monstrous imagery is elemental. Consequently, the prototype of the human monster is not to be found in teratology,[4] but in unconscious layers of a human psyche constitutionally troubled with its own physicality. We all harbour conflicts to do with the limits and structuration of bodies, because the physical changes of development bring about a series of destabilising blows to the ego. As our bodies grow we are beset by a constant stream of changes, and never aware of where these will finally lead. Primitive, conflicted unconscious fantasies about bodies and selves litter this path, as we struggle with fears about our size, the boundaries and shape of our bodies, the adequacy of our maleness or femaleness, the absence or emergence of hair and much else. To negotiate this terrain we need assistance to position ourselves on the desired side of a range of dualities; Fiedler (1978) names some of these as follows:

> [between] male and female, sexed and sexless, animal and human, large and small, self and other, and consequently between reality and illusion, experience and fantasy, fact and myth.
>
> (Fiedler, 1978, p. 24)

The extremes of the freakish body are an ever-present source of fascination to children, possibly based on needs to reposition the changing self as possessing not 'too much' or 'too little' of a characteristic (ibid., p. 27). Observing the 'hermaphrodite' stills anxieties about gender ambivalence, the bearded lady normalises the emergence of bodily hair, conjoined twins evoke conflicts regarding merger and separation, 'giants' or 'dwarfs' are a comfort to worries about size; the list continues (Marks, 1999a). In each case, monstrous extremes are a device which normalises the self. Fiedler captures the point:

> We are the freaks, the human oddities are supposed to reassure us, from their lofty perches. Not you. *Not you!*
>
> (Fiedler, 1978, p. 31)

The cultural juxtaposition of bodily difference with the imago of 'the monster' tells of how impairment signifies the dark, unconscious counterpoint to an earnest, 'untainted' ego. In the freak show, a choreographed frame was provided in which split-off, unconscious parts of self could be projected, reifying racial, ethnic and disability difference into cultural, and even existential otherness. Othering of such an intrinsic nature is a strong foundation for lasting inequality (Garland-Thomson, 1997b).

Robert Bogdan (1988) criticises Fiedler's view that 'the freak' is an inevitable consequence of constitutional human anxieties. In his view, Fiedler (1978) condemns people with unusual bodies to living as custodians of the projected 'monstrosity' of others, in a manner which distracts us from interrogating the cultural origins of othering. I return to this critique shortly. With a deconstructionist rather than psychoanalytic approach, Margrit Shildrick (2002) argues that the unitary male ideal of modernity depends on the imago of monstrosity for its re-creation, condemning both women and disabled people to 'deformity'. Her picture is one of an ideology of othering based on historical realities of power and discourse, rather than constitutional, intra-psychic aspects of human life – in fact, she objects quite stridently to the application of both Freudian and Lacanian ideas to disability (Shildrick, 2004; Goodley, 2011b). But like Fiedler (1978), Shildrick's (2002) monster has meaning not in the flesh-and-blood of biological variations, but in the *fear* of difference, mortality and shame which these hold. In this sense the 'monster' of the freak show is more a cipher than a threat in itself. It reawakens inherent contradictions to do with modernity's denial of the frailty, the animality of the body. Both the accounts of Shildrick (2002) and Fiedler (1978) have much in common with Freud's (1919) association of disorderly bodies with the psychic unease of *the uncanny*.

Hughes (2009) takes issue with Shildrick's use of monstrosity to make sense of disablism. He acknowledges that identifying how language discursively supports essentialist distinctions is theoretically important, but in his view the trope of monstrosity 'reveals little concrete about being disabled or about how to use the ontological question to enhance the cause of disabled people' (p. 401). Hughes' (2009) query is important. They may be stimulating, but do illustrative concepts like monstrosity have any use in social change? In my view, concepts which illuminate the unseen psychological transactions of unequal human relating do have something important to offer. They describe subtle aspects of disablist socialisation. If one's identity, one's self, is in part forged in the face of the othering of a hegemonic ideal, unravelling internal meanings must be part of emancipation. Exploring and naming the ways in which disabled lives are mirrored by modernist culture is, I believe, an essential part of escaping demeaning projective identifications – that is, establishing what is 'me' and 'not me'. Hughes' (2009) position does not provide for unconscious life. Instead of describing a universally human fantasy of selfhood, he sees an interest in monstrosity as 'voyeuristic fascination' (p. 403). In so doing, he glosses over a core proposition I offer with this book – namely that much of what happens in societies around disability is *mediated by fantasy*. What makes monstrosity important is that it is part of everyday life. In this sense Hughes (2009) is, in my view, not sufficiently curious about what is 'seen' in the impaired body.

Let us return now to Bogdan's (1988) objection to Fiedler's (1978) view that 'monstrous' projections onto disabled people are an inevitable side-effect of human development. As should be clear, my own position has much in common with that of Fiedler (1978). The question here is a weighty one. To what extent are visceral, apprehensive responses to prominent bodily difference intrinsic, human universals?

In the psychoanalytic model of Jacques Lacan (1977), our creation of a coherent, whole self is a process of self-delusion. To Lacan, our base existential nature is fragmented and chaotic, beginning with the infant's experience of the body as turbulent, un-integrated parts. This fragmented body ('corps morcele') is the basis for an equally unstable self. During the 'mirror phase' of development (Lacan, 1977, p. 4) the body's flailing disorder of limbs, surfaces and impulses is shepherded into an illusory wholeness, which is appropriated by the self. Here, the child has donned the unified self-identity which she sees in her reflection, in so doing denouncing the disorder at her core. The seductive illusion of wholeness provides relief, casting splinters of affect, impulse and sensation into the gloss of a new unity (Frosh, 2006). But of course this also stifles instinctual life, insulating the ego from what ultimately animates it.

The perceived integrity of the ego is thus a social construct rooted in ideology which stresses autonomy and the sanctity of the unitary self. What this means is that we all carry the creeping awareness that we are not whole, not ordered and unified, not the harmonious beings of the modernist dream. It is at this level – the level of the real – that we may carry constitutional, self-protective negative responses to the malformed body. Zizek (1991) frames the *real* as that which plays about the edge of the mirror, threatening the placid illusions of cultural life with the contorted essence of the human condition. Disability fits this description closely as the shadowy harbinger of 'a return'; disability is the devalued identity which lies dormant and ready in the bodies of all. In this sense it is a sign par excellence, holding both the threat of disintegration and the lure of enlivenment. The complex feelings evoked by disability, including guilt, hostility and obsessive control, seem readily compatible with Lacan's (1977, p. 11) unconscious store of 'imagos of the fragmented body'. The disabled body, thus, may be a resonant, animate version of the repressed, infantile fragmented body (Davis, 1997c). While this implies that its threats are pervasive, these are inversely proportional to the development of a comfort with human frailty. That is, it is primarily against the backdrop of modernity's repressions that existential troubles manifest in oppressive controls upon disability. In this sense 'disability fear' is not a simple universal, but occurs dimensionally on scales of psychological insight, and against the backdrop of constitutional struggles with difference.

As alluded to, Shildrick (2004) rejects the above application of Lacan to disabled subjectivity (Goodley, 2011b). In her view, both Freud and Lacan see self-image – ego – as the product of a foundational model of corporeality. To me, Shildrick here attributes an unlikely stance to both authors. Namely, bodily experience of women or disabled people is viewed as becoming subjectively meaningful against the standard of an intrinsic, pre-cultural ideal. This interpretation sees both Freud and Lacan as, to a large extent, ruling out the social construction of experience of the body. As should be clear, my view (with Goodley, 2011b) of Lacan's intentions is quite different – the fact that cultural ascriptions associate the disabled figure with the *corps morcelé* does not make this existential phenomenon any less universal. Further, the assumption by writers such as Niederland (1965) and his contemporaries, and more recently Wilson (2003), that Freud's view of the relationship between body shape, body ego and embodied experience was a simple, unmediated one is highly questionable. Freud's position on bodies not fitting the phallocentric ideal has, as we shall see, been a subject of earnest debate (Mitchell, 1974).

In Kristeva's (1982) treatment of the existential notion of *abjection* we see her views on what, in Lacan's terms, we might call the *real*. This is a description of conflict lying at the very core of human existence – the essence of our predicament as needy mortals in an unpredictable world – and how we use culture to digest or suture this reality. For Kristeva (1982), it is the universal catastrophe of separation from maternal care which fundamentally powers conscious selfhood and culture. The 'maternal' here refers not merely to the tangible, material 'mother'; it is a metaphor summoning an inner world of intrinsic oral conflicts to do with need, un-control and envy – a world beyond and before defensive constructions of desire. Abjection shows primordial psychological life before symbolisation; when there was 'having' and 'not having', before language's sense-making, and hence dissolution of primary experience. In the abject we find preserved the archaic matter which culture conceals, beginning with the calamity of one's body becoming separate from another. Aspects of culture which call up abjection through identity ascription, ritual transformation or religious taboo do so in order to control its dangers through separation, symbolisation or fantasied extermination. While culture depends on boundaries and categories for its repressions, the essence of the abject is its pre-symbolic nature; that is, it is unapproachable and untouched by nomenclature. As we shall discuss later, at the heart of the disability phenomenon are attacks on boundaries – relational, cultural, political, emotional. The confusion between self and other evident in disability 'chestnuts' such as altruism, guilt, abuse, control and shame resonate closely with the primacy Kristeva (1982) gives to boundlessness in her description of the human abject. Cultural responses which, to use the social model's terminology, transform impairment into disability, are the consequence.

One way of making sense of disability's role as messenger from the *real* – with both threatening and energising aspects – is through the 'carnivalesque' (or 'grotesque') quality of the unusual body (Bakhtin, 1981). The carnivalesque figure represents the right, the means, to transgress social norms, showing up the illusory nature of these in a wry or clownish manner (ibid.). Hierarchies are inverted and conventions flouted as the 'disorderly body' teasingly goads all towards acknowledging the real (Garland-Thomson, 1997b, p. 37). Here, perhaps, is an example of Douglas' (1966) lone optimistic outcome in the cultural management of anomaly, where 'matter out of place' has provoked a critical re-assessment of culture. Radical contemporary disability theatre and visual art takes up this strategy, bringing the contradictions of identity categories into vivid relief through provocative humour and discomforting imagery (Conroy, 2008; Garland-Thomson, 2009).

With this chapter I have laid some theoretical groundwork for a discussion of the psychological nature of socialisation in a disablist world. The distorting influence of defence mechanisms, human psychic aspects such as abjection and the fear of monstrosity, and cultural mechanisms surrounding stigma and liminality are useful tools in framing social responses to the impaired body. Over the next two chapters some key areas of the cultural subject matter of socialisation will be explored.

Notes

1 Object relations theory refers to a school of psychoanalytic thought pioneered by Melanie Klein, describing how personality is composed of 'internal objects'. Although arising from early formative relationships, these 'objects' are not people, but internalisations of relationships between self and other, with accompanying emotions, which are replicated through adulthood. Central is the assertion that current relationships take place on the level of tangible reality and internal fantasy, always coloured by archaic, unconscious re-enactments. A common example of an internal object might be the repeated dynamic relationship of an overly needy self and an intentionally withholding other, arising in infancy, but recreated in adult relating.

2 Put simply, the idea of cathexis refers to how parts of the self or the world become invested with unconscious emotional meaning, or, in Freudian terms, with libido (psychic energy).

3 Object constancy refers to the ability to hold significant others in mind (for example, a parent), while out of sensory contact. Its development denotes an important stage in the coalescing self's ability to independently process emotion, as the parental container has been successfully internalised.

4 The branch of biology concerned with extreme deviations from the normal development of organisms.

4 Bioethics, disability and the quality of life debate

Introduction

As we explore unconscious narratives influencing socialisation in a disablist culture, disability-related debates in applied bioethics provide useful food for thought. At issue are conflicting ways in which disabled lives are seen, by medical practitioners, the judicial system, the disability movement and popular culture. Ideas about what constitutes a worthwhile life are shown up, along with disputes over factors which shape subjective fulfilment or happiness. In terms of the socialisation of disabled people, the simple fact of having the value of one's existence openly queried is significant. The question of how experiences of self are shaped by ideology comes to the fore, highlighting those lives seen by culture as inherently, chronically traumatic. When examined from a psychoanalytic viewpoint, the sometimes over-simplified political positions taken in these debates may carry important insights about living with ongoing cultural assaults on identity. An important question is whether violent acts against the disabled community, including genocide and hate crime, represent a high water mark of ongoing cultural denigration. This chapter addresses these debates, before closing with a discussion of institutional influences on socialisation through encounters with medical care. Particularly in the case of congenital impairment, these experiences may be prominent and ongoing through formative years and beyond, drawing attention to the importance of medical discourse in shaping experiences of self.

Lives not worth living

Bioethics is concerned with philosophical dilemmas of health and illness, life and death; in particular, the relationship of medicine to nature (Asch, 2001). Medical advances have given rise to questions regarding the quality and fulfilment which lives must carry in order to be 'worth living', – to be preferable to not being alive (ibid.). Accordingly, the discipline has specific, and to some sinister, relevance to disabled people, as such lives routinely undergo bioethical scrutiny in a range of medico-legal scenarios. Adrienne Asch sums up the discipline as one which substitutes the medical question of 'can this life be saved?' with the philosophical question 'should this life be saved?' (2001, p. 299). The dilemmas underlying the medical and legal situations at hand may be expressed as: (1) what are the conditions under which it becomes morally permissible to kill, or to let die, a disabled person?; and (2) how potentially impaired must a foetus be in order to justify the prevention of its birth? (Wendell, 1989 in Asch, 2001, p. 297).

Bioethics traditionally takes the position that assessments of quality of life after treatment should be a factor in medical decisions, including resource allocation. At times this has meant that bioethicists have argued against the sustaining of life in individuals who will carry impairments (Asch, 2001). Unsurprisingly, disability studies writers have lambasted the 'medicalisation' at the centre of this position, which seems to view quality of life as an acultural function of bodily integrity. A further problem is that bioethics tends to assume a consensus on the definition of medical terms employed – the concept of health is a case in point. The defining of this familiar idea is described by Kelman (1975) as 'the most perplexing and ambiguous' issue in the study of medical social services (cited in Altman, 2001, p. 100). Thus is the tone set for the slippery, subjective and emotive nature of debate in this area.

In this brief discussion we will consider three debates in the encounter between bioethics and disability studies. These are: (1) the withholding of treatment from impaired children or adults; (2) the prenatal testing of foetuses for the presence of congenital disorders with a view to abortion; and (3) the question of assisted suicide or 'the right to die' for disabled persons. The related issue of forced sterilisation of persons with heritable impairments will be examined later in the section headed 'Eugenics'.

Withholding treatment from children and adults

A common scenario in neonatal and paediatric medicine is that in which parents have to decide whether their child should undergo treatment, where the child will be disabled after the intervention but may die without it (Asch, 2001). For example, an infant with Down syndrome may also have heart disease or an intestinal blockage. Some practitioners may counsel the parents to let the child die from the associated condition, rather than live with Down syndrome. The situation is complicated further when the treatment is invasive and/or has a poor chance of success. During the 1990s many writers in bioethics argued that it is defensible, even morally desirable to end the lives of babies who would be permanently disabled after treatment, citing suffering caused by both intervention and impairment (ibid.). One painful outcome is that of the ill child who suffers a brief and miserable life of fruitless medical interventions, compounding the anguish of parents.

The disability studies critique here centres on the social construction of conditions such as Down syndrome, spina bifida and cerebral palsy. The argument holds that assessments of quality of life are, in fact, cultural judgments masquerading as medical realities. The lack of positive cultural representations of life with, for example, Down syndrome is implicated in stereotyping and associated medical 'condemnations'. Basnett (2001) provides a telling account of a friend – like him, a wheelchair user – who was admitted to hospital with a chest infection. A junior doctor wrote in her case notes that, if required, she should not be resuscitated, due to 'poor quality of life'. In such situations nothing but stereotype informs potentially lethal decisions. As a further example, in a paper concerned with the psychological effect on parents of the birth of an impaired child, MacKeith (1973) comments: 'I do not hold the view that it is always the doctor's responsibility to do everything that he [sic.] can to save life; death is sometimes a blessing' (p. 136). In the lives of acute paediatric practitioners, where death and trauma are commonplace, it is fair to recognise the origins and positive intentions of such a sentiment. But the example does foreground the ambiguous, personal variables at play in decisions often construed as scientific and objective. Cultural imagery of disability and the ideology of segregation must surely mediate appraisals of a worthwhile life.

Princeton philosophy chair Peter Singer has drawn an especially fierce battering from disability studies for his outspoken views on the value – or lack thereof – of life with a range of physical, sensory and cognitive impairments. To Singer (1993, p. 184), 'the killing of a defective infant is not morally equivalent to the killing of a person; very often it is not morally wrong at all'. Although conceding that individuals with some impairments may maintain meaningful lives, he insists that such lives will be less satisfying than those of nondisabled people (Asch, 2001). What appears to be in evidence here is the logic of subjectivity 'written on the body', and writ large, at that. Evenly passing absolute judgments on unseen lives, Singer advocates attempting to replace the 'defective' child with a healthy one, who will enjoy life and bring more enjoyment than the unknown impaired child ever could (ibid.). With such charged, divergent positions at play, and the unknown quantity of practitioners' personal exposure to disability, the meanings of impairment presented to parents who are often in crisis are a powerful, confusing jumble. The medical encounter here is far from value neutral (Marks, 1999a). Instead, it carries chance fragments of a kaleidoscope of cultural and intra-psychic meanings.

Prenatal testing and abortion

The growing availability of prenatal testing presents parents with the dilemma of whether to bear children who will live with impairments (Asch, 2001; Gill, 2010). Asch (2001) writes:

> …the vast majority of [bioethics] theorists and health professionals … argue that prenatal testing, followed by pregnancy termination if an impairment is detected, promotes family well-being and the public health.
>
> (Asch, 2001, p. 305)

In the context of a pro-choice position on abortion, one approach simply views the impairment question as one amongst many confronting people debating the feasibility of parenthood. But Sinason (2002) points to systematic policy variations applying to disability, such as the UK's waiving of an upper limit for abortions in the case of impaired foetuses. In an international survey of geneticists, Wertz (1995) found that 54 per cent endorsed what some may term eugenic goals; that is, the reduction of the number of carriers of genetic disorders in the general population. Reasons given related to pervasive negative attitudes towards disabled life, and the 'destructive' impact of a disabled child on family functioning. Although not objecting to abortion per se, disability studies critics here, too, point to the cultural origins of the idea that a disabled child cannot provide the fulfilment parents yearn for (ibid.). Some voices from the disability movement argue that the desire to prevent the birth of impaired foetuses is an expression of broader cultural antipathy towards persons with those impairments, not just unborn, but living – the so-called *expressivist critique.*

In her psychoanalytic work with learning disabled patients, Valerie Sinason (1992; 2002) has uncovered evidence of the profound psychological impact of knowing that only a lack of technology allowed for one's birth. Persons with a range of impairments live with the knowledge that, had parents or professionals known of their nature before birth, the pregnancy would probably have been terminated. Sinason writes:

> The deepest and most painful psychoanalytic theme that comes from long-term work is that learning disabled people can experience extreme annihilatory fear because it is hard (or impossible) to separate out the idea of amniocentesis or abortion of unborn learning disabled foetuses from a death wish towards learning disabled children and adults.
>
> (Sinason, 2002, p. 39)

The essence of the expressivist critique holds that policies and practices aimed at preventing impaired births 'express' the broader population's desire – perhaps unconscious – that persons with such impairments did not exist. Learning disabled people, who are central to this debate, are seen as targets for the most wretched of projections, relegating their ascribed identity in many societies to a status below full humanness (Sinason, 1992; Parmenter, 2001). But across a range of heritable impairments, disabled people routinely undergo genetic counselling explicitly aimed at preventing the birth of others just like them. Rod Michalko (2002) tells of being haunted in young life by the knowledge that 'my type of person' – a blind person – 'was not welcome in my homeland' (p. 46). Reflection on the reasons for this led him to prevailing cultural imputations of life without sight. He writes:

> What was it about me and my life that recommended not reproducing it? Why should I be prevented from happening again? The answer is simple: blindness is a condition that deprives people of most, and sometimes all, of their eyesight and, in turn, eliminates most, and sometimes all, of their ability and even pleasure.
>
> (Michalko, 2002, p. 50)

As an example of the extreme expressivist position, Saxton (1998) views prenatal testing to prevent disability as 'the greatest insult', which declares that 'some of us are "too flawed" in our very DNA to exist' (cited in Asch, 2001, p. 308). A vital question here regards the effects on psychology and identity of the knowledge that 'there are people who go to great lengths to avoid the birth of someone like you' (Glover, 2006, p. 5). In response to combative political positions such as that of Saxton, Shakespeare (2006, p. 87) largely dismisses the expressivist argument, framing it as a histrionic 'plot discourse' which ascribes illusory, sinister intent to reproductive health policy. Shakespeare's (2006) position is a hyper-rational one, emphasising that 'there is no government plan to eliminate disabled people', and adding that it is often parents themselves who actively choose to terminate (ibid.). Although slightly modifying his stance later, here he frames the issue as a mistaken 'eugenic threat', not an ongoing experience of social denigration. Whilst his position on parents' choices is undoubtedly true, it is equally true that medicine and culture have a symbiotic relationship, and that parents' views on the possibilities of disabled life have complex ideological and personal origins. The dearth of exposure most people have had to nuanced narratives of functional disabled lives means appraisals probably rely heavily on fantasy. But more importantly, the fact that reproductive health policy contains no deliberate conspiracy does not change its potential meaning in the lives of disabled persons. It is not difficult to see how anyone might feel harmed by the not unrealistic knowledge that they are in some way an accident, unwanted or inferior. A critique of social policy which focuses on intentions but not effects will never be satisfactory. Without doubt, a host of dreadful health care policies have been implemented with the best possible intentions, but little understanding of meanings these bring to individual lives. All of this does not mean that genetic testing and counselling are bad and should be scrapped; not at all. Shakespeare (2006) is correct to dismiss this splitting logic, which, among other problems, has a politically regressive, 'pro-life' position as its natural end-point. Instead, it must be possible to integrate an awareness of hurtful messaging into the way genetic services are practised and thought about.

Shakespeare (2006) continues his cool-headed argument by pointing to contradictions in the assumption that 'if amniocentesis had been available, I would not have been born'. There would, he writes, be no 'I' to be born, as the 'I' concerned would not exist. A more 'rational' view states that 'this technology might prevent people like myself from being born' (p. 89) – an idea which may still be distressing, but has less 'personal resonance' than the idea of one's non-existence (ibid.). The problem is that the issue's essence cannot be dealt with adequately in intellectualising terms, as it is rooted in irrational and unconscious layers of experience. Shakespeare (2006) seems reluctant to allocate thought-space to the persistent tissue of denigrations surrounding disability in broad society, which may be seen to crystallise in reproductive health policy. The bioethics debate, in this schema, is not the problem, but simply a terrain of engagement surrounding an issue of deeper import: the complex, cultural territory of identity, trauma and selfhood. In placing prenatal testing among a range of innocuous reasons why one might not have been born – if one's parents had not met, if they had used contraception, and so forth – Shakespeare (2006) mistakenly equates free-floating aspects of life experience with those which are applied with specific identity-meanings. This is similar to asserting that the experience of being poor is the same whether or not one inhabits a racist state in which poverty is a function of demeaning, racialised exclusions. In the South African apartheid state the deprivations suffered by black people were couched in an explicit logic which connected undeserving to colour, to identity. Similarly, the knowledge that efforts are afoot to prevent the existence of others 'like me' must imbue 'my way of being' with a debasing evaluation. Under apartheid, thus, poverty tracks back to undeserving and undeserving tracks back to blackness; the struggle, the affliction, is ultimately within. Here, as in disabled lives, the experience of deprivation and marginality are tied to identity, to the nature, the essence, of one's being. The reason for poverty coincides with the reason for amniocentesis; and it is in the internal realm that the dreary ramifications of these social realities grow. As mentioned, Shakespeare later alters his view to include more recognition of the potential negative messaging of prenatal diagnosis (Shakespeare, 2008). As in so many disability-related debates, emotive investments of participants – beginning, here, with simplified, vilifying utterances from the disability movement – have set a tone of impoverishing oppositionality rather than nuanced engagement.

Whilst impairment prevention is not wrong, we do need to explore the human meanings which attend such activities. If the expressivist logic was taken to its extreme it might support objections to such self-evidently humanitarian initiatives as polio vaccination or the clearing of landmines, as these may be viewed as devaluing disabled life (Shakespeare, 2006). But the absurdity of these ideas should not distract us from the cultural and personal meanings attached to prenatal genetic services.

An important ideological question is whether terminating, for example, a Down syndrome pregnancy embodies validating discriminatory elements of society from whom parents may wish to protect their unborn child. Terminations reduce the extent to which society will be confronted with its prejudices through greater integration of difference. Impairment prevention, in effect, may be an acquiescence to threats to dominant *enjoyment*, depriving culture of the means to overcome the impoverishing implications of separation. One result is that some disabled people live with ongoing messaging that their lives are 'not worth living' – experiences which might enliven the more insecure, fragmented parts of any psyche. At play here are questions about the basis of human experience, of selfhood. Occupying a world in which one's experience is repeatedly constructed as wretched will, at least in part, *create* experience in this way. Abject identity associations mean that a positive experience of self must flout cultural expectations. This requires apprehending one's selfhood somewhere other than in the mirrors of the social world. Of course, familial bonds are crucial in the formation of the self. I do not construct the disabled individual as a one-dimensional product of disablist culture. But disablism and medicalising modernity are real. Self-worth, if it is to be found, must develop in spite of these realities.

Assisted suicide and the right to die

An important distinction in this emotive area is between assisting suicide in the final stages of terminal illness and the voluntary euthanasia of non terminally ill persons with impairments. The crux of the contrast is between enabling dying persons to die, and the legal facilitating of disabled people to end their lives (Shakespeare, 2006). In the second case what seems to occur is that miserable cultural assessments of life with, say, quadriplegia, muster discursive forces favouring the termination of life. A number of landmark judgments in the USA have pronounced on requests for assisted suicide from severely impaired persons, in the process gathering a telling sample of social constructions of disabled lives. The question presented to the courts is, in essence, whether these lives are worth living.

In the now famous case of Elizabeth Bouvia, a woman living with severe cerebral palsy and arthritis, such a request for assisted suicide was made in 1983 (Asch, 2001). Bouvia asked the court to grant permission for hospital staff to sedate her and withdraw tube feeding in order that she starve to death. The American Civil Liberties Union agreed to represent her case, centring their argument squarely on her impairment – her 'intolerable affliction' which caused her to endure a 'pitiful existence' involving the 'indignity and humiliation' of personal assistance with bodily functions (ibid., p. 311). In 1986 the California Supreme Court upheld this account, stating that 'she herself is imprisoned, and must lie physically helpless, subject to the ignominy, embarrassment, humiliation and dehumanising aspects created by her helplessness' (ibid.). It is important to note that Bouvia's was not a case of terminal illness; with appropriate care she may have lived for many years. Crucially, what was missing from the assessment of her condition and request was an evaluation of her psychosocial circumstances and mental state (Gill, 2004).

Had a non-impaired Elizabeth Bouvia checked into a hospital and refused feeding, she would likely have been diagnosed with suicidal depression rooted in multiple social stressors. Yet, three psychiatrists reviewed her decision as reasonable, and not influenced by psychological morbidity (Herr and Phil, 1992). Because of her impairment Bouvia's suicidality was not seen as a function of her mental state, negating the ethical obligation to provide psychiatric treatment for mood disturbance. More disquieting still is an assessment of the life stressors borne by Bouvia in the years directly prior to her request to die. During this period she experienced marriage and divorce, the miscarriage of a wanted pregnancy, her mother's illness, the death of her brother, many forced moves due to familial problems, unreliable personal assistance and withdrawal from university study after being informed by her dean that her disability would preclude her from succeeding in postgraduate social work training (Asch, 2001).

Bouvia's case shows up experiences of exclusion and deprivation which, in so many disabled lives, are piled on top of universally human life-struggles. The terrain of disability (rather than impairment) seems wholly to have been ignored by the ACLU and the judiciary in their assessment of Bouvia's case, although it seems beyond doubt that a severely impaired person such as herself would be well acquainted with prejudice. But besides these concerns, a glance at the purely psychosocial stressors which beset her life suggests that most humans under such circumstances may contemplate the escape of suicide (Herr and Phil, 1992; Gill, 2004; 2010). Beguiled by her impairment, judicial authorities and mental health professionals alike somehow forgot that through adulthood Bouvia's life had features commonly seen as positively meaningful in the modern West. She had lived independently, completed a college education and begun postgraduate study, married, had a sex life with her husband resulting in pregnancy and planned motherhood. At work here is a medicalising sleight of hand which attributes distress to the 'immutable realities' of impairment, while ignoring both psychosocial adversity and disablist disadvantage.

United States courts displayed a similar impairment bias in the case of Kenneth Bergstedt, arguing for a differentiation between the suicidality of impaired and nondisabled persons. The court viewed the latter as benefitting from psychiatric rehabilitation in addressing their 'potentially reversible pessimism' regarding quality of life (Herr and Phil, 1992, p. 6). A cultural view of the inevitable futility and wretchedness of impaired life is unmistakable here. Coleman (1998) describes civil rights proponents of assisted suicide for disabled people as 'white, well-off, worried and well' (cited in Gill, 2010, pp. 31–32). Her point is that from positions of privilege it is difficult to have insight into marginal lives, and the key influences which shape these. Instead, what shows is the spectre of severe impairment, and fantasies about its inevitable and definitive implications for quality of life.

The case of Larry McAfee shows a dramatic disregard of material deprivation in shaping impaired experience (Herr and Phil, 1992). McAfee was granted his request of assisted suicide by judicial authorities who, remarkably, made no mention in the judgment of the appalling social circumstances from which he wished to escape. Due to the severity of his physical impairments, McAfee was turned away from all residential care facilities in his county, and consequently forced to take up residence in an intensive care unit for the final eight months of his life, although he was not ill or unstable. A condition known as *ICU psychosis* has been identified, involving severe emotional disturbance resulting from the 'timelessness' of the environment; there is no privacy, no darkness, intermittent crises and constant activity (ibid.). The Georgia Supreme Court agreed that McAfee's ventilator should be shut off with no mention of what was, in fact, an awful failure of the social care net. Here, in the words of Herr and Phil (1992, p. 8), 'the state that had denied McAfee the right to live a meaningful, independent life did not contest his fight to die'. The same logic was applied in the case of David Rivlin, a quadriplegic man who requested assisted suicide to escape life in a nursing home which provided no reasonable possibilities for a meaningful life (Gill, 2010).

The issue of respecting the autonomy of disabled people – as all citizens – in life and death decisions deserves recognition. But when death is chosen as the only escape from appalling but remediable social circumstances, it is 'perverse and unfair' to construe such actions as an expression of healthy self-determination (Bickenbach, 1998, p. 128). Unfortunately, as in the prenatal testing debate discussed above, this issue has often been engaged with through crude binaries. Activist positions have at times been unhelpfully combative and overstated, contributing to what Gill (2010) terms the 'straw man' simplification of disability rights objections to assisted suicide. This portrayal, in her view, distracts attention from important knowledge the disability lobby stands to contribute to bioethics debates. Resonating with my own position above, Gill (2010) stresses that disability rights arguments carry experiential knowledge which is difficult to communicate across social and identity divides. The real threats to a fulfilling life posed by institutionalisation, discrimination, poverty and abuse experienced in disabled lives place the devaluing judgments of assisted suicide advocates in a very different light (ibid.). These structural forces, as Gill (2010) observes, remain an obscured and threatening social reality to those occupying positions where autonomy and privilege are beyond question. Conwell and Caine (1991), in a study of medical records in cases of suicide, found that more than 90 per cent of individuals ended their lives during the course of a diagnosable mental disorder. There is no reason why this principle should not apply to disabled people. Suicidal depression is a life-threatening but often treatable condition, presenting an ethical obligation to provide psychological and psycho-pharmacological treatment. The common-sense attribution of emotional distress to the 'constancies' of impairment almost certainly results in under-diagnosis of mood and other disorders in disabled persons. Our attention cannot resist being drawn to poignant fantasies about the lived nature of impairment, rather than the 'banal' real-life concerns of housing, assistive care, medical services and emotional support (Herr and Phil, 1992).

In closing this discussion, consider the black, sardonic words of Bickenbach (1998), as he satirises the contradictions of cultural assessments of a 'liveable' life:

> It is telling that … there is never any suggestion that the right to physician-assisted suicide should extend to people who do not have a severe disability. Implicit in the judgments themselves … is precisely the prevailing prejudicial social attitude that having a disability is a sensible reason for committing suicide. Perhaps proponents of physician-assisted suicide would be steadfast in their view even if it meant that qualified doctors could patrol school grounds waiting for despondent but mentally competent seventeen-year-olds who, having failed geography or being unable to find a date for the prom, might want to use their assisted-suicide services.
>
> (Bickenbach, 1998, p. 130)

Eugenics

In envisioning the psychic undercurrents which give life to modernity, Frosh (1989, p. 233) writes of a balance between the age's 'two faces'. On one hand we find 'multiplicity, contradiction, flow', and the 'celebration of heterogeneity'. The flipside of these intents, perhaps enlivened by more primitive psychic impulses and defences, reflects 'rigidity, domination' and 'totalitarianism', manifesting in the dehumanising divisions of fascism and the global scourge of racism (ibid.). Disability has not been exempt from the destructive excesses of the latter. Davis (2002) presses us to never forget that it was the physically impaired and 'feeble-minded' who were the first to be despatched to the death camps by the Nazis. It was only after the murder of between 200,000 and 300,000 impaired persons that the attention of the vanguard of the 'final solution' moved on to dealing with 'racial undesirables' (Ravaud and Stiker, 2001). As we consider the 'dark intentions' which some suspect to be part of modern bioethics, the question before us concerns whether a fascist undercurrent is discernible in modern society more broadly, carrying echoes of a totalitarian drive to obliterate difference. In so doing, Shakespeare's (2006) cautions against a plot discourse are relevant. He is correct: prenatal testing, for example, is not evidence of a broader conspiracy to exterminate disabled life. But denying that such destructiveness exists as part of human complexity is also a distortion. Frosh's (1989) words above bring us back to psychoanalysis' key strength – a comfort with the human constant of ambivalence.

The term eugenics was coined by Francis Galton in 1883, spawning a movement aimed at translating scientific knowledge on heredity into social policies to prevent the proliferation of 'degenerate' human stock (Trent, 1994). It will surprise many that early proponents of eugenics spanned the political spectrum, and included progressive liberals. But it was the movement's links with reactionary ideology which assured its longevity. Advocates of racial purification believed that eliminating 'inferior' human stock would put an end to such problems as poverty, crime, unwanted children, insanity and intellectual impairment (ibid.). This burgeoning movement coincided with the twentieth century's ever-growing medicalisation of disability, as bodies marked with the corrupting significations of impairment and colour attracted what Foucault (1979, p. 54) termed the 'racisms of the state'. When not in the base manifestation of genocide or enforced sterilisation, these controls took the form of an ideology of measurement, positioning all in relation to statistical expressions of normalcy (Fujiura and Rutkowski-Kmitta, 2001). It was Charles Darwin's theory of natural selection which provided the backdrop for a construing of disabled people as 'evolutionary defectives', to be purged through the just balances of nature (Davis, 1997a, p. 14).

As we trace proliferation of the scientific (or *scientistic*) measurement and categorising of humanity through the twentieth century, a corresponding, but hidden and hegemonic 'nondisabled' identity was being crystallised. As an analogy, consider McRuer's (2006) description of the coalescing of heteronormativity:

> ... it was the 'homosexual menace' that was specified and embodied; the subsequent policing and containment of that menace allowed the new heterosexual normalcy to remain unspecified and disembodied.
>
> (McRuer, 2006, p. 1)

Like the heterosexual, the nondisabled figure came to 'masquerade as a non-identity, as the natural order of things' (ibid., p. 79). Slowly, forces of a new, bureaucratised totalitarian sameness set upon disability difference, showing up deviations as errors of nature, as 'glitches', rather than expressions of the spectrum of diversity (Davis, 1995). Pernick (1997) views the history of the eugenic movement as an essential precursor to present-day evaluative judgments about disability. The hideous pinnacle of murderous intent towards disabled people – the Nazi extermination during World War II – reflected eugenic principles not at all unique to the Third Reich. German racial purification was, in fact, founded upon the British and American eugenic arguments cited above. At the height of the genocide in 1941, prominent British biologist Julian Huxley was publicly bemoaning the lack of eugenics-based social policy in Britain (Hubbard, 1997). More remarkably, unlike the mass murder of Jewish people, no prosecutions were launched against those responsible for the disability genocide in Germany (Gallagher, 1990 in Marks, 1999b). In 1933 Germany had begun the forced sterilisation of mainly intellectually impaired persons, eventually implemented on as many as 400,000 individuals. The policy was modelled on similar programmes already in place in California (Braddock and Parish, 2001). Between 1907 and 1949 approximately 47,000 intellectually impaired persons were forcibly sterilised in the USA (Braddock and Parish, 2001). As in the Nazi extermination, these procedures were performed by medical practitioners. Post-war and far more recent accounts of legalised and illicit sterilisations have emerged in countries including Spain (Bosch, 1998), Japan (Asch, 2001), Australia (Cordner and Ettershank, 1997), Denmark (Braddock and Parish, 2001) and Sweden (Hughes, 2002a).

As we have seen, some disability studies critics view the modern availability of genetic counselling as a sanitised version of the eugenics movement's attack on the disabled population. Hubbard (1997) argues that counselling services, through the use of liberal rights discourse, present pregnant women with a double-bind disguised as free choice. In this view, the prospective mother who chooses to forego prenatal testing, or not to terminate her pregnancy after a positive result, is tacitly saddled with responsibility for whatever the impairment means to her child, herself and her family. An important consideration is that degree of impairment is typically difficult to establish prenatally. In the convenient, euphemistic distortions of a modernist dream of autonomy, the woman concerned has 'chosen' this child, this life. By consequence she is liable for the pain that may ensue – and not just physical pain, but the anguish engendered by society's possible shunning of her child. In practice, the prevailing logic directs this responsibility to her, leaving discriminatory culture untouched (ibid.). In this line of argument, the logic of the selection and extermination of lives remains, though veiled in a rights-based discourse of women who 'elect' to terminate troubled pregnancies. Zizek (2004) clearly articulates how, under the illusory neutrality of human rights discourse, violence is reframed as volition. What are, in fact, the effects of power become viewed, within 'university discourse' (p. 388), as the self-evident implications of empirical realities. In this sense, nothing is 'done to' the women Hubbard (1997) describes, yet they come away personally culpable for the painful ramifications of an unequal society. In opposition to Shakespeare's (2006) assertion that it is often parents themselves who choose termination, Hubbard (1997, p. 199) states that this is so because 'society promises much grief to parents of children it deems unfit to inhabit the world'.

For Shakespeare (2006), any relating of genetics research to eugenics is irrational. In tangible terms, the death camps of Germany are clearly light years from the cool, sterile rationality of a genetic consultation room. But the question is whether we are able to trace the faint outlines of related intra-psychic currents underpinning each, while taking care not to stereotype health workers. Eugenic ideas assumed wild and heinous expression in Nazi Germany, but it seems plausible that unconscious motives for disallowing difference are (at least qualitatively) common across nations and times. At this juncture we again see disability studies' need for a psychological frame of reference. In my view, it is a lack of psychological conceptualisation which prevents Shakespeare (2006) from reaching the root of disability studies' furious critique of modern genetics. Without a psychological lens it is difficult to envision a deep wound, which tells of the unremitting experience of being seen as intrinsically damaged. Instead, the debate rages about theory and history, rather than examining how the arena of bioethics provides a focus for the expression of manifest cultural denigrations which continue unabated in the fabric of social life.

Hate crime

Recently, awareness of hate crime directed at the disabled community has increased markedly, and research contributions to the area have begun to emerge. It remains uncertain whether this increment reflects shifts in incidence or levels of reporting. Frustrations relating to the recent economic downturn in Great Britain (as elsewhere) have been connected to a number of horrific incidents of group-based violence against disabled individuals, including several murders (Roulstone et al., 2011). Such crimes may depict the high water mark of ongoing, unconscious aggressive impulses towards the disabled minority, existing on a continuum with both everyday prejudice and eugenic fantasies. A psychoanalytic consideration of some cases suggests a combination of two irrational motivations. First, the satisfying of urges for domination through sadism is familiar as a defensive response to inner feelings or memories of humiliation or disempowerment. In the sadistic act the relationship of abuse is inverted, as vulnerability and terror are projected into the other, who is consequently punished for his or her 'weakness'. The other aspect is one we have already seen: a paradoxical envy of the disabled figure, who is hated for, in fantasy, possessing a position of privilege or care.

Although no data are yet available in my country, South Africa, this thumbnail analysis fits painfully well with three other forms of sadistic violence with which we are acquainted. I consider the designation 'hate crime' an appropriate description for this violence. Over recent years, and particularly during 2009, widespread incidents of collective, violent xenophobia were directed at asylum seekers from such countries as Somalia and Zimbabwe. The fantasy here was of 'gold-diggers' who were exploiting the local economy to the detriment of citizens who, after 17 years of democracy, remain in the grip of grinding poverty. The other two forms of violence both involve rape. First, 'corrective rape' is a hate crime directed at lesbian women, who may be gang-raped as 'corrective' punishment for their sexual orientation (Potgieter, 2006). The last hate crime in this disturbing list is the rape of infants and very young children (Richter, 2003). In each of these scenarios, the combination of extreme violence, the sadistic inversion of a relationship of disempowerment, brutal othering and echoes of hateful envy mirror descriptions of disability hate crime. If one combines group-based psychotic defences and associated authoritarian impulses with the unconscious meanings of the disabled figure, the reality of disablist hate crime should not surprise us. Without the defence offered by adequate policing and litigation in developed countries, the developing world's disabled population is likely to be subject to such abuses on a large scale.

Disability and the medical encounter

As we saw in the previous chapter, a discourse analytic view of disability (Foucault, 1976; Stiker, 1982), based on interrogation of how the body is culturally produced and regulated, treats rehabilitation interventions as normalisation (Turner, 2001). In this view, rehabilitation functions primarily to restore the social order through subduing difference – that is, exercising social control on politico-cultural dissidents. To Stiker (1982), the multitude of damaged bodies produced by the horrors of World War I were the initial catalyst for rehabilitation science's ultimate expansion into a global industry. Notions of 'replacement, substitution and compensation' were foundational to this new vision. But the vision that reduced both body and society to entities subject to scientific control was a fantasy. Stiker (1982) writes:

> The image of the maimed person and of the society around him [sic.] becomes prosthetic. Replacement, re-establishment of the prior situation, substitution, compensation – all this now becomes possible language … the war … was nothing less than a catastrophe … But catastrophe does not generate aberrancy. Catastrophe can be the object of repair … Culpability and moral obligation are linked with the idea of catastrophe; we can and must repair, re-establish, restore, in other words, efface, expiate, redeem … speaking of rehabilitation envisages disability as a lack to be filled, almost a lack to overcome … This is a notion different from cure. Cure is a removal and relates to health. Rehabilitation is situated in the social sphere and constitutes replacement for a deficit.
>
> (Stiker, 1982, p. 124)

At work were parallel fantasies, where the restoration of 'broken' bodies supported a vision of idealised safety, familiarity and home. In each case the imagined control, functionality and uniformity was illusory – a fantasy of a prior time of human and social wholeness, of harmony. Stiker (1982) asks us to consider whether a hope of re-realising this mythic state fosters health care practice too preoccupied with repair, with cure. The disabled figure, in such circumstances, fills the invidious position of an awkward, irredeemable intrusion on medicine's project. Dealing with chronic difference has never been part of biomedicine's brief. In fact, Ravaud and Stiker's (2001, p. 507) strict discourse analytic view regards rehabilitation as primarily aiming to 'efface any difference'. Devices, prostheses and technologies of rehabilitation, thus, are seen not as primarily for attaining functional and fulfilling ways of being, but more for causing individuals to act more like others (ibid.). The disabled body is directed back towards the cherished normative ideal of self-contained autonomy, to which its own 'normal' state is an insult. Rosemarie Garland-Thomson describes the dimensions of this insult:

> ... the incomplete, unbounded, compromised and subjected body, susceptible to external forces: property badly managed, a fortress inadequately defended, a self helplessly violated.
>
> (Garland-Thomson, 1997b, p. 45)

In applied settings, Rioux (1994) observes that rehabilitative success is typically gauged by how closely clients come to approximating the 'normal'. Evaluation research tends to be functionalist in nature, and assumes congruence between the ideals of providers and consumers, thus sidestepping some weighty ideological issues. The defining of 'needs', for example, is a complex question (Fraser, 1989; Finkelstein, 1998; Handley, 2000). Theorists defending social service models point to disabled clients who want assistance in becoming 'as normal as possible'. A sensitive balance is required between respecting individual choice and the reality of a social world in which all, impaired and not, are steeped in ideology which disdains difference. Finkelstein (1998) urges that we make sense of the stated needs of impaired clients in terms of their disability-related beliefs. Seeing suffering as a result of impairment informs a need for normalisation, while emphasising discrimination implies a political need for securing citizenship rights (ibid.). Since health professionals are often influential authority figures in disabled lives, the needs discourses they carry are of great significance (French and Swain, 2001). Traditionally, needs and corresponding services have been determined by health workers, positioning disabled people as passive recipients with little opportunity for control (ibid.). Rinck and Calkins (1996), for example, found that disabled people acquiesced to professional decisions in institutional settings, fearing the loss of privileges or care.

Robert Scott's (1969) monograph is an eloquent description of how rehabilitation may dictate the 'correct' way to live one's disability. The trappings and deportment of the blind man he describes – the guide dog, white cane and docile, melancholic demeanour – are facets of a closely scripted role which shape the individual into a culturally palatable package. In his study, an indication of rehabilitative success was 'the degree to which the client has come to understand himself and his problems from the worker's perspective' (p. 14). From a psychoanalytic point of view, this preferred role may be interpreted as a product of defences engaged in response to anxious fantasies evoked by a particular impairment type. The guide dog certainly assists a mass of sight impaired persons worldwide with mobility; but just as certainly it functions as a reassuring container of projected 'blindness fantasies' carried by observers. The common incidence of earnest or angry protestations at disabled persons choosing unconventional methods – also noted by Scott – is testimony to this. The idea of fearful unconscious resonances being managed through applying social controls is basic to a critical, psychological understanding of disability normalisation. A consequence is that identities are contested, not least through nondisabled professionals subtly or overtly advocating what is 'appropriate and normal' behaviour in the lives of disabled clients (French, 1999, p. 21). Noteworthy, too, is the familiar image of disabled individuals or organisations objecting to impaired lifestyle choices which flout their own conventions. Perhaps, as in Scott's (1969) analysis, this is a result of the 'success' of disablist socialisation.

The extended, sometimes lifelong influence of health professionals in disabled lives brings immense responsibility, through the modelling of attitudes about the constraints and possibilities of an impairment (Hordon, 1994). Importantly, health professionals are mainly exposed to disabled people in vulnerable, help-seeking roles, potentially reinforcing stereotypes of dependency and frailty. Irrespective of degree of experience, health workers staffing settings such as casualty wards or rehabilitation centres tend to greatly underestimate the life satisfaction of disabled people (Bach and Tilton, 1994; Shakespeare et al., 2009). In Asch's (1998) view, doctors and bioethicists have real influence on disability-related life decisions, yet cannot provide useful information if they remain sceptical about disabled people leading fulfilling lives (in Miller, 2006). Disconcerting evidence suggests that health workers' attitudes towards disabled people roughly reflect those of the broader population, showing up as predominantly negative and based on stereotyping (Johnson, 1993; Biley, 1994; French, 1994b; James and Thomas, 1996; Scullion, 1999). But more hopefully, some studies indicate that the presence of equal-status, non-therapeutic contact impacts positively on attitudes of professionals towards disabled people (French, 1994b; Eberhardt and Mayberry, 1995; Basnett, 2001; Shakespeare et al., 2009). Basnett (2001), himself both disabled and a health professional, sees the individualising view of disability enacted by most health practitioners as part of an institutional legitimation of roles, which thwarts the development of critical social consciousness in health care settings.

One demeaning aspect of medical socialisation is the phenomenon of 'public stripping', in which disabled patients, at times naked, are used as objects for medical tuition. This practice, which appears disturbingly widespread, is now recognised as institutional abuse (French and Swain, 2001). Sutherland (1981) provides the following first-person account:

> My memory is basically of a whole series of experiences of being very coldly and formally mauled around. It's very alienating. It's as if you're a medical specimen ... I was never told that I was nice to look at or nice to touch, there was never any feeling of being nice, just of being odd, peculiar. It's horrible. It's taken me years and years to get over it.
>
> (Sutherland, 1981 in French, 1994a, p. 103)

Coleridge (1993) believes that the impact of medical-institutional socialisation on the self-image of disabled people is underestimated. For some, childhood may have meant constant involvement with health practitioners, when 'play, enjoyment and discovery were replaced by stress, medical examinations and developmental programmes' (French and Swain, 2001, p. 738). The repressive constricting of healthy psycho-sexual development may be a further side-effect of familial–medical preoccupations with childhood impairment (McRuer and Wilkerson, 2003). Against the backdrop of lives of assessment and therapy, Goodley and Runswick-Cole (2010) describe how the play of disabled children may be seen more as a marker of functional level or an instrument of intervention than simply what it is – play. There is something subtle and powerful in this description of selves created in otherness, where the imperative to 'progress' towards a different state of being dwells very close to the core. As we shall see later, childhood impairment can also disrupt healthy risk-taking and exploratory play, due to parents' and professionals' worries about safety. Instead, children may be limited to relatively controlled activities in segregated environments, where play is monitored as something purposive, rather than lived as intrinsically meaningful (ibid.).

Biomedicine's emphasis on cure, as already argued, sidelines development of emancipatory knowledge about living with impairment in a disablist world. The considerable pressures on health professionals to cure show up the chronically 'defective' body as a failure, a blight (Sinason, 1992). Intra-psychic defences correlated with the Cartesian medical stance must, to some extent, reflect its dualisms. Here, disability appears as an intolerable 'absence', squeezing away the thought space necessary to imagine novel, 'neo-normal' lifestyles. Sinason (1992) describes health practitioners' responses to the incurable in terms of an unconscious defensive manoeuvre of 'going stupid'; 'not just because it is painful, but because it is unbearable to see damage and not be able to repair it' (p. 36). In a similar vein, Main (1989) calls attention to 'hallowed' clinical viewpoints or methods which, in fact, function to manage practitioner anxiety. For Main, defences erected against feelings of helplessness in doctors are of primary importance in the study of health and illness, expressed in ways as diverse as 'laughter, forgetfulness, aloofness, scotomata, denial' and much else (pp. 207–8).

As should be clear, my own position carries much empathy for health practitioners. After most have received little training in emotional and psychosocial aspects of disease and disability, professionals are exposed to a combination of demanding working conditions, strict hierarchies and ongoing vicarious trauma, as well as prejudiced generalisations about oppressive practice. There is little question that very much continues to be wrong with the response of modern medicine to disability. But if we are to ask health workers to open new and reflexive 'thought space' to differing views on disability, it is essential that other stakeholders reflect, too, on the very real quandaries facing the health profession. A legacy of disciplinary boundaries, notably between social and health sciences, places many practitioners in extremely invidious positions in dealing with emotional trauma, discrimination, poverty, abuse and much else. Gliedman and Roth's (1980) statement quoted earlier, that most psychological knowledge of health professionals is accumulated through trial and error should, I believe, be read with an attitude of compassion for workers and patients alike.

Health professionals who have not been adequately prepared for the 'messiness' of emotional and psychosocial aspects of disability are, as noted by Sinason (1992) and Main (1989), likely to respond to it with defensiveness. Asch and Fine (1997, p. 251) describe how practitioner needs for normalisation may lead to disabled patients assuming an inauthentic, placating role. Michelle, a 17 year old respondent in their study, told of how she wore her prosthetic arms only on visits to her doctor, as they were a clumsy hindrance. While 'perfectly comfortable' with others seeing her under-developed arms, she could not expose these to her doctor. Modern Western culture, reflected in biomedical desires for cure, prizes what Frank (1995, p. 78) terms the 'restitution narrative'. This is in evidence in diverse cultural contexts, from television advertisements for cold remedies to moralising parables about the consequences of an unhealthy lifestyle. In each case the story shows how things 'get better' when one follows social protocols, and 'tells' one's illness in a conciliatory, cure-striving manner. Social or occupational default is the unacceptable outcome of a body poorly managed. In this cultural fantasy all is curable, or at least avoidable; it is only human dereliction which permits matter out of place (Douglas, 1966).

Although controversial, the theme of loss is perennially associated with disability – we shall examine it closely later. But no matter one's ideological position, it is reasonable to suggest that the functional deficits which follow an adventitious impairment will, to many, embody experiences of loss. Further, marginal lives subject to discrimination will certainly involve loss. It is the intractability of loss which makes it the antithesis of cure, of progress. Consequently, its presence may evoke avoidant, distorting defences in health care relationships. Hinshelwood (1987) sketches such avoidance against the backdrop of residential care for learning disabled persons, pointing out how in clinical encounters despair is often not recognised, while anger is over-emphasised. In one possible scenario the client attempts to communicate despondency, which appears pre-consciously to the practitioner as the spectre of loss, perhaps calling forth echoes of guilt over material and power inequalities (ibid.). But the aversive unconscious response is experienced as coming from the client, who is consequently seen as wishing to cause harm. The incipient guilt of the clinician is important here, in informing an experience of 'blameless persecution'. What was despair therefore comes to be viewed as hostility, perhaps evoking a counter-aggressive, disciplining response (ibid.). Finally, the client is left with an enactment of the all-too-familiar experience that 'others cannot withstand my despair', driving such emotion underground. The stereotype of the troublesome, ungrateful, uncooperative or manipulative service consumer is plainly evident here.

As we have seen, medical training falls short in preparing professionals for the ambiguities of disability. But parallel to training is the question of personality profiles attracted to the 'reparative' vocations of medicine. Marsh (2006), for example, characterises persons drawn to training in surgery as 'the fixers'; 'interventionists' who 'need to be the active agents in resolution of situations to obtain personal satisfaction' (p. 121). The indefinite, intractable nature of permanent impairment would, one imagines, be a very difficult challenge to this sort of mind. Such personality substrates must also be understood in interaction with the quite brutal demands of training regimens, involving exhausting working hours dealing with trauma, pain and death. Rather than providing psychological skills to manage this onslaught, medical institutions too often carry a quite authoritarian and judgmental chain of command, based on the split-off vicarious trauma of those who went before. In my view such practitioners are victims of history and institutional circumstance who deserve our empathy, and are typically doing the very best they can with little personal support. It is imperative that disability studies engages constructively and openly with health disciplines, towards building relationships which make the most of what health services can offer in disabled lives. Exclusion and prejudice remain real, but the response to them requires a new, measured and even-handed sense of purpose.

A final issue in this area is that of adequate representation of the disabled community in the ranks of health disciplines (Lawthom and Goodley, 2006). In mental health, for example, several sources attest to institutional resistance to disabled persons being trained in professions such as clinical psychology (Asch and Rousso, 1985; French, 1988; Bliss, 1994; James and Thomas, 1996; Stannett, 2006) – I add my own experience to this list. The assumption in some psychoanalytic work that impairment implies psychological disturbance has led to disabled persons being viewed as unsuitable for psychotherapy training (Asch and Rousso, 1985). Besides psychological wellness, a further concern cited is the potential disruption of the therapeutic relationship caused by visible impairment (Bliss, 1994). Bliss (1994) responds to this issue by pointing out that it is only disabled clinicians like herself who are able to be fully aware of impairment's implications in the clinical frame. Some accounts argue that visible impairment may, in fact, be a therapeutic asset which functions as evocative 'grist for the mill', deepening psychological enquiry (French, 1988; Levinson and Parritt, 2006). But the key issues regarding inclusion of disabled practitioners here, as well as in other health professions, are the following. First, it must be incontrovertible that disabled persons are best placed to empathise with the predicaments of others with bodily differences, in mental health services as well as other health care domains. Note, though, that this does not imply that disabled people are by their nature capable of such empathy. Inhabiting a social category does not equate with consciousness of the layered, often paradoxical nature of oppression. Personal insight, in conjunction with political conscientisation, is the foundation of empathy.

The second issue flows from this, and relates to the broad need for a shared narrative of group consciousness, emerging from the exploration of personal experience. The importance of sifting through and examining the phenomenology of impaired life in disablist society cannot be overestimated. This is the business of transcending internalised silences, opening the way for positive identification. With identity categories such as race it is self-evident that mental health professions – that is, professions concerned with finding voice – should be demographically representative. It is difficult to see how the same principle would not apply to disability, in mental health as well as all other professions concerned with the needs and care of disabled people. Professional participation is an essential route towards threading knowledge of the realities of disabled life into the philosophy and technique of health delivery.

5 Exploring the cultural shaping of socialisation

The psychological positioning of disabled lives

Introduction

This chapter explores cultural substrates which shape disability-related social institutions, and hence disabled socialisation. The resilience of disablist prejudice, and of othering in general, is at the very heart of the modernist ideal and the narcissistic drives of the capital market. As was briefly discussed in Chapter 3, the idea of narcissism refers to our tendency to defend against feelings of inadequacy through self-aggrandising. This can be an extreme, destructive psychological problem, but occurs in all in a more benign form. We all have ways of helping ourselves to feel more adequate, attractive, in control and valuable. Modern commodities, with their associations of prestige and success, may function as reassuring psychological resources here.

The chapter begins with a consideration of this cultural backdrop, including such issues as autonomy, the bodily ideal and the appropriation of artistic and charity representations of the disabled figure. In each area we focus on the psychological usefulness of cultural mechanisms of othering for the dominant majority. What this illustrates is the differential psychological positioning of disabled lives, as a result of alienation from material and cultural power. After this we bring the discussion inward to the world of psychological development. Tracing the shaping of disabled identity in the family, debates on the psychological impact of congenital impairment are an important point of departure. As before, an examination of traditional psychoanalytic work in this area reveals a decontextualised view of disability, often involving a grief model of adjustment to the birth of a disabled child. In critiquing this work, we examine theoretical ideas about how bodily difference may impress itself on psychological development, exploring how ideology intervenes in shaping experiences of embodiment. Further difficult questions about the emotional reverberations of disability in families and the growing availability of corrective surgeries are considered, as part of the conscious and unconscious cultural soup of meanings which shape the disabled identity. The understandable sensitivity around theorising the family has created unhelpful divides in research work. I explore these problems, hoping to facilitate freer debate in this very important area. Among many other consequences, prejudice in the socialisation of disabled people feeds into the problem of creating a valued, coherent disabled political identity – one with which a majority of impaired individuals would want to be associated. We explore some impediments to this, through attempting to relate ambivalence among disabled people to cultural influences on subjectivity. This discussion also illustrates some important shortcomings in traditional approaches to minority identity politics.

Culture and prejudice

Narcissism, normalcy, modernity and the market

> If such a thing as a psycho-analysis of today's prototypical culture were possible; if the absolute predominance of the economy did not beggar all attempts at explaining conditions by the psychic life of their victims … such an investigation would needs show the sickness proper to the time to consist precisely in normality.
>
> (Adorno, 1951, p. 58)

Adherents to the materialist social model view would baulk at Theodore Adorno's call for a 'psychoanalysis of culture' in investigating prejudice, viewing whatever may come to light as trivial and diversionary. But as we have seen, traditional Marxian priorities appear dry and unsatisfactory in the face of a growing recognition of the role of culture and discourse in inequality. Although such voices from within disability studies (e.g. Paterson and Hughes, 1999; Corker and Shakespeare, 2002; Shakespeare, 2006) would not deny for a moment that exclusion from the world of work is a core aspect of disablist oppression, the growing view is that it is essential to analyse how culture is implicated in meanings which rationalise and reproduce discrimination. The key issue is this: if we assume that the self is, to some extent, a precipitate of cultural meanings mediated through language, it is essential that we attend to the significations which surround us. In this sense, communities are no less significant sites for the negotiation of power – for example, in relationships around disability – than are institutions (Borsay, 2002). Frantz Fanon's (1952) work on racism is useful for our purposes, as it traces how social practices are translated into ideological givens which, in turn, reproduce psychological phenomena such as feelings and complexes at the individual level (Frosh, 1989). Exploration of these functional threads, linking ideology, cultural practices and subjectivity, must be at the heart of a model of how oppression works.

The relevance of Adorno's (1951) words relates to how cultural and psychological aspects of disablism remain invisible to most, woven into the groundwork of the everyday practices and assumptions that compose 'normal' life. In the words of Lennard J. Davis, 'while we may acknowledge we are racist, we barely know we are ableist' (Davis, 2002, p. 148). Demonstrating this, Coleridge (1993) describes a journey of discovery into his own subtle prejudices. He remarks:

> Even someone starting out with full sympathy and the intent to champion the cause of disability finds himself falling into the very trap that created the problem in the first place.
>
> (Coleridge, 1993, p. 21)

If culture had little influence on the marginalisation of disabled people, it would follow that oppression would be relatively consistent across contexts (assuming that there was similarity in modes of exchange). This seems not to be the case. Archaeological and historiographical evidence suggests that the harshness of disablism is more situation-specific, and hence the product of local cultural mechanisms (Scheer and Groce, 1988; Braddock and Parish, 2001). The theoretical picture suggested in this book would view these cultural influences as situation-specific, but also as local, varying manifestations of a more universal undercurrent of intra-psychic struggles with physicality. In considering disabled life in mediaeval or ancient times, a first principle is that physical and cognitive difference was more the rule than the exception (Stiker, 1982; Mitchell and Snyder, 2001a). In the modern world ideals of control and resolute autonomy serve to reify the illusion of essential difference between the whole and the broken – a distinction which would previously have been far less discernible. For example, during and after periods when Europe was tormented by plagues (e.g. the Black Death, 1347–51), Stiker (1982) argues that the massively widespread nature of disease de-emphasised impairment-difference more than in any other epoch. In this picture we see the context-dependent nature of disability signification, where the universality of human frailty looms so large as to make a mockery of modernity's pretensions.

In what follows we examine theoretical perspectives on the nature of Western late capitalist modernity, paying special attention to the role of narcissistic psychology in safeguarding its illusory, fleeting identities. A point of departure is that narcissistic meaning-making is so central in market economies as to locate individuals in identity hierarchies, based on differential access to the material means for creating narcissistic distinctiveness. In other words, to convincingly maintain capitalist ideals of autonomy, mastery and status – all likely ingredients in narcissistic self-representations – one needs the commodities and trappings of modern materialistic life. We require the material means to passably bolster our self-identities towards the narcissistic cultural ideal; the luxury cars, sophisticated lifestyles and pristine bodies of the idealised phantasm of the modern age. These resources make the illusion of control plausible – control of destiny, of biology, of the self and the world. The import of all of this for disabled people is, I believe, twofold. First, the material deprivation suffered by disabled people in most societies brings with it the reality of alienation from the cultural means to approximate the narcissistic ideal. Capital accumulation and, in particular, successfully autonomous life are deeply interwoven with this narcissistic ideal, and as deeply alien to the compoundly impoverished lives of most disabled people. Recognising this does not reduce the denigrated disabled identity to a product of material exchange. Instead, it underscores the mutually constitutive nature of political economy and psychology, where even as modernity propounds its illusion of control, it needs the disabled figure to personify disarray. Modernity is not just about 'having', it is about 'being'. This leads us to the second implication of the 'culture of narcissism' (Lasch, 1978; 1984). It is a culture founded on the reification and denigration of out-groups. Visibly disabled persons, to be sure, fall squarely into the category of shameful misfits who are the bane – as well as the needed other – of the aggrandising self. Upholding the human rights of disabled people, consequently, exists in chronic tension with the machinery of narcissistic culture.

Bauman (1997) paints a picture of modernity which has 'a dream of purity', 'a vision of order' and 'a world clean and hygienic' at its centre (Bauman, 1997 in Hughes, 2002b, p. 573). The imperative to endlessly purify existence with superior 'beginnings' positions disabled people as a rude, intractable disfigurement of the age's noble intents. But this 'order making' is indistinguishable from the 'announcement' of new abnormalities, drawing new lines and setting apart 'ever new strangers' (ibid.). The crisp categories of modernism quell the impinging, chaotic voice of disability – of humanness. The ghettos, institutions, retirement homes and terminal care wards of modern societies, write Dass and Gorman (1985), are the product of a culture which pays to keep suffering away. But this safety from the troubles of the world brings, over time, feelings of being 'dry, empty and alone in our insulated havens' (ibid., p. 57).

Christopher Lasch's (1978; 1984) provocative picture of modernity's narcissism presents an image of atomised, self-adoring humans incapable of giving to or receiving from one another (Treacher, 1989). Lasch (1984) argues that the self-absorption, individualism and rampant materialism of contemporary culture points to an emptiness at the heart of modern lives (Frosh, 1991). In this world the visual reality of surfaces is everything, as paranoia drives insatiable, conspicuous consumption (ibid.). But simultaneously alienation arises as a result of dwindling possibilities for the recognition of self and other, as objects are all that remain. More precisely, what remains are projected aspects of self appearing in fantasy as objects – a single plane on which everything exists only to gratify or thwart the desires of the 'modern man' (Lasch, 1984). Immediate gratification is elemental; the 'momentary illusion of personal well-being, health and psychic security' (Lasch, 1978, p. 7). The sculpting and adorning of the body – it, too, an object of fantasy – give obsequious materiality to the silent self. Murphy (1987) refers to this bodily obsession as:

> …part of the immortality project of a secularised middle class that no longer believes in redemption of the soul and has turned instead to redemption of the body.
>
> (Murphy, 1987, p. 113)

There is little inclination in this abrupt world to admit the painful effects of authentic relating, although it is on these that the 'development and sustenance of selfhood depends' (Richards, 1989 in Frosh, 1991, p. 66). In a world of impermanence the synthetic self must be constantly re-conjured, and sanctified through defamation of the other. Difference is reformulated as the damage of the other, temporarily shoring up illusions of value and power.

It is important to recognise that narcissistic culture – as, arguably, all culture – is shaped by what has been lost. The narcissistic manoeuvres with which we create, augment and adorn our facades are ways of managing what we could not have, or cannot be. In Freud's (1923, p. 29) words, 'the character of the ego is a precipitate of abandoned object cathexes', where 'cathexes' may be loosely understood as emotional investments. He goes on to say that the ego thus 'contains the history of those object choices' (ibid.). In a sobering corrective to modernist hopes, Freud describes an ego desperately attempting to dampen the reality of loss through re-creating itself in aggrandising guises, aiming to assume something of the features of the lost object. The connection between commodities of narcissistic culture and an impoverished internal world seems clear. But let us focus more closely on relating disability symbolism with prejudices based in narcissistic psychic functioning. An individual, developmental view would pose questions regarding early infantile experiences of misattuned parenting and distress, later forming the substance of disability projections to do with dependency, shame and rejection. At the cultural level, ongoing projection, projective identification and introjection solidify these fantasies into familiar meanings, embedding their depictions in institutions and policies. The phenomenon of segregation is a key marker here, as a colossal enactment of difference which facilitates projection.

We saw in a previous chapter that 'traditional' psychoanalytic work construes disabled people themselves as prone to narcissism. To understand this one must begin by recognising that it is authoritarian and depriving treatment which fosters narcissistic pathology in all populations. The question then becomes one of how visible impairment may distort relationships – in the home, the school, the community – in systematic ways which incubate such treatment. The narcissistic frailties of influential figures in disabled lives may lead to rigid, splitting and authoritarian responses – the re-infliction of unconsciously held deprivations. The wealth of experiential accounts of institutionalisation of disabled people gives ample, painful colour to this form of treatment. In short, narcissism begets narcissism. Its presence in those shaping the socialisation of disabled lives limits the attuned mirroring which supports development of an integrated self. These concerns will be revisited later.

Bollas (1987) describes the 'normotic personality', a strongly narcissistic profile which synergises closely with the materialism of late modernity. Normotic tendencies – not at all uncommon – involve occupying a life-world which is 'abnormally normal', preoccupied only with the 'thingness' of objects, and 'fundamentally disinterested in subjective life' (ibid., p. 136). In this subjective space nothing is real beyond the material, which is mastered with precision and security. Rationality is the key to freedom, while emotion and imagination are steered well clear of. Narcissistically oriented defences such as rationalisation and intellectualisation are prominent, based in a cultural milieu emphasising wealth as the route to personal power. As noted above, this emotionless state may emerge from inadequate early mirroring and validation of one's inner life. Refuge from deeply embedded abandonment has required annihilating compassion for oneself or others (ibid., p. 136). The emotional 'matter out of place' within this psyche is mirrored by the disorderliness of the impaired 'misfit' in the community. Both must be reformed, neutralised and assimilated, as states of mind are substituted with commodities – commodities which are often inaccessible or unusable to impaired persons. Systematically depriving impaired people of these defensive resources primes such individuals as receptacles for unwanted characteristics. Lives of exclusion and deprivation, in concert with cultural denigration, position some disabled people as chronically exposed to what, in the modern world, lies beyond the veil of avid material distractions.

One demonstration of the differential access to such distractions available to disabled people is in the field of design. Pullin (2009) compiles a critique of the design of disability-related products and devices which exposes glaring contradictions in how society wordlessly constructs, and creates, disabled life. While the gadgets and accessories of the world of mainstream consumption are endlessly updated to be more distinctive, compact, chic, clever and elegant, design in the disability world is characterised by grey functionality. In contrast to the fickle, shifting aesthetics of the mainstream design industry, disability assistive technology is dominated by an engineering, solution-focused emphasis, where virtually no designers have artistic training. Opportunities for bodily adornment and aesthetic self-expression in the nature of devices in daily use are virtually absent (ibid.). Here, it seems clear that the disabled figure is positioned as out of the running in the game of internal and material narcissistic accumulations. Aesthetic trappings designate value in the world of consumerist glamour; as certainly, assistive technology design denotes the body which is viewed as no longer part of the race.

Disablism is, it seems, so interwoven with modernist cultural mores such as autonomy, the free market and the narcissistic gaze that it is difficult to imagine how real change might take place. The fragmented, disappointing outcomes of rights-based approaches have convinced some authors that oppression will continue until the 'very basis of the rules of the market' are questioned (Russell and Malhotra, 2002 in Sheldon, 2005, p. 124). Shakespeare and Watson (2001) concur, adding that the splintered and impotent influence of mainstream concepts such as democracy and citizenship has been further undercut by the growth of the global market, limiting the likelihood of national-level investment in equity-based reform. Disability prejudices run rampant in the free market, allowing (among much else) for the immense distortions we see in access to employment. McDonough (1997), for example, found weak correlations between individual impairment attributes and employment disability. What such evidence shows is that discrimination bars disabled people from a range of feasible occupations (Abberley, 2002), although some impairments will reduce output in certain types of work. French (1993a), for example, describes how sight impairment will regularly reduce speed of productivity despite assistive technology and a facilitative environment. Against the modernist worship of the market, she describes the consequent impasse as follows:

> Other more profound societal changes, for example paying disabled employees the same amount as able-bodied employees for less work if their working speeds are slow, would more successfully reduce disability, but enormous attitudinal changes within society, and within disabled people themselves, would need to take place before this could be put into practice without causing even worse problems in terms of resentment, guilt and lowering of self-esteem.
>
> (French, 1993a, p. 20)

It is the individual who is coerced into the preferred ways and shapes of capitalist modernity, never the converse. As a rather macabre demonstration, Frank (2006) describes what he terms 'technoluxe' medicine. This marketplace includes such services as the exclusive podiatry of New York, where a woman may pay to undergo foot surgery in order to make her feet look good in the latest designer shoes. The foot is transformed to fit the shoe, not the other way around. Here, it is those possessing most resources to channel into their bodies whose bodies accrue the most capital (ibid.). Frank (2006, p. 74) describes this 'boutique medicine' discourse as a 'Prozac-like language of transformation and life change', calling forth the body as a commodified analogue of the self.

The Western notion of the autonomous individual is so familiar, so hegemonic, that it may appear acultural. This being is constructed as the exclusive architect of his or her nature and biography, solely culpable for social and economic success or failure (Rose, 1989). Discourses measuring human qualities are put to work here, re-rendering socio-political inequalities as just desserts. Success in this world hinges on control and the independent implementation of self-interest; marginality is the destiny of the undeserving. These pronouncements made by the oracle of the market are tinged with more than a little morality, delineating not only destiny, but self (Bartky, 1990). Impairment's contradiction of capitalist principles, such as those described by French (1993a) above, identify the disabled figure as, at least in fantasy, the basket-case of the market.

The framework of social liberalism legitimates market forces by downplaying human difference in favour of an illusory level playing field (Shakespeare and Watson, 2001). This Utopia is a myth. But even if it were possible, differing abilities would persist. The 'universal, abstract, disembodied individual' of this ideal world of work is, in actuality one who is 'male, white, heterosexual and nondisabled' (Lister, 1997 in Shakespeare and Watson, 2001, p. 558). Because of the assumption of fairness, the grievances of individuals marginalised by the market are viewed as:

> ... the rantings of biased, partial and selfish special interest groups that wish to seek favour for their own particular grouping at the expense of the mainstream.
>
> (Young, 1990 in Shakespeare and Watson, 2001, p. 558)

Beyond the simple rationalising of the market, Zizek (2004) regards neoliberal discourses of democracy, human rights and equality as a self-deceiving sham. Democracy and human rights create an ideological platform from which power may be enunciated as 'neutral knowledge', rather than domination (p. 383). This is an ideological master which, in Lacan's terms, has hystericised itself. What this means is that the perpetuation of injustice has become cloaked in a helpless, even self-righteous abstention to scientific representations of 'the state of things' (Zizek, 2004, p. 383). This 'hysterical' position is analogous to one who claims powerlessness, but in fact manipulates through the very illusion of subjectification. Disability inequality thus may be 'regrettable', 'tragic', but is not something inflicted. Instead, we are all helpless before the inherent justness of the market, or the authority of democratic bureaucracies. In Zizek's picture we wring our hands momentarily, turn away, and continue with the business of accumulation. According to Lacan, hysterics who demand a new master – that is, who deny the performative reality of their own power – will get one (Zizek, 2004, p. 388). That appears to be what has happened, as all – at least in unconscious hysterical enactment – fall prostrate before the just and unassailable pronouncements of democracy and science.

One such 'new master' for a society finding refuge in hystericisation is equality. In the USA the coming to prominence of the illusion of a society of equal opportunities may, at first, have left citizens insecure about how to prove their worth – a function which was previously fulfilled in an undisguised form by class lineage (McWilliams, 1994). As early as 1800, the answer to this dilemma began to crystallise as the 'just' accumulation of observable material assets, placing the emergence of narcissistic materialism far earlier than some theorists believe (ibid.). To demonstrate the tensions of this transition, McWilliams (1994) refers to E. M. Forster's (1921) character Leonard Bast, a modern man who 'knew that he was poor'. Forster (1921) writes:

> Had he lived some centuries ago, in the brightly coloured civilizations of the past, he would have had definite status, his rank and income would have corresponded. But in his day the angel of democracy had arisen, enshadowing the classes with leathern wings, and proclaiming: 'All men are equal – all men, that is to say, who possess umbrellas'.
>
> (*Howards End* – E. M. Forster, 1921, pp. 45–46)

Garland-Thomson (1997b) conceptualises the counterpoint to disability-difference as the *normate* – a veiled figure only discernible in the outlines of the bodily deviants who flank, and hence constitute it. This normate body is the prototype for Foucault's (1979, p. 184) 'principle of coercion', exercised through technologies which measure, classify and regulate. To Garland-Thomson (1997b), the normate self is informed by four interlocking ideological principles: self-government, self-determination, autonomy and progress. Modern society is entrusted to this noble agent, dismissing eccentrics as non-contributors to the human project. Davis (1995) persuasively unravels the modern notion of normalcy, which arose with the advent of statistical tools such as the bell curve. He points out that the concept of 'normal' emerged as late as the nineteenth century – the English word appears around 1840 (Davis, 2002). Prior to this schemas of human value centred on divine, rather than corporeal ideals. Before celestial standards all were positioned on a continuum of imperfection, with no normal curve to mark out deviance. Later, the homogenising of bodies coincided with the rise of nationalism, the standardisation of languages and the emergence of 'national types' (Davis, 1995; 2002, pp. 105–6). The age of unitary identities, commodification-based narcissism and the veneration of progress had begun. 'Ableist' bias emerged, by consequence, not as a feature of a bigoted few, but as part of the very fabric of enlightenment (Davis, 2002).

Rod Michalko (2002) remarks on the odd arbitrariness of meanings ascribed to human differences; some are happily subsumed within normalcy (height, eye colour), while others locate the bearer as an outlier. Diseases or mutations implicate identifiable 'causes' such as genetic defects or bacteria. But curiously, non-impaired biology simply happens 'naturally'; or – better – *supernaturally*. Science, says Michalko (2002), cannot attribute cause here, as factors it named would themselves require a cause, rendering an unfathomable, ballooning regress. There can be little debate that 'normal human biology', 'normal human variation' and 'nature' itself are interpretive, metaphoric entities, sculpted into credible descriptors by definitions of pathology. It is understandable that medicine requires these delineations in order to provide services. But what is at issue is their application and assimilation as unquestioned cultural givens. Biomedicine should accept responsibility for a critical reappraisal of categories of normalcy. Instead, it appears that modern life is formulated around difference, and difference seems inseparable from value.

Artistic and literary representations

Depictions of disabled lives in literature and cinema tend to replicate the normate hegemony, creating disabled characters as distant and objectified (Shakespeare, 1999). Typically, impairment is portrayed as a character's central feature, to be used as a fulcrum for a moral fable or tale of redemption – what Mitchell and Snyder (2001b, p. 47) term an 'opportunistic metaphorical device'. In short, the disabled figure is a means to an end, which draws identification and emotional discharge from the audience through using impairment as an existential signifier (Garland-Thomson, 1997b). Cinema stereotypes such as the 'noble warrior', the 'charity cripple', the 'curio', the 'freak' and the 'Pollyanna' abound, while impairment which is incidental to the plot is rare (Darke, 1998, p. 181; Shakespeare, 1999). Disabled people as background extras connote movie scenes which are not intended as depictions of 'normal life', but instead 'heighten an atmosphere of exoticism, perversion, evil or fantasy' (Shakespeare, 1999, p. 164). Aptly, Mitchell and Snyder (1997; 2001b) term this over-signification of the disabled figure *narrative prosthesis*. Continuing this metaphor, the disabled body 'serves as a crutch upon which literary narratives lean for their representational power, disruptive potentiality, and analytical insight' (Mitchell and Snyder, 2000 in Davidson, 2003, p. 58). Even more conspicuous, though, is the fact that most disabled film characters are portrayed by nondisabled performers (Marks, 1999a). Marks (1999a) muses that this is so in order that, while the disability drama offers a passing catharsis to the viewer, it is reassuring for him or her to know that it is 'only pretend' (p. 128). The disabled character, thus, is used as a container for the projections of an audience who enjoys even greater insulation from their unconscious lives through the knowledge that Al Pacino is 'not really blind' and Daniel Day Lewis is 'not really paralysed' (ibid.).

For Marks (1999a), there would be discomfort if the artist remained disabled after the curtain, as evidence would remain of the fear states originally evoked by the impairment. This ambivalence, in my view, mirrors the positioning of disabled people across society; spurned, yet needed – the objects of both aversion and prurience. In his book *The cinema of isolation* Martin Norden (1994) links celluloid disability stereotypes in various eras of film to the political realities of the time. For example, post-World War II representations show a rehabilitative and normalising view, relating to the high numbers of impaired veterans returning home – among them screen writers and directors. Decades later, the legacy of McCarthyism and the Cold War created disability in cinema as a freakish, dangerous symbol, a contaminating threat to cherished homeland norms (Norden, 1994; Darke, 1998). Frequently a disabled character is 'cured' during the drama, highlighting a perennial tension between the 'erotic, complete body' and the 'uncanny, incomplete body' (Davis, 1997c, p. 66). The narrative, thus, works to re-evoke and resolve the projected conflicts of the latter.

Most troubling is the constant stream of television and film carrying blatant, egregious disability stereotyping which raises virtually no audible objection (Davis, 2002). The industry belief appears to be that there is little to learn about disability which an ordinary, sensitive person would not intuit (ibid.). Ideas like politics, oppression or systemic disadvantage are far from this colloquial view; disability is not seen as requiring interrogation or self-reflection. In photographic art disabled people have traditionally been virtually absent (Hevey, 1997). While over recent years an interest in disability imagery has grown in the visual arts, appearance of the disabled figure remains very much the exception (Garland-Thomson, 2009). Still, when combined with the emergence of radical disabled performance art mentioned earlier, this development is not insignificant. In the photographic mainstream, however, Hevey (1997, p. 332) attributes the absence of impairment to a reading of the disabled figure as 'socially dead'. By this phrase, Hevey means simply not having a role in society worthy of documenting. If present at all, disabled subjects are most likely to be symbols of otherness (Davis, 1997c). Hevey (1992) tells of a haunting resonance between medical photographs of disabled people and racialised colonial images. In each the 'patients' and 'blacks' stand frozen and passive, waiting to be 'done to', while 'doctors' and 'whites' fill authoritative and coolly confident attitudes (p. 53). What is absent across these media is a disabled figure who is nuanced and normatively complex, living life and negotiating human struggles; with hopes and disappointments, fears and strengths, falling in and out of love, finding and losing faith and so forth. Instead, the disabled figure appears as a portent which gives safe, vicarious life to the unthinkable before being reassigned to invisibility. Avery (1999) summarises:

> ... our novels and films, religion, art and myths are replete with images of the tortured body, the body distorted by pain, the Picassoesque figure that cries out in anguish and terror. But less often explored is the psychic pain caused by the disability experience, the effects of the social construction of stigma that situate the anomalous body as subaltern.
>
> (Avery, 1999, p. 116)

I concur with Mitchell and Snyder (2001b), who believe that narrative representations must affect how disabled individuals conceptualise, and hence live, their lives. As in the narrow, dehumanising messaging of disability design (Pullin, 2009), the disabled life is portrayed as a problem to be solved, narrowing imagination's potential for creating new ways of social life. There is little question that meanings found in film and print reflect public logic about what disability is, and what is to be done. As audiences project conflicts into the disabled body, it is inevitable that, to some extent, disabled individuals will be drawn into doing the same.

Charity discourse

Across most nations, a tradition of charity-based support for disabled persons, at times informed by religious doctrine, is an ever-present contributor to cultural ascriptions about disability. Such organisations often aim to provide for disabled people excluded from social and economic life, and abandoned by the state. In this sense, charitable services go some way to addressing profound need in a host of domains. But some argue that in the process of providing, charity discourse entrenches oppression through construing individuals as passive objects of benevolence, rather than entitled citizens. Pity and kindness become the unstable foundations for service provision, while lives fall increasingly under the influence of 'expert' and 'philanthropic' decision-making (Rioux, 2002). A central theme of this book is the need to understand unconscious aspects of the disability story, but also to show acceptance and empathy for self and other in the midst of this muddle. There can be little doubt that useful, even life-saving charitable disability work is performed around the globe by individuals with the best intentions; as with health practitioners, it is unfair and destructive to stereotype or pathologise these workers. Instead, we should aim to facilitate deeper understanding and change through collaboration, in order to build upon rather than dismiss what charity organisations may provide. This does not mean shying away from honest critique; not at all. But what is required is the fostering of relationships which allow such critique to be constructively integrated. It is, to begin, incumbent on disability studies to try to honestly comprehend the complex histories and legacies of charity organisations, and the consequent predicaments of those in authority who face demands for transformation.

While providing appropriately for some needs, and less appropriately for others, it is not unfair to say that charity typically does little to alter political realities. It may, in fact, inadvertently support inequality (Coleridge, 1993; Jack, 1995). If development is equated to people assuming control over their own lives, much charity-based disability work probably does not qualify as 'developmental' (Coleridge, 1993). A critical truth is that the survival of a significant proportion of charity organisations depends on conceptions of disability as dependency and damage, which induce pity and altruism (Marks, 1999a). This need to diminish disabled people in the ken of the public seems inevitably at odds with efforts to eradicate prejudice, contributing to a cycle of exclusion (ibid.). At one extreme, fetishised images of charity advertising have been linked to the purported role of pornography in gender oppression. In both cases body parts are the focus for eliciting an othering response, and the relationships in which the images are created, interpreted and dispersed are beyond the reach of the subject (Barnes and Mercer, 2001). The act of giving, against this backdrop, is not a gesture of unity but a reaffirmation of separateness (Murphy et al., 1988). The radical critique of Ravaud and Stiker (2001) views the primary function of charity organisations as collaborating with organs of state in enforcing identity distinctions. One must 'qualify' for charity support, through donning a disabled identity, perhaps involving a host of wordless ascriptions which this entails (ibid.; Scott, 1969). All such institutional categorising, these writers add, militates against acceptance of the other 'in his or her irreducible difference', narrowing the potential for novel, multiple ways of being human (Ravaud and Stiker, 2001, p. 496).

As already argued, if disabled persons do act as ciphers for shameful parts of others, instinctual impulses towards this group will likely be of a hostile nature. Aggressive urges may, through reaction formation, be experienced consciously as a mix of shades of guilt and altruistic, reparative intentions. The pay-off of this coping strategy is substantial, allowing guilt over hostility to resolve into an act which positions one as both powerful and generous (Shakespeare, 1994). Young (1994, p. 131) characterises the political functioning of projective identification as the 'mapping' of internal processes onto groups and institutions, in a manner which allows us to 'experience the virulent as though it is benign and part of the definition of a good social order'. Charity organisations certainly reassure us with knowledge of social cohesion and generosity to 'unfortunates', while obscuring the political roots of inequality. The common, paternalistic assumption that disabled people are generally treated with kindness (Davis, 2002) is a familiar, cherished myth. I term this the *fantasy of filled needs* – the idea that in our society 'things are in place' to provide for 'those who cannot provide for themselves'. The global truth of deprivation in disabled lives remains as unbelievable as it is obscure. The groundless idealisation of unseen services bears testimony to social realities which are both un-thought and unable to be thought.

In the Kleinian picture of infancy, managing constitutional aggression is a central struggle (Klein, 1959). In fact, anxiety surrounding aggressive impulses gives rise to the ego's earliest defences (Klein, 1948). The common idealisations of disabled people as plucky, spiritual, inspiring or gifted are, in part, reformulations of hostility, with charity discourse providing a sanctioned means for discharge. The reshaping of internal hostility into public virtue is captured, for Longmore (1997), in the American disability charity telethon. The telethon, to Longmore (1997), is a moral allegory, a ritual of 'cleansing and renewal' (p. 140). The moment of largesse forms an indispensable barricade against the spectre of self-interested conspicuous consumption; the solution is 'equally conspicuous contribution' (ibid.). At a manifest level everyday reality appears in carnivalesque, ritualised inversion, with the 'unfortunates' assuming centre stage. But more intrinsic is the moral restoration of those who give, or simply observe (ibid.). In this world, as across the charity spectrum, impairment alone causes suffering, negating any need to interrogate society or self. In the telethon temporary redemption is found from the guilt-ridden excesses of consumption, as well as refuge from the more haunting co-occurrence of freedom, opportunity and equality with the horrors of social suffering. David Hevey (1992) encapsulates:

> Charity advertising ... represents the highest public validation of the isolation of disabled people. It presents a solution to the 'problem' of disablement by a disguised blaming of the victim. It fails to find a solution because it is itself the problem ...
>
> (Hevey, 1992, p. 51)

Zizek's (2004) analysis is characteristically economical and penetrating. To him, charity is a crude 'humanitarian mask', fashioned in an attempt to staunch the contradictions of the ethics of autonomy at the core of capitalism (p. 388). The 'ruthless pursuit of profit', which is capital's only intent, leaves its masters subject to 'a super-ego[1] blackmail of gigantic proportions' (ibid.). Neoliberal justifications for social inequality across a range of axes seem, on close scrutiny, ever more sinister.

After reflection on modern Western cultural responses to impairment, we return now to the arena more traditionally associated with socialisation – the family. The intention, though, is to follow a thread which traces the concentric layering of disablist ideology as it settles in both disabled and nondisabled subjectivity.

Disability and the family

Attachment and infancy

A discussion of the effects of early attachment relationships on disabled subjectivity is largely limited to incidents of congenital impairment, reducing generalisability. Yet, I believe there is much to be learnt about disablist ideology broadly through examining the titrated, sensitive relational world surrounding the birth of a disabled infant. Further, while a family's experience of a child becoming disabled is complicated by a host of variables not considered here, I believe that this discussion can help our understanding of such scenarios.

Most of the small number of psychoanalytic contributions to congenital disability in families employ concepts borrowed from grief and bereavement theory (e.g. Burlingham, 1961; Solnit and Stark, 1961; Pinkerton, 1970; MacKeith, 1973; Drotar et al., 1975). These writers draw on Freud's (1923) work on mourning, viewing an impaired birth as an experience of object loss – the loss of the 'longed-for, healthy child' (Solnit and Stark, 1961, p. 524). Parents are expected to traverse a stage-wise mourning process if there is to be any hope of healthy relating to the child (Drotar et al., 1975). Drotar and co-workers describe possible features of these stages as overwhelming shock, irrational behaviour, uncontrollable tearfulness, helplessness, denial, disbelief, anger and anxiety (ibid.). Distressed mothers may, in this picture, experience violently negative feelings towards self and baby, including hatred of the impairment, self-blame and 'not caring if the baby dies' (ibid., p. 711). The trauma of the discrepancy between the imagined child and the actual, impaired baby is viewed as a major threat to early relating (Solnit and

Stark, 1961), potentially leading to a family milieu of 'chronic sorrow' (Drotar et al., 1975, p. 710). MacKeith (1973, p. 133) reported 'protection' and 'revulsion' as two primary maternal reactions to an impaired infant, co-existing in complex relation to one another, and to consciousness. In work with mothers of blind infants, Burlingham (1961, p. 122) describes feelings of 'injury, of hurt pride, of guilt, and of … depression' potentially leading to withdrawal, and even an irrational death wish towards the child. From a psychiatric viewpoint, Fisman and Wolf (1991, p. 213) found that the birth of a child with a pervasive developmental disorder has 'a significant effect on family members', including disrupted parenting, marital discord and maternal depression.

As we shall see, psychoanalytic theorists have used the same 'bereavement model' in approaching adjustment to adventitious disability. In both scenarios the approach has been heatedly rejected by social model writers, arguing that a grief model reduces socio-political adversity to the psychological problems of people who have not come to terms with impairment (Abberley, 1993; Finkelstein and French, 1993; Oliver, 1995). Further, it ignores the broad lack of social services geared to meet the complex needs of families with a recent, congenitally impaired addition (Ferguson and Asch, 1989). Consequently, work in this area from psychoanalysis and psychology has been rubbished as part of the medical model. Ferguson (2001, p. 375) and others see the psychoanalytic view as malign in its persistent 'pessimism', characterising parents, almost without exception, as overcome with shock, disappointment and revulsion. Ferguson, the father of a congenitally impaired son, finds such accounts a destructive, misleading sleight upon real lives, placing parents in double-binds where any response is read as pathological (see also Tregaskis, 2006). Clearly, observations of prominent researchers in this tradition (e.g. Solnit and Stark, 1961; Solnit, 1989) seem oblivious to concerns about disability construction. For example, they make the odious and now anachronistic recommendation that parents not be forced to see their impaired newborn before his or her institutionalisation. There is no examination at all of possible internalised aversive feelings about disability within parents or society at large.

The tendency of 'traditional' psychoanalysis to seek causal links between impairment and psychopathology is mirrored in the accounts of childbirth above. Again, impairment is everything. In a uni-directional functional relationship, unchanging bodily realities are seen as the cause of predictable social and psychological givens. Some writers may see this assessment as unfair, but a passing reference to relational factors makes no dent in the dominant logic. This criticism need not question the felt experience of impairment within parents or disabled people of any age. What is being questioned is the attributing of every aspect of experience to impairment.

As discussed in the previous chapter, the leap from body to psyche is negotiated through the concept of the *body ego* – the earliest representation of the ego, arising as a 'reflection' of bodily structure and sensation. Freud (1923) writes:

> The ego is first and foremost a bodily ego; it is not merely a surface entity, but is itself the projection of a surface.
>
> (Freud, 1923, p. 26)

Orbach (1994, p. 166) describes the body ego concept as a 'rather undeveloped notion'. It is this indistinct idea which is elemental to positions which excise impaired bodies (and minds) from the world of ideology, from the world of social responses. Yorke's (1980) stated position is an informative example:

> If … we had considered cases in which early disabilities, such as congenital blindness, deafness, or deformities leading to early restrictions of motility, had continued into later life we would have found that deviations, defects, and arrests of development were intimately interwoven with the disability itself and ensured, inter alia, that the ego … would be an abnormal one.
>
> (Yorke, 1980, p. 191)

Besides the cause–effect logic of the impact of congenital impairment on psychology, the space made available for the grief of parents presents their responses as independent of contextual factors, including engagements with health professionals (see Dreger, 2006). While the personal histories of parents may be seen as mediating adjustment processes to some extent, the reality of 'what must be dealt with' is assumed to be constant. Again, the irresistible equating of a defective body with a wretched existence is in view, disguising an exploration of what happens between people in shaping the socialisation of disabled lives. Interestingly, writers drawing on Freud's (1923) utterances in buttressing essentialist positions may be unaware of his later shift to emphasising the importance of maternal care in enhancing the body ego (Freud, 1933). Disability studies critics, in my view, do Freud a similar injustice (e.g. Corker and Shakespeare, 2002; Goodley, 2011a; 2011b). Raphael-Leff (1994) stresses that psychological representations of the body do not 'just spring from within', instead being psychosocial products of time and place (p. 13). Experience of the body is, thus, never purely solipsistic. Instead, 'we "learn" our bodies through the hands, faces and minds of significant carers and their bodily ministrations' (p. 16). Psychic representations of the body are also multiple, and shift as social situations alter their salience. The picture of impairment meanings at play here is fundamentally fluid, and shaped by intersubjective experiences borne of overt and invisible cultural assumptions. Raphael-Leff (1994) elaborates:

> Indeed, right into adulthood, a web of associative connections link the flesh of our permeable bodies in our most intimate moments to the bodies of others. Even in the privacy of masturbatory acts and within the secret realms of bulimic activity or self-mutilating solitude, their imagined responses guide erotic fantasy or relentlessly dictate cruel standards.
>
> (Raphael-Leff, 1994, p. 17)

Later in this passage she describes how the bodily self of fantasy is shaped by cultural meanings and aesthetics which are 'as effective to psyche as Chinese foot-binding is to flesh' (ibid.). The 'malformed' infant body thus only becomes imbued with difference through mirroring responses, typically tainted with disability-related anxieties.

Lussier (1960; 1980) recounts how a psychotherapy process with a congenitally disabled boy showed up his assumption of a functional relationship between impairment and psychic disturbance. The boy, Peter, had under-developed and non-functioning arms; Lussier assumed that the psychotherapy would surround negotiating loss to do with not having a healthily functioning body. The grief model of disability, as well as the idea of a presocial body ego, can both be seen in his approach. But as therapy progressed, profound social (specifically parental) factors underlying his distress began to emerge. Peter's mother seemed ashamed of his impairment, and thus, in effect, of him (Lussier, 1980). In early childhood his mother would carefully cover his arms when they were in public, and showed little ability to comfort him on occasions when he was stared at (Lussier, 1960, p. 433). Over time Lussier felt that Peter was communicating to him that his body was 'a complete unit, self-sufficient, integral, not mutilated' (Lussier, 1980, p. 180). Instead, it was his maternal mirroring which had left painful impressions on his sense of self, stunting his emotional growth and ability to separate. Movingly, Lussier (1980) concludes:

> ... the boy, as shown throughout his analysis, seemed to have been much more in need of the confidence of his mother in him than in need of normal arms.
>
> (Lussier, 1980, p. 179)

Clinical impressions are that in early life Peter had received a fragment of accurate validation from someone – perhaps a relative or teacher, or an alternate emotional part of his mother. This mirroring allowed him to later re-find his 'whole' bodily self in work with Lussier, separate from his mother's shaming ascriptions. With a subtle similarity, Balikov (1960) reported working with three nondisabled children born to blind parents, who lived an isolated family life. Remarkably, the children grew into appearing and behaving as if blind – for example, feeling their way around nursery school with their hands and feet, and reporting 'not seeing' objects before tactile exploration (Balikov, 1960). Of course, this is an extreme example, with complex overtones of behavioural modelling as well as possible unreported comorbid psychiatric problems, yet the demonstration of experiences of bodily function as a product of learning remains.

Critical debate around the grief and bereavement approach to birth of a congenitally impaired child is, unsurprisingly, emotive. Key participants in this debate are parents themselves who, of course, have ongoing relationships with loved family members. This reality quite understandably puts parents, with the support of many writers from disability studies, wholly at odds with researchers interested in making sense of the impact – often seen as aversive – of an impaired birth. Ferguson, from his personal experience, describes this position as follows:

> As a father, I do not love my son in spite of his handicaps, as some abstracted, idealised version of reality. The object of my affection is the flesh and blood Ian whom I dress every day, put in a wheelchair, and struggle to talk to in

> words he can understand. Disability complicates the relationship but does not necessarily damage it.
>
> (Ferguson and Asch, 1989, p. 114)

What all stakeholders face here is an example of destructive, split debate in the disability arena, where unseen social injustices are expressed in a furious rejection of empirical enquiries into the familial sanctum. Recognition of these injustices must be a point of departure for this debate. Vast numbers of parents have suffered immeasurably under a lack of social service support, experiencing discrimination of both their loved ones and themselves. It is not surprising that researchers preoccupied with how impairment harms the family are experienced as a further persecution. The impasse is quite understandable, but somehow needs to be overcome if we are to create an integrated thought-space for considering the fundamental issue of congenital impairment in families.

The core of the points I make below is that, in this splitting engagement, all participate in silencing aspects of the issue at hand, including professionals, parents and activists. Let us begin our discussion with Lindemann's (1981) words, expressing disgust at psychoanalytic assumptions about disability in families:

> How can we call such a daughter a 'burden'? On what basis do textbooks repeatedly claim that parents of children with disabilities 'cannot make an honest attachment to their real child until they have withdrawn their affection from the normal, wished-for child'?
>
> (Lindemann, 1981 cited in Olkin, 1999, p. 92)

Quoting Solnit's (1989) description of 'sad, resentful, discouraged' parental reactions, Yuker (1994) implores us to 'stop studying the presumably horrible negative effects of a child with a disability on parents and siblings' (Yuker, 1994 in Olkin, 1999, p. 92). Ferguson (2001, p. 375) – an influential voice in this debate – similarly scorns psychoanalytic findings, emphasising that parental reactions are 'inescapably embedded within a sociohistorical context'. To Ferguson, the 'horror stories' and 'tragic connotations' of psychoanalytic writing are slanderous to parents, and reflect a profoundly destructive intellectual attitude, employing a logic which simply reverses an earlier, even more crude view (ibid., p. 376). Whereas religion previously understood disabled infants as damaged by the misdeeds of ancestors, now it is the impaired child who brings suffering to the family (see also Barnes and Mercer, 2005a). Whether family researchers focused on attitudinal categories (such as guilt, denial, displaced anger or grief) or behavioural aspects (including role disruption, marital discord or social withdrawal) it was consistently assumed that disability 'distorted the connection between child and parent in ways that were both intrinsic and harmful' (Ferguson, 2001, p. 379). Parents showing dissatisfaction with the support of health professionals faced this being interpreted as displaced anger directed, in fact, at their child (ibid., p. 380; see also Heifetz, 1980; Turnbull and Summers, 1987). Harris and Wideman (1988) – themselves working from a psychoanalytic viewpoint – slate such use of theory by professionals as a mechanism to contain their own welling anxieties, rather than to illuminate patient experience.

The vociferous objections of Ferguson, Olkin, Gill and others to the construction of families with disabled children as miserable and disturbed make sense. Imagine the possible contextual stressors at work. Having a young child with a severe impairment may bring direct and indirect prejudice, physical demands, financial strain, chronic uncertainties regarding service provision and much else. As an aside, Calton (2010, p. 849) emphasises the influence of class on access to material coping resources, which make it more possible for wealthier parents to accomplish 'modern ideals' of integration for their impaired children. Facing all such adversity, the vast majority of parents quite simply want the best for their children, and are deeply committed to attempting to achieve that vision.

The continual experience of extreme stress and uncertainty brought by physical aspects of impairment, along with the pain of seeing one's child suffer prejudice, may at times position parents in life-worlds of ongoing trauma. But in the critique of Ferguson and others a paradoxical danger arises from the need to contrarily re-author the story of disability in families. The question of what, in fact, amounts to empathy for parents is not a politically simple one. As we shall see, a hallmark of disabled life in prejudiced society is the constructing of experience, identity and self in opposition to dominant stereotypes. The question of how subjectivity is shaped in congenitally impaired children is an especially important one. We cannot risk overlooking, for example, the potential influence of unconscious relational dynamics in families. Disability studies and disabled people will be done a disservice if we allow a rebuttal of prejudiced assumptions to derail an exploration of how real, human struggles, which *do* occur, impact on the early development of self. This, in my view, is what is in danger of happening. The words of Miller (2006), who has achondroplasia,[2] provide an interesting contrast to the critique from disability studies:

> The birth of a disabled child to able-bodied parents is often met with disappointment, or even anger, due to the loss of the idealised child … The birth of a disabled child often leads to a period of grief.
>
> (Miller, 2006, p. 218)

The simple authenticity of these words rings true – the proposition that the birth of an achondroplasic infant would, to most parents, be a complex, evocative and difficult experience. But to some, such observations are difficult to allow, as these confirm stereotypes. Unexpectedly, the need to overtly value families may at times be an impediment to compassion: idealisation is not empathy.

As in the split between the helpless invalid and the 'supercrip', families are as unseen in the idealisation of virtues as in the denigration of pathology. Empathy takes place when difficult, nuanced and contradictory realities are speakable; when things don't make sense (personal, environmental, historical), and a place is made for that confusion. Emancipatory political narratives have difficulty in holding such complexity, inevitably placing subtle sanctions on what experiences are ideologically permissible. This silence adds to the already substantial emotional sensitivity of ongoing relationships with impaired children. There are human individuals, not theoretical abstractions at play here, and the emotional risks are consequently great.

One service framework for parents informed by social model principles is family-centred practice (FCP). Quite appropriately, this approach positions families as 'key decision-makers, central to and experts in the wants and needs of their child' (Dodd et al., 2009, p. 173). In an interesting, perhaps ambivalent critique of its application, Dodd et al. (2009) describe how FCP may lead professionals to expect families to 'always be proactive and energetic in the pursuit of care for their child' (p. 179). These writers found that at times parents simply did not have the personal resources to be 'empowered' or take on new rehabilitation techniques, as they struggled to balance competing responsibilities. This work moves somewhat towards a 'real-world' picture of family life as the emotionally fraught, unpredictable and layered business that it is – disabled offspring or not. One female respondent described her guilty, painful shift from an exclusive, self-depriving focus on her impaired daughter to a more balanced lifestyle, involving her own needs and those of her other children (ibid., p. 179). In this self-denying predicament one wonders: have constructions of the 'empowered' family become imperatives felt by the practitioner? As FCP may make it hard for parents to acknowledge difficult material and physical struggles, materialist disability studies discourse may do the same for the emotional world. Dodd et al.'s (2009) work resonated with the experience of a colleague of mine. As the mother of a son with Down syndrome, she had participated in self-help group meetings for parents. Her experience was that the helpfulness of the groups was restricted by an 'optimism discourse', which allowed little or no space for painful or conflicted aspects of parenting. This optimism was, perhaps, analogous to the drive in FCP to hand over power and responsibility to parents who may, quite understandably, feel wobbly and unsure about their 'empowerment'. An empathic stance would allow struggle in these parents, no matter its accompanying personal or material narrative.

McLaughlin and Goodley (2008) describe their 'nagging concern' that parents are often spoken for on behalf of those who 'stress the need to remain certain about identity and truth' (p. 318). The consequence is that simplistic conceptions of parents' responses are created, failing to recognise how 'certainty and uncertainty' are used as parts of strategic coping (p. 317). Although it is not clear, one imagines that it is health professionals whom these writers see as inappropriately speaking on behalf of parents. But here too, a subtle disability movement discourse may be at work, defining bounds of identity and experience. As in the work of Dodd et al. (2009) above, a turn to complexity is discernible here, although the position still may be understood as needing to substantiate, or even idealise, parents' responses *on principle*. The valuing of uncertainty, although viewed here as purely strategic, may open the door a crack to the imponderables which make family life what it is.

Rocque (2010) provides qualitative data on how mothers of children diagnosed on the autism spectrum mediate their child's relating to the world. These mothers show creativity and resourcefulness in the face of the pain of their child enduring hostility and exclusion. It is a picture which captures the very real conflicts we face in theoretically approaching disability in families. There is no question that such families deserve our compassion, in lives full of experiences which leave one feeling under attack by the world. The extreme, and quite natural need for support leads to reflections on familial dynamics being experienced as an affront. The dilemma is a profound one, but one requiring both sensitivity and clear purpose. A danger is that we fall into a split between the 'good' family and the 'bad' world of discriminatory communities, diagnosing psychologists and the like. This leaves us unable to think clearly – freely – about either. This point of departure is one from which we stand to learn very little about disabled subjectivity. Taking up the role of go-between for one's autism-spectrum child is, itself, a manifestation of disablism's influence on formative relationships within the family.

I believe it is possible to explore this psychological experience in a nuanced way without being a 'collaborator'. Ryan and Runswick-Cole (2008) would, I imagine, disagree. These writers take exception to the interpretation of mothers as 'constraints' within the lives of their impaired children. For the bleak history of psychoanalytic and psychological research into this area described above this critique is well justified. But there is no mention in their work of the need for a new, balanced enquiry. Instead, the call is that we move beyond 'static positions and stereotypical representations and understandings', presumably towards a new, more beneficent orthodoxy based on mothers' experience of 'what are described by feminist scholars as oppressive mothering ideologies and disabling environments' (p. 199). My worry is that orthodoxy remains. Among other writers, Veck (2002) is criticised for such 'stereotyping' – for other reasons, I critique this work later. Veck's (2002) disabled respondent gives a first-person account of his experience of mothering, which was in some ways an aversive one. This, it seems, is not permissible. I am left wondering whether Ryan and Runswick-Cole (2008) believe that the best we can hope for is to replace one stereotype with another.

In a social work text on working with disability in families, Burke (2008) seems, by comparison, disarmingly at ease with the jumble which is parenting. With a practical approach a range of evidence is reviewed, showing up hope, dread and much in between. The reality of altered expectations within parents, stress and anxiety, complex family dynamics, the emotional predicaments of siblings, restriction of family activities and a range of other issues are named. The intent here is not primarily to examine psychological concerns, but the data provided clearly identifies such issues as real and relevant topics of study. Burke (2008) emphasises that emotional reactions to an impaired birth are not stereotypical, but highly varied. Responses span all between joy and grief, and typically appear as admixtures of these feelings and others. The simple reality of complexity – of *mixed feelings* – in all relationships should come as no surprise, but may be obscured through discursive controls. A further, fascinating counterpoint to the dominant, de-psychologising view of families within disability studies is provided by Singh and Ghai (2009). These writers speak candidly of difficult emotional aspects of disability in families, including parental shame or overprotectiveness, hostility in siblings and feelings of worthlessness. It is both puzzling and encouraging that such issues as children feeling blamed by their parents can be spoken of here – within the international journal most closely identified with the social model. The research originated in India, potentially defusing something of the prickliness of the issues on fuzzy, 'cross-cultural' grounds. It seems unlikely that such a study, if originating in Britain, would have found its way to print in an historical materialist dominated publication.

In the previous chapter I framed the discussion of psychoanalytic work on disability as a challenge to reject totalising ideological judgments, in favour of an approach which builds disciplinary and conceptual relationships. In his critique of psychoanalysis, Ferguson (2001) refers specifically to the study by Drotar et al. (1975) mentioned above. He views this work as a blatant pathologisation of parents, whose emphasis on their child's ability is dismissed as 'denial'. I accept this critique, but there remains much that is moving and authentic in the accounts of the 20 couples interviewed by these investigators. Further, a close reading of these competing lines of thought shows up psychoanalysis' unique value in finely describing emotional states. This offers important knowledge about the conscious and unconscious relational milieu in which disabled children develop. Ferguson's (2001) ardent de-pathologising position cannot help obscuring this relational world. As before, there is a baby in this cloudy psychoanalytic bathwater.

We come here to an example of how a psychoanalytic view can radically re-orient debate through upsetting binaries. Winnicott (1947) reframes the idea of parents' difficult, ambivalent feelings towards an infant as a wholly normative, even necessary part of child-rearing. The presence of aspects of ill feeling within a mother towards her new-born is, in this view, nothing short of rationally, naturally appropriate. We need not be afraid or ashamed of such feelings. Among much else, the baby has been 'a danger to her body in pregnancy and at birth', 'an interference with her private life', a cause of pain to her nipples, and the reason for immense fatigue (ibid., p. 201). In short, the baby has replaced her needs with the priority of his or her own. In many important senses parenting involves allowing oneself to be used in fulfilling continual infant needs. To Winnicott (1947), the mother is treated as 'an unpaid servant, a slave', who must love her child 'excretions and all' (p. 201).

This corrective to uni-dimensional, romanticised notions of motherhood draws attention to maternal struggles, providing an accepting space for natural feelings of resentment, fatigue, anxiety or disappointment. In an approach which rejects binary logics, these feelings are not evidence of not loving one's baby. In light of the immense, guilt-inducing cultural judgments regarding 'good mothering' inflicted on women, such feelings are often repressed or viewed as evidence of failure, with potentially far-reaching effects. It is instructive to see how Read (2000), from within disability studies, interprets Winnicott's (1947; 1974) intentions regarding empathy for mothers in a diametrically opposite way. Where, in my understanding, Winnicott stood for allowing mothers to have and express the difficult emotional ramifications of their role, Read (2000) places his work not far from the centre of a psychoanalytic conspiracy to defame motherhood. Winnicott's (1974) idea of the *good enough* mother is not, as Read (2000) maintains, intended to identify all mothers as, by definition, failures. Rather, it underscores how difficult the task is, and that, by definition, it cannot be performed perfectly. Drawing heavily on Badinter's (1981) reactionary anti-psychoanalytic position, Read (2000), in my view, misses a constructive opportunity to explore what her own mother-centred position and that of Winnicott (1974) have in common.

As we have seen, it is an axiom of psychoanalytic thinking that feelings which cannot be consciously acknowledged will tend to become enacted. Thus it is that for Winnicott (1947), a culture of acceptance of difficult or unmentionable feelings about parenthood has real implications for the psychological well-being of children, and hence adults. Ferguson (2001) and others, through needing to disavow pathologising ascriptions, risk de-legitimating the actual, felt experience of parents responding to untold external and internal realities. If we acknowledge that disability reliably provokes human struggle to do with difference, the experience for parents adjusting to the unexpected birth of a congenitally impaired infant should be no different. In the early, merged relationship between parent and infant unconscious exchanges are as important to developing selfhood as are conscious ministrations. Anyone who has parented an infant is aware of the difficult task of emotional holding. In these delicate circumstances it is hard to see how the reverberations of feelings about bodily difference could be seen as anything other than an important topic of study. But this study should be undertaken in a manner which promotes empathy for parents, rather than threatens it. It is an odd and unfortunate paradox that in terms of disability studies critique, parents are particularly unentitled to complicated feelings if their children are disabled. With the best intentions, this discourse may selectively deprive parents of disabled infants of the space needed to process emotional meanings around a birth, and further into childhood and beyond. Complex dynamics of guilt and self-recrimination are possible outcomes of such repression, potentially impacting on growing relationships and limiting compassionate, open engagement with parents' experience.

Broader psychoanalytic ideas on child-bearing are a useful context for this debate. Sinason (1992) describes how pregnant women naturally carry a range of unconscious fantasies regarding their bodily state and the imminent birth. If one accepts the ideas of Fiedler (1978) and others regarding universal human preoccupations with bodily monstrosity, it follows that the drastic changes of pregnancy provoke strong unconscious fantasy. These anxieties may surround 'what' one is carrying, how it will represent one to the world, issues of entitlement or ability in parenting, fears to do with that extra glass of wine or cigarette, feelings about the sex that led to conception, and so forth (Sinason, 1992, p. 258). For all, each stage of parenting calls forth projections. According to Sinason (1992), when a 'healthy' baby is born, these fears tend to be released, through an experience of having been disconfirmed. But if an impaired child appears, some mothers may experience this as a confirmation of something of the anxieties which came before, evoking a personal set of feelings about both self and baby (ibid.). Potential emotional effects for a father are analogous. Besides the material challenges of caring for an impaired child, the most healthy of parents may still face unseen, inner struggles to do with the meaning of the birth. Raphael-Leff (1994) describes the rich, meaning-laden bond between mother and infant, emphasising the profound, complex evocativeness of all maternal relationships, not just those with congenitally impaired infants. She writes:

> A mother's palpating hand, charged with affect, reflects her relation to male and female bodies, as well as the positive or negative forces unconsciously invested in her baby and feelings towards her own feminine bodiliness and fecundity, her unconscious representations of maternity, sexuality and gender … To a mother, the baby may at first signify completion of her own fertile identity; alternatively, representing some facet of her internal world she or he is greeted as a beloved or hated reincarnation for a significant figure in her emotional life. She or he may be invested with an idealised female baby-self or ascribed repudiated aspects of the mother's self-image depending on her unique psychohistory.
>
> (Raphael-Leff, 1994, p. 23)

The capacity of parents to contain painful emotions, and not expose these to their infants, is an important part of promoting healthy development (Rustin, 1991). To do this it is essential that parents not be obliged to deny their feelings, but instead find accepting relationships where these may be expressed and digested. The concept of *maternal reverie* (Bion, 1962a) describes the intense, 'tuned-in' awareness mothers have of their infants – emotional care which fosters the development of integrated selfhood (Rustin, 1991). The mother's (or father's) task here is to receive the infant's difficult feelings, while remaining secure and caring (Holmes, 1996). Resisting the urge to rebut the distress, the mother takes it inside herself, processing it on the infant's behalf (ibid.). To perform this role of growing the self through allowing the baby to 'be', the mother herself requires emotional containment. If she does not receive enough support and acceptance in managing her natural maternal anxieties – such as those described above – her resources for containing her infant will be affected. Further, part of reverie involves the mother's empathic imagining of the child's experience and needs, which rests on positive identification. Anxiety-ridden feelings of 'differentness' possibly associated with an impaired birth may disrupt this, undermining a mother's trust in her intuitive 'knowing' about what her baby needs (Lussier, 1980; Harris and Wideman, 1988). The intention here is not to judge mothers; precisely the contrary. Instead, it is to affirm that, in a world full of shame-ridden, negative disability meanings, it is absolutely normal for mothers of impaired infants to grapple with these difficulties. Such mothers are in an impossible fix, between personal fears, guilt-ridden maternal imperatives, political correctness, misattuned health care relationships and probably much besides. They need and deserve space, acceptance, support and an empathic recognition that to feel fear or shame surrounding disability is a normative point of departure for all.

Through lacking a psychological framework, disability studies has been unable to systematically investigate the socialisation of its constituency. If we are to understand inter-generational links, and thus the links between the individual and the social, concepts from attachment theory are indispensable (Kraemer and Roberts, 1996). Although beginning with early formative relationships, these ideas readily apply to all influential figures in development, tracing the construction of feelings about self and other which extend through life (ibid., Erskine and Judd, 1994). Self-worth, insight into personal pain, the ability to articulate subjective states and the capacity to work and love are all intimately connected to our experiences of attachment. A political movement aiming to fully understand oppression – to fully understand itself – must explore these realities. If not openly addressed, common anxieties and projections surrounding impairment may disrupt attachments in identifiable ways. For example, it is important for all babies to be allowed an early experience of omnipotence – a fantasy experience of being in control of needed resources and carers. The management and later, gentle trimming back of this experience influences the development of healthy, realistic agency. These tasks of growing up may interact with a confusion in disablist culture between agency and dependency (Harris and Wideman, 1988) – we are culturally unsure whether disabled people are capable of 'nothing' or capable of 'anything'. The culture of autonomy makes it natural for mothers to carry fears regarding a disabled infant's potential for independence and survival in an unwelcoming world. Trusting an impaired child's capacity to grow and cope with the incremental process of separation may be particularly hard for such mothers. The delicate balance between care and intrusion, trust and support, is immensely difficult for all mothers, and further complicated here.

A second essential experience for the infant is that of the mother (and thus the world) surviving his or her aggressive impulses, showing that she is both sufficiently accepting and robust to contain her baby's difficult or destructive feelings. A key proposition of this book is that part of the psycho-social predicament of disabled people involves a 'de-realisation' of experience, borne of the ongoing deflecting or ignoring of subjective reality by an anxious, unready world. One can see how such dynamics may begin in families, with parents quite naturally struggling to contain complex feelings about their infant's nature and future, which make it harder to provide him or her with an authentic experience of acceptance. I suggest that for a proportion of the disabled population, experiences of another being truly able to 'stand' one's subjective reality, and provide moments of precious, attuned validation of self, are rare.

It may be useful to reflect at this point on a handful of parents' accounts of the discovery that their baby is congenitally impaired. Rinaldi (1996) matter-of-factly points to ever-present cultural imagery prizing the 'unmarked-beautiful-healthy-intelligent-"regular"' child, constantly reminding parents of the discrimination and struggle which is likely to be their child's social destiny (Rinaldi, 1996 in Avery, 1999, p. 116). A realistic fear for parents of children who are visibly different is of painful interpersonal experiences which injure the self, and upset fulfilling psychosocial functioning (Parens, 2006). Finding internal trust which allows for healthy separating under these circumstances may be thorny and challenging. Abelow Hedley (2006) provides a moving account of the early stages of family life after the birth of her daughter, who has achondroplasia:

> Everything was confusion: how to react, how to proceed, what to do. As the frantic days unfolded it seemed that all we could focus on was how to repair the flaws, and we would listen to anyone from a faith healer to a surgeon if we thought there was a 'fix' for her in it … There are dangers both social and emotional in being different and a certain amount of safety in being normal.
> (Abelow Hedley, 2006, p. 43)

An aspect of earlier psychoanalytic accounts of congenital impairment which is especially offensive to disability studies critics is the suggestion that parents may carry a painful fantasy of an unborn 'whole' and healthy child. More recently, Sinason (1992) tells of a psychotherapy patient, Steven, whose mother spoke of him 'not as a boy', but as a 'shadowy representation of the not-properly-mourned healthy twin of himself he should have been' (p. 131). After Sinason commented on how Steven had grown over the holidays, his mother responded with sadness, saying 'yes, he would have been so tall' (ibid.). She writes: 'Her real speech was for the other Steven, the healthy one who has never lived or died and has not been put to rest' (ibid.). It is not at all surprising that parents are offended by work which reduces their experience to this, although Sinason, I believe, does not do so. Her description here is simply one of a deeply troubled, unhelpful maternal relationship; not at all novel to psychotherapists anywhere in the world. Disability challenges us to make real conceptual and relational space for difficult feelings, while not stereotyping or disrespecting ongoing lives, relationships and material struggles.

Considering the taut, often guilty constraints on grief sketched above, it is likely that many parents are given very little opportunity by themselves or others to express feelings of loss. Feelings which are circumvented tend to go underground, becoming more likely to disrupt relationships in unconscious ways. Disabled children surrounded by unspoken emotional currents may develop in an identity limbo, subtly aware of their presence as a disappointment or accident. This may lead to an appeasing hesitancy around expressing their own difficult experiences (see Bowlby, 1979). These ideas may put the radical positions of the expressivist critique in a slightly different light. Central here is the reality that, because of segregation, most parents will have had limited exposure to disabled people, much less to integrated, fulfilled disabled lives. Imagined futures, consequently, may be filled with anxious fantasies. In each of the situations touched on above parents' experiences must be normalised, allowing for honest processing of whatever anxieties, losses or projections may be at play, in order to limit these being unconsciously borne by their children. All parents will unconsciously give some of their own conflicts to their children in projection. The business of being a parent is doing one's best to limit this. In engagement with disability, our unconscious worlds are much more alive, more present and require more careful attention.

One implication of parents developing an entitled, honest voice will be the spread of development research paradigms which explore non-normative pathways. Most development theory rests on observation of nondisabled children (Asch, 1984; Watermeyer, 2002a). Conversely, psychological development research on congenital impairment focuses excessively on 'naked' physiological factors, rather than intersubjective ones. Kenneth Wright (1991), for example, provides a psychoanalytic account of the role of sight in early attachment. Wright (1991) falls into the medicalising trap of viewing congenital blindness' and its impact on selfhood as a presocial given (see Omwake and Solnit, 1961 for a similar example). Here, the role of sight in developing healthy, integrated selfhood is positioned in a manner which condemns those who cannot traverse the normative path (due to blindness) to a fragmented, immature internal world (Watermeyer, 2002a). Research observation which excludes disabled life creates theory which is not only descriptive of development, but also has normative implications, potentially expelling and pathologising those with differing somatic pathways. A candid literature which describes the internal and relational experience of parents of congenitally impaired children will, I believe, advance more equitable and inclusive models of psychological development.

The words of Harris and Wideman (1988, p. 119), reflecting on accounts gathered from parents of congenitally impaired children, capture the tone of my position. What they found was 'an absolutely human mix of love, grief, sadness, hatred, depression, and hope'. These are the sorts of honest, nuanced accounts of life around disability which are so lacking in Hollywood movies. Disabled people and parents must be encouraged to express experience, without sanctioning or silencing from medicine or disability studies. We need not shy away from realities of trauma and ambivalence. A common, regrettable picture is of the silence and withdrawal of support which so often follows a congenitally impaired birth being worsened by an empowerment discourse which places a moratorium on expressing emotional difficulty. There is no question that relational distortions based on difficult unconscious resonances with impairment can have profound effects on the emotional development of the congenitally impaired child (Watermeyer, 2002a). This can be recognised without apportioning blame. Instead, it should usher in an empathic discussion of the emotional realities of parents who may hitherto have feared being shamed for their feelings. Harris and Wideman (1988) underscore how important such exploration is:

> To minimise this process, along with its trauma and its transcendent aspects, is to diminish the large and substantial emotional work of which parents of disabled infants are amply capable.
>
> (Harris and Wideman, 1988, p. 120)

What Harris and Wideman (1988) warn against is the split between the social and the psychic which disability studies seems at times prepared to allow. This position risks undermining the usage (and even availability) of psychological services by parents of congenitally impaired infants. Disability studies must set the tone in making space for examining both material and existential levels.

The body, ideology and surgery

As medical science advances, and in many cases becomes increasingly capital-driven, its procedures seem ever more entangled with the bodily dictates of narcissistic culture. Against this backdrop, a range of surgeries to normalise children with congenital differences has arisen. These interventions do not save or prolong life, but are performed for aesthetic reasons, to create bodies which appear more normal, less disabled (Miller, 2006). Such surgeries include limb-lengthening for achondroplasia, gender assignation for intersex conditions and cranio-facial surgeries for cleft lip and palate. Entering this debate more recently are medical procedures which, similarly, do not prolong life, but are argued to reduce physical difficulties with personal care, such as growth attenuation interventions for severely, multiply impaired children.

Because these procedures are not medically essential, questions to do with the cultural intolerance of difference are central in deciding whether to opt for surgery. Quite naturally, many parents hope that achieving a more normal appearance will protect their child from discrimination, and facilitate a more positive development of self. But the shared, unconscious nature of disability-related anxieties means that it is often unclear precisely whose needs are at stake. As we have seen, there is evidence that visible impairment can make the emotional tasks of early parenting harder, presenting disruptions to attachment relationships (A. Freud, 1952; Lussier, 1960, 1980; Burlingham, 1961; Fisman and Wolf, 1991; Wright, 1991; Sinason, 1992; Watermeyer, 2002a; Asch, 2006). Paraphrasing an earlier comment, if society in general finds impairment emotionally evocative and disquieting, there is no reason why parents should be any different. For example, studies focusing on children with cleft lip or palate have found reduced levels of play, touch and smiling interaction with parents (Rogers-Salyer et al., 1987; Walters, 1997 in Asch, 2006, p. 238). Mothers' responses to their infants in these observations seemed troubled, at times limiting early involvement and bonding. In a disturbing 6-year study involving more than 1,200 Israeli families of children with atypical bodies, Weiss (1994) found some form of overt rejection in four fifths of families (Weiss, 1994 in Asch, 2006, p. 238). Interestingly, Adrienne Asch's (Ferguson and Asch, 1989; Asch, 2001; 2006) position on such research seems to shift, giving increased credence in later work to research which finds parental-relational difficulties arising from impairment. In an earlier publication co-authored with Ferguson she rejects such work as a sleight on struggling parents, which also endorses stereotypes such as over-protection, denial and drives to 'fix' impairment (Ferguson and Asch, 1989). Examining relational circumstances around corrective surgery has, I believe, much to teach us about what disability provokes in families, throwing light on the dilemmas highlighted in Asch's work.

Kittay (2006, p. 90) judges operations which lengthen limbs or reshape genitals as typically 'intrusive, painful, time-consuming, emotionally wrenching, minimally helpful in improving the body's functionality … and expensive'. Genital surgeries create 'only a crude simulacrum of normalcy' (Frank, 2006, p. 80), and may in fact impede function (Kittay, 2006, p. 90).

Limb-lengthening surgery to 'normalise' achondroplasic bodies is an especially long-term and severely invasive undertaking. Sanford (2006) tells of her 6-year process of multiple surgeries, beginning at age 11, and leading to her gaining 11 inches in height and a more normatively proportioned body. She also sustained complications including bilateral tears to her tibialis tendons, and as many as 60 scars (ibid.). From the outset the programme caused severe pain, as well as, ironically, periods of mobility impairment. With reference to the latter, she writes:

> After being subconsciously aware of the world's practical preferences for people of average size, I was now acquainted with its intolerance for the nonambulatory.
>
> (Sanford, 2006, p. 34)

Sanford's candid, moving account shows how the intervention subtly devalues her identity, framing her as someone unable to feel whole without a 'normate' body. Her uncertainty about whether the benefits of the procedure outweighed its costs remain. In the case of genital surgery for intersex conditions, decisions are often made by parents and doctors before the child concerned is old enough to be consulted (Frank, 2006). Because these interventions create only cosmetic changes, individuals may find themselves alienated from people with normal genitals, as well as from their own, familiar bodies (ibid.). Considering psychological aspects of limb-lengthening, Sanford (2006) regards it as 'dangerous' for parents to base decisions for surgery on the idea of ameliorating damage to their child's identity. The danger is that the intervention becomes framed as a panacea, drawing the child away from intrinsic identity development, and leaving him or her 'ill-equipped to face the challenges posed both by the procedures and by the rest of her life' (p. 29). Instead, parents should give priority to fostering a strong, grounded and entitled self-identity, irrespective of later decisions on surgery (ibid.). At times professionals may advocate surgery to 'improve' troubled parent–child relationships stemming from appearance (Asch, 2006). In these instances surgery may embody a hurtful concretisation of unconscious feelings of unacceptance in the child, damaging the self-worth it was intended to cultivate (ibid). Trust in being loved and lovable may be threatened by this, within a self already subjected to a world obsessed with surfaces.

A slightly different set of questions is presented by the recent debate over growth attenuation interventions. In 2004 the parents of Ashley, a 6 year old girl with severe, global developmental deficits, asked that she undergo a set of procedures to improve her and her parents' quality of life (Parens, 2009). Ashley could not walk, sit up or use sign language, and doctors expected that her neurological and cognitive functioning would not improve (Asch and Stubblefield, 2010). Ashley's parents very much wanted to carry on caring for her at home, but faced problems regarding how her continued growth would make this ever more physically difficult (ibid.). Medically attenuating (restricting) Ashley's growth would make her easier to lift and move, making it more possible for her to live among her loving family (Parens, 2009). Ashley's growth was attenuated through a combination of high doses of oestrogen, a hysterectomy and the surgical removal of her breast buds (Gunther and Diekema, 2006). The hysterectomy was performed in order to remove the distress which some intellectually impaired women experience due to menstruation, as well as the risk of impregnation by a sexual predator (Parens, 2009).

Gunther and Diekema (2006), in their assessment of the ethics of the decision, emphasise the difficulty of caring for people with conditions such as Ashley's. All bodily needs and functions must be fulfilled by carers, who are usually parents, and these tasks become measurably more difficult with adolescence and adulthood (ibid.). Arresting growth at an early age makes continued care in the home more possible. Recalling arguments to do with assisted suicide from an earlier section, Asch and Stubblefield (2010) question whether and why the 'only options' open to Ashley's parents were growth attenuation or institutionalisation. They point to the fact that non-ambulatory adults with and without intellectual impairments live in community settings, implying that contextual factors to do with adequate service provision must be investigated. A further, highly controversial issue is whether parents' requests for non-medical intervention should be acceded to on the grounds that their child has an intellectual impairment, and thus cannot take part in decision-making (Parens, 2009). Here, too, Asch and Stubblefield (2010) take exception to the utilitarian position (Gunther and Diekema, 2006; Diekema and Fost, 2010), arguing that there is no way to be sure that Ashley remains unaware and unharmed by the procedures. In short, Ashley may be more self-aware than we presume, and experience feelings and implications of the interventions which she is unable to communicate. It is virtually impossible to accurately gauge the intellectual awareness of a non-verbal, severely learning disabled person who is unable to point. Quite correctly, Asch and Stubblefield (2010) note that 'there is a long history of underestimation of cognitive abilities of people appearing to be profoundly cognitively impaired' (p. 47). Parens (2009) accepts this critique, but, as we shall see, then settles on a compromise position which views parents as being best placed to understand implications for their child, and hence to make decisions. For Ashley, it will remain unknown whether her experience of embodiment has been altered.

Earlier I countered the idea that bodily 'distortions', through their reflection in the body ego, will directly impact on ego functioning. Although an intersex condition, for example, may evoke disgust in members of the community or family, the 'embodiedness' experienced by the child is, to him or her, normal; any other bodily shape or function would probably feel unnatural. This is not a denial of difference in subjective embodiment, but an observation that where such difference exists it is – like all embodiment – a social accomplishment. We recall Raphael-Leff's (1994) description of how we 'learn our bodies' through the symbolic communications of others (p. 16). Lussier (1980) was, it seems, taught this by his patient Peter. His conclusion:

> The body one cathects from birth on, as it is and as it is perceived by the child, not the body as it could or should be, is what matters psychologically. Any child is destined to invest, to cathect the body he has, as it is, which will soon become a basic part of who he is and this is the body that the mother has to acknowledge, to incorporate, to fuse with, in order to grant it psychological existence for the child, a safe, secure, existence. Mental health grows on this soil.
>
> (Lussier, 1980, p. 181)

An aversion instinctively felt towards bodily malformations may distract us from the fact that changing a child's body, especially in the early years, will alter that most basic patterning of experience – sensory awareness of the body (Asch, 2006). Besides the bewilderment or fright of unexpected changes, I wonder whether the assault on bodily integrity may bring unconscious fantasies of punishment or sadistic treatment. Lussier (1980) found that the surgical fitting of prosthetic arms was felt by his patient as castration – as a mutilation of the body he had always known. In a world in which normalcy is assumed to be prized by all, these observations are a thought-provoking corrective. Traditional psychoanalytic accounts often associate disability with a fantasy of castration (e.g. Niederland, 1965), which is presumed to emanate from presocial body ego distortions. If castration experiences are present, one may ask whether these result from an impaired body, or an intrusive cultural and medical world of demands for normalisation. At their extreme, narcissistic culture and for-profit medicine may form a menacing combination.

Sanford's (2006) story of decision-making around her limb-lengthening surgery begins with her parents suggesting it at age 10; she said she was 'not interested', seeing no point in changing who she was. Since she did not see her achondroplasia as a disease, it could not be cured – in fact, to 'cure' her would be to 'remove all physical evidence of an enormous piece of my identity' (pp. 34–35). But extended family, teachers and acquaintances – all of normal stature – quickly became enthusiastic, speaking of a 'great opportunity' (p. 30). As we have seen, she later changed her mind. Besides the influence of family and friends, the manner in which surgical possibilities are presented by health professionals is critical (Engel, 1993; Mouradian, 2006). Traditionally charged with the responsibility to cure, physicians may be impressed and animated over new techniques, fostering medical encounters where 'correction' is assumed to be everyone's priority (Morris, 2006). The potential for surgery to undo important parts of self associated with embodiment, or with the experience of being born different to others, may be overlooked (ibid.). Instead, after diagnosis the typical question is not '*should* something be fixed?' but '*when* should it be fixed?' (Aspinall, 2006, p. 15 – my emphasis). Surgeons, as we have seen, are primarily trained in medical procedures, rather than analysis of psychosocial implications (Marsh, 2006). Across a host of disability-related interventions, including surgery, occupational therapy and physiotherapy, prosthetics, psycho- and pharmacotherapy and much else, children are routinely subject to life-shaping decisions made by well-meaning parents and professionals who do not consult them (French, 1994a). The promise of even partial cure seems endlessly seductive.

It is common for individuals to discover only in adulthood that they were born with an intersex condition, and that their genitals were surgically altered. Some accounts describe young lives haunted by an indefinable awareness of difference. Later, perhaps during early sexual experiences, such persons discover their reproductive organs to be different to those of others, and begin, with pain and rage, to piece together how parents 'chose' their shape and gender identity (Frank, 2006). Evident in such choices by parents is the bewilderment of a mix of personal, emotional responses, prejudiced cultural imperatives, the clamour of well-intentioned professional proscriptions, and the simple hope that their child will grow into a happy, well-adjusted person. As already said, such parents need and deserve our empathy, particularly in the form of non-directive psychological care, in order to make some sense of this painful jumble. Abelow Hedley (2006) describes her quandary:

> I am a mother see-sawing between the nagging desire to alleviate some of my daughter's difference, to feel we are doing something – and the strong belief that I have to protect my daughter against those marauding, seductive, and unattainable notions of normalcy.
>
> (Abelow Hedley, 2006, p. 44)

Such dilemmas place parents squarely in the crucible where bodies meet culture; where subjectivity and embodiment feel the deep impressions made by the dictates of culture. It is culture which, in Zizek's (2004) words, has hystericised its authority as statistical norms and 'human nature'. Parents may be torn between feelings of bowing to society's unwillingness to re-own its disavowals, and the struggle of how to gather trust that their child will withstand shaming and discriminatory treatment. Tugging towards 'correction' is the hegemonic cultural view of difference as intolerable; as something we all just want to 'go away'. As already noted, Parens (2009), after much experience and reflection, has come to the 'boring but fundamental ideal of truly informed decision-making' (p. 22). This involvement applies to cognitively able children as well as parents. Noteworthy to him is that children's views are both highly variable and sophisticated in their understanding of using medical procedures for social ends. This level of nuance and reflection shows in a quotation from Isabel, a pre-school age girl deciding whether or not to have surgery to make her face appear more normal:

> I want to [have surgery] because I don't want to look so different that people stare, or think that I have a developmental problem … I still want to look like me and I was afraid that surgery would change who I was … My mom told me it didn't matter if I decided to have the surgery or not. She said what I looked like on the outside could never change the person I am on the inside. That made me feel better … [but the surgery] will make it easier for people to get to know me instead of just looking at my outside.
>
> (Parens, 2009, p. 22)

Parens (2009) describes with admirable honesty how accounts such as this have helped in moving beyond his own splits. On the one hand, the splitting position views those who express affinity for their own, unusual embodiment as in psychological denial. Alternatively, those who opt for surgical correction may be judged as collaborators with oppression, who suffer from 'false consciousness'. Each of these views is an intrusive judgment on unique lives. A crucial point is that a politicised approach which simplistically prohibits using medical means as a response to social problems will harm some of the people it intends to help (ibid.). Asch (2006) urges that all appearance-altering surgery be delayed until children are old enough to participate in decision-making, believing that this models to children that 'character, not outward form, is what ought to count' (p. 237). Where cognitive impairment is not present, applying this principle is simple. In the case of profoundly learning disabled children or adults, Parens (2009) recommends allowing parents to decide, but in the context of a close, unequivocal examination of their reasoning. 'Respecting parents', he writes, 'does not mean thoughtlessly acceding to their wishes', but instead 'asking them hard questions' and 'engaging them in a process of becoming truly informed' (p. 23). Parens' (2009) deeply thoughtful, yet pragmatic position makes an empathic space for parents who are fallible, who have their own histories and life struggles, and are in the midst of crisis. This view resonates closely with my own – that is, one critical of how idealisation is at times mistaken for empathy.

Asch and Stubblefield's (2010) analysis returns repeatedly to the risk that surgical procedures or growth attenuation may be experienced as 'a failure to love and embrace the child with the characteristics and capacities she has' (p. 47). In closing this discussion, Sanford (2006) captures the parent's conundrum:

> ... the lines are so blurry, where cosmetic meets psychosocial meets medical necessity ... she would bloody well get the very message I know we must never send: we love you, you're perfect the way you are ... now change.
>
> (Sanford, 2006, p. 46)

Guilt

The association of disability with guilt – within impaired persons, as well as 'in the air' wherever disability images are found – is familiar across cultures, as well as in psychoanalytic writing. Lane (1992, p. 11) describes how American mothers experience 'inexplicable guilt' on discovering that their infant is deaf. The origins and relational implications of this guilt are complex. Persistent cultural and religious beliefs tell us that disability is punishment for moral laxity (Lane, 1992; Sontag, 1997; Avery, 1999; Barnes and Mercer, 2005b). We explored earlier how unconscious narratives of impairment often contain anxious feelings of loss of control, upsetting omnipotent fantasies of vigour. The flipside of this universal, defended position is the inference that when the body fails it must be because of our own doing (Murphy, 1987). As with any emotional trauma it is often psychologically easier to accept blame for, say, the impairment of a newborn, than to grapple with the fearsome truth that events in the world are random, and we have no control (Turnbull and Summers, 1987; Sontag, 1997). In relation to congenital deafness, Lane (1992, p. 12) muses that self-blame not only restores a sense of 'cosmic' control, but also justifies the ostracisation of deaf persons, by constructing this as somehow their own fault. In this way, the broader population is enabled to deflect guilt over the palpable reality of inequality.

MacKeith (1973) – a psychoanalytic family researcher of the ilk rejected by disability studies – asserts that parental guilt may be based on a combination of feeling responsible for an impaired birth, and defensive reactions to difficult, hostile feelings towards the child. There is some logic here. Mothers in general very often suffer bouts of guilt at not feeling a ready, 'automatic' attachment to their baby. When the baby carries unexpected difference, these normative feelings may easily be amplified. But the predicament is thorny for these mothers. It is, as argued above, culturally and politically even less admissible for mothers of impaired infants to carry ambivalent feelings. These feelings may thus be re-channelled into additional motivations to care, still carrying a flavour of blameworthiness. Having said this, Ferguson's (2001) protestation that any parental behaviours tend to be reframed as signs of pathology remains an essential corrective. Nevertheless, in my view, the assumption that difficult or aversive feelings towards an infant are unnatural or blameworthy is simply wrong. This is an assumption at the core of the denigration of women and the work of motherhood, maintaining a culture of self-recrimination which does not benefit healthy relating. The social inadmissibility of these conflicts actually contributes to the risk of 'acting out' in the form of abuse or neglect (e.g. Friedrich and Boriskin, 1976). Disability studies critics, in their attempt to defend parents against persecution, may instead propagate a collective code of silence. It is not only the more extreme, unconsciously fuelled feelings about an impaired infant which evoke guilt. Many parents may see common-sensically normative responses of shock, grief and disappointment as signs of 'bad parenting', or bad-ness. Where it applies, a social modelist proscription of politically inconvenient feelings can leave parents with nowhere to go. Very resonant here is Shakespeare's (2006) vehement rejection of the 'expressivist' accusation that parents who choose to terminate an impaired foetus are necessarily prejudiced. A subtle awareness of growing up as a disappointment or a 'trouble' to one's parents is familiar in clinical work with disabled people. I feel sure that the absence of a normalising space for parents' conflicts must relate to this. While I wholeheartedly agree with Ferguson (2001) that all parent–child relationships are unique, and in some sense sacred, it is not heresy to say that most adults would not choose the stress, anxiety, emotional pain and physical work which may accompany raising a disabled child.

One way in which unprocessed guilt may, over time, subtly distort relationships is in the arena of psychic boundaries (Watermeyer and Swartz, 2008). In relational networks surrounding impairment feelings of 'survivor guilt' over perceived functional deficits are elemental (Sinason, 1989; 1992). For Sinason (1992) guilt may cause us to avoid recognising difference, due to the painfulness of perceived damage. She provides the example of a residential setting for learning disabled persons, where a care worker's guilt at being non-impaired becomes enacted in an idealising collusion, leading to the unhelpful, even controlling belief that the resident is capable of anything. Some variant of this may be found in parental relationships, complicating the already thorny challenge of separation. As we will see later, the ambivalence of others engendered by guilt may create life-worlds of confused and confusing relational boundaries around the disabled individual. Murphy (1987), from his own experience, remarks as follows:

> Indeed, a mutuality of guilt is the very life-stuff of the paralytic's family, just as it is, on a smaller scale, central to the cohesion – and turmoil – of all modern families.
>
> (Murphy, 1987, p. 92)

Sinason (1992) construes the 'loss' at the root of the guilt of the other as a real representation of lived difference. In other words, she sees the conflict as an inability to confront actual suffering or deficit, rather than a struggle with fantasies about difference. In my view this is a partial regression to the modernist problem of the social model, seeing impairment as an uncontested, presocial reality. Without denying actual difference, I believe that in these interactions fantasy is central, especially around evocative issues such as learning disability. Fantasies about deficit, not deficit itself, are what shape relationships. Recognising this is an important step towards the principle of the self-definition of experience by disabled people. The fact that the observer's imaginings may resemble aspects of the disabled person's actual experience is purely culturally informed coincidence. The profound unconscious mediation of interactions around, say, learning disability, means that ideas about experience are often more influenced by fantasy than by talking and listening. In order to hear the other, fantasies (perhaps guilt-inducing) about what it is like to be impaired in that way must be explored, owned and withdrawn. The identifications (both positive and negative) with impairment which we all carry mean that a pull towards mindlessly deciding what disabled life is like, is virtually irresistible. We need to empty our minds in order to allow our expectations to be surprised, and to learn.

The assumption that 'to be disabled is to suffer' ironically may place pressure on disabled people to display happiness, in order to rescue others from unease. Sinason (1992) relates the words of a mother of a multiply impaired son:

> I try to keep him happy … Because I brought him into the world with all of his difficulties, so if I can't keep him happy what is the point?
>
> (Sinason, 1992, p. 141)

With painful clarity, guilt appears here as an imperative to cheerfulness. In some way this son seems required to protect his parent from guilt, and perhaps aversion, over his impairments. One finding of Drotar et al.'s (1975) problematic, but not valueless study, was that some relationships between mothers and disabled children carried anxieties leading to 'closer than normal' (p. 714) relational bonds. This observation carries a clear pathologising slant; but it would be nonsense to ignore how situational stressors, discrimination and impairment-related anxieties impact in a very real way on healthy separation. To contradict this is, as already argued, to position these relationships outside the broad trawl of family mental health. Relational boundaries, interwoven with dynamics of guilt in familial socialisation, as well as the 'real world' of dependency, must be at centre stage in exploring the shaping of disabled subjectivity.

It appears to me nothing short of natural that family members and others may feel guilty about being able to share in things denied to a disabled companion.

Mingled with this may be guilt arising from hidden resentment at how the disability impacts on them, both practically and emotionally. In clinical work one regularly encounters siblings whose selves are forged on a 'survivor' identity, fostering guilty, self-denying drives towards reparation (Burke, 2008). Correspondingly, a disabled family member may feel guilt over needing assistance, moulding a stilted, grateful role. Or, more apparent may be guilt over not feeling sufficiently appreciative, instead being in touch with resentment over unnecessary exclusion. In the lives of disabled people in modern society, the subjective experience of unfairness is a touchstone. But as we shall see in more detail later, the need to be grateful undercuts the ability to express negative feelings, such as rage, hurt or frustration. This 'protectionism' easily becomes a socialised habit, militating against the development of an articulate, entitled disability movement (Watermeyer and Swartz, 2008; Watermeyer, 2009). In short, be it in the family, the school, the workplace or the community at large, disability is a hothouse for the distortions, silences and manipulations engendered by guilt. Without stereotyping, we must investigate the real ways in which this shared 'disability complex' may confuse, sully or hijack love, kindness and authentic contact.

The late Mairian Corker (1994), in describing the world's response to her deafness, shows how she could not but be shaped by meanings she made of her treatment. Such meanings may take up an unconscious residence, as the very stuff of self. She writes:

> To stand a chance of furthering myself I was told that I had to be prepared to climb the precipice, suffer the cuts and bruises to my sense of humanity in silence and cope with my broken ears. Only then could I attain the prize awaiting me at the top. I dutifully climbed, feeling hollow inside, and was hurt ... I realised that I was being offered the stick without the ice-cream 'for my own good' (Miller, 1987). The precipice became a different kind of symbol. It meant that I became my broken ears and that there was nothing in between. The chasm which had opened up between who I thought I was and who I actually was, was of such enormity that my roots had become shrouded in the mists of the past. I had, in effect, lost myself.
>
> (Corker, 1994, p. xvi)

The tangle of deprivation, guilt, duty, atonement, repression, stoicism and shame described by Corker (1994) is surely not unusual. At the heart of the predicament may be a dim, unconscious suspicion that one is by one's birth a cause of pain, a trouble; the bringer of distress, not joy, energy and hope. These worries are clearly visible in the previous section's accounts of children considering corrective surgery. Silence itself is the danger here. In the midst of silence whatever fantasies pertain are allowed to settle as truth. It is silence, in some form, which is at the heart of Corker's (1994) moving description above. A fantasy that the love and belonging one receives is somehow conditional exists somewhere in all children. The unspoken meanings of disability easily find purchase and unconscious confirmation in such fears. There must be important realities about disabled subjectivity to be uncovered here.

Identity politics and the movement

A pivotal area in which disabled people's constructions of self and other play out is in attempts to mobilise a united group affiliation. Although the disability lobby is relatively visible in some countries, few would disagree that, overall, progress has been disappointing. A comfortable majority of the world's disabled population is either unaware of disability politics, or chooses to have little to do with it. In what is to follow I attempt to connect this difficulty to disabled socialisation, and present some ideas on a possible reconceptualisation of disabled groupness. This leads to a discussion of the unique contribution which the awkward category of 'disabled' has to make to identity politics.

Galvanising a disability movement requires promoting a 'disabled subject' – a reified disabled identity – as the bedrock of its politics. Solidarity entails a degree of 'essentialising'. In a previous chapter we examined the tension between this strategic essentialism and an equally strategic constructionism, which resists oppression through undermining its categories (Garland-Thomson, 1997b). Inevitably these two strategies must, in part, work against one another. Mustering a united front requires the masking of diversity. While this is problematic to some, social model writers point out that constructionist approaches reduce the materiality of disablism to the ephemeral level of thought processes (Priestley, 1998), making a carefully 'essentialist' strategy indispensable (Oliver and Barnes, 2008). This dispute forms the backdrop to the sluggish development of unity under a disabled identity. Many disabled people seem to find themselves between a rock and a hard place on the issue of group identification, creating an ambivalent, splintered community.

Members of marginal minorities such as racial or ethnic groups often share geographical, linguistic, occupational, cultural or religious associations, laying the groundwork for political allegiance (Scotch, 1988). By contrast, the history of disabled people reflects severe social and political isolation, with most growing up in families as the single disabled member. Thus, a majority of those not subject to the even greater, insulating constriction of institutionalisation, will live out entire lives surrounded predominantly by nondisabled persons (ibid.). Notably, this is a predicament shared by sexual minorities (Samuels, 2003). Throughout the world disabled people are over-represented among the poor, minimally educated and unemployed – those whose voices are heard the least in modern society. The common construction of disability as a secluded, profoundly individual experience is, in all likelihood, a lived and unquestioned reality to most. But even those shown the opportunity for political mobilisation often baulk at the idea of self-identifying as disabled. Charlton (1998, p. 78) is unsurprised that oppressed people hesitate to identify with their status, since 'all the signposts in their lives point them away from this kind of consciousness'. Who would choose to advertise the identity which had been the fulcrum of one's shunning by society? For people living with overwhelming social adversity, inviting victimisation through openly identifying themselves may seem crazy. In much of the world the 'disabled community' exists only in the imagination of a handful of activists; there is no history, no identifiable culture, and a constituency which is scattered and hard to reach (ibid., p. 79). Exclusion from education and community concealment are massive obstacles to the development of a 'web of affiliations' (ibid., p. 79), leaving commonalities hidden under differences in impairment.

As researcher and clinician I have commonly experienced disabled individuals taking up critical and distancing positions in relation to others with impairments (Low, 1996). Self-descriptions may be prefaced with the qualifier that one is 'not like other disabled people' who may be 'too dependent' or 'malingering' (ibid.). Lane (1992) observes simply that colonised peoples seek to fit the categories stipulated by their colonisers, undervaluing their own. Feelings of hostility or rage may thereafter become directed at one another rather than the oppressor group (Glover, 2006). Pride – so essential in forging a minority front – is 'no easy thing to come by', as disability has been 'soaked in shame, dressed in silence, rooted in isolation' (Clare, 1991 in Sandahl, 2003, p. 44).

At baseline, the category of 'disabled' is, to say the least, an unstable one (Davis, 2002). Social oppression, writes Susan Wendell (1997), may well be the only thing that disabled people have in common. Whatever the commonality, what is certain is that it will co-exist with extreme diversity, in experiential, political and physiological terms (Vernon and Swain, 2002). Convincingly making the case that a category including such variance actually has intrinsic coherence is all but impossible (Davis, 2002). 'Disability' ostensibly straddles human states from bipolar mood disorder to diabetes, quadriplegia to facial scarring, achondroplasia to chronic fatigue syndrome. The list has hardly begun. Social model writers, consequently, are probably justified in their worry that a too-close examination of personal aspects of disabled lives will show up more divergence than unity. This quandary is at the heart of this book – the contention that the social modelist solution of an homogenising, structuralist analysis may actually work against personal integration, self-knowledge and measured entitlement, through imposing a silence and orthodoxy from within. The need to defend an 'essentialist' disabled category in opposition to an equally constructed nondisabled category carries a welter of contradictions (Tregaskis, 2004; Crowther, 2007). Zola (1989), for example, observes that the universality of ageing creates an ineffaceable link between these two groups (Zola, 1989; Williams, 2001). So, if disabled people are indeed a 'minority group', it is a peculiar minority that putatively includes all of us – if not now, then at some not too distant time (Williams, 2001).

As was alluded to in the previous chapter, Swain and French (2000; 2008) seek to build positive identity through what they term an 'affirmative model' of disability. They describe this as follows:

> It is essentially a non-tragic view of disability and impairment which encompasses positive social identities, both individual and collective, for disabled people grounded in the benefits of lifestyle and life experience of being impaired and disabled.
>
> (Swain and French, 2000, p. 569)

This well-intentioned political 'solution' to the denigration of disabled life involves the fashioning of an alternative, expressly positive image, one which may attract the identification of a hesitant impaired population. The difficulty is that like other forms of disability movement orthodoxy, it seeks to overturn an oppressive binary by colluding with it. The risk of this sort of engineering is that it will replace demeaning imputations with stoic imperatives, leaving disabled people, and society as a whole, no closer to an integration of that part of humanity which the disabled imago holds. Instead, we have a drama of competing stereotypes, possibly tugging already battered individuals still further from internal truths. In their later thoughts on the issue, Swain and French (2008) deal with some of the more vivid simplifications of the approach, but the essential difficulties remain.

Shakespeare (2006) characterises the pitfalls of the social modelist drive to solidarity as follows:

> A strong political identity, which should be a means to an end, has become an end in itself. Rather than looking outward, the disability movement has often turned inwards. Rather than building bridges with other groups or seeking the integration of its members within society, the vanguard of the disability movement has often been separatist, promoting a notion of 'us' disabled people against 'them' non-disabled oppressors. (Holdsworth, 1993; Branfield, 1998; 1999). [We must] … offer an alternative to the prison of identity politics, which leads to the politics of victimhood and the celebration of failure.
>
> (Shakespeare, 2006, pp. 80, 82)

Shakespeare's (2006) criticism is timeous. Significantly, he expressly does not diminish the importance of group solidarity, describing it as an essential 'means to an end'. Accurate, empathic validation of experience is much needed in fostering self-acknowledgment and psychological integration. For me, it is a question of the tone with which solidarity is promoted. A truly inclusive, open and accepting position which builds relationships across identity lines is very different – both externally and psychologically – from one based on in-group idealisation, antagonism and expectations of abuse from the world. No-one, on reading this book, would by now doubt my recognition of the appalling, abusive circumstances suffered globally by a substantial proportion of the disabled community. And from this beginning point, growing new relationships based on trust is hard; it may even appear irrational. But this is the crux of how relations of inequality remain so deeply embedded, and re-enacted. Hard though it is, all must change. Shakespeare's (2006) views on the 'inward-looking' problems of the social model movement are taken up in a rather heated exchange between Crowther (2007) and Oliver and Barnes (2008) in *Disability and Society*. For me, this engagement confirmed the depth of ideological splits at play. On the one hand, writers such as Shakespeare, Crowther and myself urge that the disability movement overcome separatism, build interdisciplinary relationships and focus real energy on forging alliances which facilitate the renewal and modification of services and organisations. The tone of Oliver and Barnes (2008) remains combative. While I fully understand their outrage, I believe that separatist politics based on the apportioning of blame simply cannot lead us to a more caring society.

A compromise between the vanishing uniqueness of the social constructionist self and the depersonalised materialist subject is proposed by Charles Taylor (1989). The self here is continually shaped as we locate ourselves – mainly unconsciously – 'in social narratives', which are typically not 'of our own making' (Somers, 1994, p. 606). This picture of self, embedded in what Taylor (1989, p. 36) calls 'webs of interlocution', is one conceptual way of reintroducing ontology into the materialist subject. Representations of being, rather than an epistemology concerned only with action and materiality, are seen here as elemental. What this creates is space to allow close group affiliations when salient, but a caution against reducing individual lives to groupness. There is no single solution to what is, after all, a problem – or gift – of diversity.

Examining a range of minority political groupings, we see in the work of Nancy Fraser (1995; 2000) that the pitfalls of reified identities and separatism are not unique to the disability lobby. The picture she paints is a melee of othering and counter-othering. To Margaret Somers, the new categories spawned by minority interest 'create a new shade of universalism that contains its own inevitable exclusions' (Somers, 1994, p. 613). The drive to reify identity may, to Fraser (2000, p. 108), create a state of affairs in which the 'politics of recognition' actually displaces the 'politics of redistribution'. In my own words, this signals the prizing of a 'deserving', 'oppressed' minority identity over the principles which define a society which cares for all. Social model activism certainly sets out to prioritise material redistribution. But from there, according to Shakespeare (2006, p. 80), it may morph into 'an end in itself'. In response to the dilemma described by Fraser (2000), some have chosen to abdicate from identity politics altogether, seeing only a perpetual tussle for exclusive legitimacy (ibid.).

Fraser (2000) does not recommend that we abandon identity politics wholesale, nor does she believe that 'recognition struggle' is always destructive. Some strategies are less dangerous, and address injustices not amenable to redistributive remedies alone (Fraser, 1995). In fact, if carefully managed, action for recognition can 'promote interaction and cooperation across gulfs of difference' (Fraser, 2000, p. 109). There is an important message for the disability movement here. The at times strident reifying of disabled and nondisabled groupness is both a cause and an effect of the resistance to integrating the psychological layer of disability experience. A politics based on what we all share reduces, rather than aggravates, the political and subjective sense of danger provoked by internal, human struggle. Disability struggle is human struggle, no more, no less. Disabled people are, as we have seen, simply subject to a more direct experience of the universal strains of shame, guilt and abjection that dwell in the human condition. In Fraser's (2000) view, what is required is an account of recognition which is sufficiently flexible and courageous to accommodate complex identities, rather than enforcing narrow in-group values (see also Bickenbach, 2001).

Tracing the human experience of disablism and impairment, while continuing to interrogate the structures of inequality, re-presents disabled lives as not only normal, but well placed to throw light on areas of humanness concealed by modernity. Developing personal insight into social struggle will uncover in-group differences, but also universal commonalities. This does not mean scuppering identity politics. It is more a business of augmenting and finessing its simplifications, allowing voices less disrupted by ambivalence or orthodoxy. In Fraser's (1995, p. 69) words, we must 'conceptualise cultural recognition and social equality in forms that support rather than undermine one another'. Hughes (2009) remains nervous about a philosophical position on disability which applies a 'universalist ontology' – that is, the idea that frailty is not an exception to the human condition, but what defines it. His concern is that the real-life, material struggles of disabled people will fade into the background, subsumed under a mistaken idea that, in fact, all people are oppressed, disadvantaged and mortal. His position is understandably pragmatic, but assumes that the cause of material inequality cannot be furthered within a more inclusive identity environment. As a South African, I am struck by the commonality in predicaments of a range of marginal groupings in our country, connecting the disability movement with the HIV/AIDS lobby, the so-called landless people's movement, the lesbian, gay, bisexual and transgendered community and many others. All have similar ideals, and much to gain through overcoming a legacy of segregated interest. We have not begun to tap this potential.

Drawing on Hegel, Axel Honneth (1995, p. 14) envisions a post-identity politics society, in which ethics and solidarity are not sought in the clamouring of competing minorities, but in the principle of the freedom of all. This society will embark from a 'framework of ethical bonds' rather than the 'acts of isolated subjects' (ibid.). Honneth (1995) paints the vision as follows:

> As he [Hegel] puts it, the 'existence of difference' is what allows ethical life to move beyond its natural initial state and, in a series of rectifications of destroyed equilibria, ultimately leads to a unity of the universal and the particular … For only if the world-historical course of the 'budding of ethical life' can be conceived of as an interpenetration of socialisation and individuation can one assume that the organic coherence of the resulting form of society lies in the intersubjective recognition of the particularity of all individuals.
>
> (Honneth, 1995, p. 15)

The language of psychoanalysis is a place to begin theorising this 'interpenetration', tracing links between ideology, socialisation and subjectivity. The 'healthy' political recognition advocated by Fraser (2000, p. 113) is, analogously, one based not on 'group-specific identity', but on the status of individual members of all groups as 'full partners in social interaction'.

Contrary to those intent on building positive, distinctive identities, Davis (2001; 2002) proposes that the disability lobby embraces its nature as a porous and contingent category. The threat to the 'minority identity community' posed by disability's woolliness is, for Davis, one reason why other lobby groups have at times given disability a wide berth. Disability, it seems, risks spoiling the contrived neatness of categories of victim and oppressor, revealing the built-in self-destructiveness of identity politics (Davis, 2001). Disability is perfectly placed to drive a critique of identity studies, showing up the dream of inclusiveness for massing minority interests as a forlorn one. The list of these interests will always grow longer, leading to the meaninglessness of particular identities (ibid.). As 'alterity' becomes subsumed under 'identity', the latter becomes increasingly meaningless, eventually 'so broad a category that it cannot contain identity' (ibid., p. 537). As identity politics comes increasingly to explain everything, it will ultimately explain nothing. Besides this is the problem of its typical aspirations, expressed as 'equity' in access to the entitlements of an illusory modernist Utopia.

Fascinating to me is the fact that group identity remains the single area not assailed by postmodern deconstruction (Davis, 2002). No-one has dared to attack the sanctity of one's existence as, say, black, lesbian or female (ibid.). Now enter disability, the identity which – par excellence – invites just such critique; the sort that threatens the orthodoxy at the heart of separatism. Through its disruptions, disability may ultimately unite all other identities, replacing postmodernism with what Davis (2002, p. 14) calls *dysmodernism*. The instability of the disability category is capitalised on, coming into view as a subset of the instability of identity as a whole, and ushering in the 'dysmodern' era (ibid., p 25). Here is an identity able to baffle convention by holding out a hand to humanity, saying 'all are welcome', or, perhaps more correctly, 'all are already here'.

There is an intriguing synergy between Davis' critique of identity and the Lacanian picture of identity as an escape from internal fragmentation (Lacan, 1977). Lacan's model of the manic optimism with which we suture our fragmented inner parts seems analogous to the proliferation of identity politics, which is equally fearful of what the recognition of commonality may hold. The drive to identify what we are inevitably involves dissociating from what we are not. If we are, indeed, the same, then what inheres in our 'sameness'? For Lacan, of course, it is all that is unthinkable. But in our political world one cause for careful optimism is that recognising common human fallibility brings with it a natural humility.

Of course, I am not naïve enough to believe that modernist narcissism will not remain, but a key question for those concerned with social change is where, strategically, to place our philosophical investments. Real inclusivity can only be based on commonality.

Note

1 The super-ego, in Freudian theory, is a psychological structure which enforces rules and morals on the ego – an idea similar to the *conscience*. Depending on formative relationships, the super-ego may be rigid and hyper-critical of the self, or less prominent in emotional functioning.

2 Achondroplasia is a disorder which limits bone growth, resulting in short stature. It is the most common of congenital conditions sometimes referred to as dwarfism.

6 Oppression, psychology and change

Initial conceptual reflections

Introduction

In this chapter we begin by assessing recent attempts to integrate personal and psychological aspects of disablism into social model disability studies. It should be clear that, for me, the limitations of the social model for theorising disablist socialisation and subjectivity rule it out as an exclusive way forward. But as we try to develop new theoretical nets for interpreting the disability world, it is sensible to begin with what the social model view has provided in this area over the last decade. This is the work of theorists who believe that an integrative approach can be achieved, while holding onto the essence of social model politics. From here we move to an exploration of the under-theorised idea of *internalised oppression*, drawing on psychoanalytic views of racism. This discussion leads logically to the issue of *mirroring*, which is at the centre of this book's model of how inequality is maintained through disablist socialisation. The final two sections of the chapter present beginning points for our thinking on how internal change may happen. First, perspectives from development studies are explored, including group-based strategies of conscientisation. Subsequently, I discuss the ideologically charged relationship between disability and mental health care. Over time, all of these issues must be interwoven as part of a new, integrated model of the psychological nature of life with disablism.

Psycho-emotional aspects of disability

The idea that disability and disablism always have a personal, internal and emotional narrative is a self-evident truth. Consider Gill's (2001) words on the prominence of psychological struggle in disablist oppression:

> One does not venture far into an exploration of the disability experience before noticing that isolation, invisibility, tension, and struggle are recurring topics whenever and however disabled persons are asked about their lives.
>
> (Gill, 2001, p. 351)

I have already argued that by neglecting these realities the social model tacitly endorses concealment of emotional and physical pain, shame and other aspects of struggle not easily reducible to 'disabling barriers'. This silence has a painful and ironic resonance with the veiling of subjective life characteristic to the social struggle of impaired people. Wendell (1997) describes this 'social silence' as follows:

> Coming into the public world with illness, pain or a de-valued body, we encounter resistance to mixing the two worlds; the split is vividly revealed. Much of our experience goes underground, because there is no socially acceptable way of expressing it and having our physical and psychological experience acknowledged and shared.
>
> (Wendell, 1997, pp. 266–67)

Beneath the materiality of 'barriers' are the internal layers of disablism, which I term *emotional oppression.* Material stifling of the voice of disabled subjectivity in the 'real' world brings a corresponding smothering of parts of self on the internal plane. As we shall see, the socialisation of disabled people is full of demands by an apprehensive, unready world to silence experience. If we are to conceptualise embodied, impaired subjectivity in a disablist world, a key question is how this ideology of silence, through socialisation, shapes selfhood. A psychological framework of contextual and embodied disablement is essential if we are to approach disablism not as a set of simple, structural entities operating on 'dumb', homogeneous persons, but as dynamic processes in which selves undergo formation, interpellation,[1] resistance and much else.

Some writers in the social model tradition have attempted to integrate the psychological nature of disability into their framework. Most notable of these is Carol Thomas (Thomas, 1999a; 2002), who includes her construct of 'psycho-emotional aspects of disablism' in an 'extended' social model view (Thomas, 1999a, p. 46). She defines this *psycho-emotional* layer as follows:

> ... other dimensions of socially imposed restrictions ... those which operate to shape personal identity, subjectivity, or the landscapes of our interior worlds and work along psychological and emotional pathways ... not only a concern for 'what we do' and 'how we act' (are prevented from doing and acting) as disabled people, but also a concern for 'who we are' (are prevented from being), and how we feel and think about ourselves.
>
> (Thomas, 1999a, p. 46)

Quite correctly, Thomas (1999a, p. 48; 1999b) warns us against seeing personal struggle as a consequence of impairment, or as 'private troubles' without political relevance. She provides two examples of these aspects of oppression: first, spending most of one's time at home due to feeling ashamed of a facial disfigurement; and second, not disclosing one's epilepsy to a girlfriend or boyfriend for fear of rejection (Thomas, 1999a, p. 48). As discussed earlier, Thomas (1999a, p. 48) views such struggles as 'mixed in' with *impairment effects,* which may, too, carry psycho-emotional implications. These aspects combine in her 'social relational definition of disability' (Thomas, 1999a, p. 156), incorporating something of the intersubjective, emotional forces operating on disabled individuals, while still holding firm to the structuralist core of the social model. Following Thomas, Reeve (2002; 2006) operationalises these developments in studies focusing explicitly on psycho-emotional phenomena. She embarks from a Foucauldian position, interested in the 'gaze' and 'surveillance' which disabled people suffer, presumably from both inside and out. In my view, though, both Thomas and Reeve are hamstrung by a dissociation from psychological concepts (see also Veck, 2002) – not surprising, considering the Foucauldian approach. Psychological constructs are hardly seen in this work. It is not clear whether this is a result of disciplinary boundaries, or the belief that psychological ideas are too contaminated with 'individualism' to be of use. Thomas' (1999a, p. 74) deep mistrust of 'psychologists and others' mentioned in Chapter 2 returns to mind. In both sets of work, and despite Thomas' (1999a) admirable efforts, attachment to the disability–impairment binary means there is no suitable home for psychological phenomena.

Barnes et al. (2002a, p. 10), from the social modelist 'centre', describe Thomas' (1999a) contribution in approving tones, referring to 'practices that undermine the psychological and emotional well-being of people with impairments'. What is interesting about this description is how it locates the subject of study as external to the individual – as something which 'comes in from outside'. No-one would deny that oppression is, at least initially, just that. But what also needs conceptual attention is the impressions left by these forces – what happens on the *inside.* This means theorising psychological personhood in the face of disablism, examining subjectivity in a manner which addresses the internalisation of a distorted and distorting social world.

Analyses such as those of Reeve (2002) and Veck (2002) provide a conceptual structure which leads us to the individual, but then stops short. Such analyses frame the internal worlds of disabled people as homogeneous, with no personal life-narrative, no conscious and unconscious meaning-making and no temporal change – in short, as faceless passives trapped in discourse. There are no tools to help us become privy to who dwells in the face of disablism, and what his or her world view may be. Consequently, these accounts present as somewhat blandly ideological and lopsided, without descriptions of function *within* the individual able to hold up the argument. The watchfulness about pathologising is understood, but the outcome feels inherently partial and unsatisfactory. Goodley and Lawthom's (2006) contribution, though showing important initiative in the area, carries similar difficulties.

In Veck's (2002) work, the author's stated aim is 'connecting relational and psychological processes of exclusion'. The paper introduces us to the experience of a visibly physically disabled mature student, Ray. But again, it is difficult to find explanations which may be termed 'psychological'. At issue is Ray's behaviour, which is described by university staff as 'difficult'. Veck advises the need to understand psychological responses, but seems unwilling to think in a psychological way. I wonder whether the crux of this reluctance is a fear that Ray may, if scrutinised, indeed appear to the reader – the world – as a difficult person. More provocatively, it may come into view that interpersonal conflicts are not easily reducible to prejudiced responses in that moment, but also involve relational dynamics of which, through socialisation, he has become a part. If anyone remains surprised that lives of exclusion, denigration and distorted relationships shape personalities, at times in maladjusted ways, I find it difficult to understand why. Is it not in the nature of personality, of trauma, of complicity that the sequelae of social abuse are to be found? We need to get to grips with Ray's 'difficultness', trusting that a layered internal exploration will reveal the sense in his behaviour, including unconscious communications, self-destructive enactments, harmful introjects and the like. I have no doubt that we will find a painful wealth of material in the ways Ray has, over a lifetime, been responded to by the world. The key is that the psychological phenomena that we see are at every stage explicitly connected to aspects of the social world – to socialisation, identity, discrimination and distortions in relationship. The politically correct representation of the disabled community as a homogeneous group of hapless, well-intentioned people carries, for me, disquieting resonances of paternalistic, idealising racial stereotypes. Examining complex subjectivities means getting to the heart of oppressive social forces, be they structural, symbolic or interpersonal. We need psychological conceptualisation which is linked to disablist ideology, as disseminated through a host of channels – from the family to the school to the society at large.

Paradoxically, the great strength of the psychoanalytic approach is its recognition of uncertainty. The story of disability theory is, for me, one of attempts at reducing immense human complexity to politically expedient grand narratives, with some helpful outcomes, and a host of limitations. A political voice is potent and influential when it appears to 'know' some ultimate social truth. But if our work is theorising social reality for the purpose of understanding, rather than strategy – as I believe it is – we find not only nuance, but also paradox and inconsistency. Hoggett (1992), in his psychoanalytic model of social engagement, argues that authentic relating to the world and the self is only possible if we are willing to acknowledge limitations and disappointments, and, most importantly, that which we do not know. With this permission, we move to a discussion of three topics relevant to the engagement between psychology and disability studies, beginning with the notion of internalised oppression.

Internalised oppression

> For what is being suggested is that the real persuasive power of the social environment, its most enticing hold over our lives, resides not in what it explicitly says to us, but in the way it enters unbidden and unnoticed into the foundation stones of our psychic structure.
>
> (Frosh, 1991, p. 2)

Stephen Frosh (1991) positions unconscious internalisations at centre stage in channeling how we choose to live our lives. Ideology composes the refractory code through which we perceive self and other, producing a world in which oppressive distortions present as unremarkable normality. Interestingly, Frosh's position finds support from voices within the disability movement. In his international study, Coleridge (1993) made the startling finding that a majority of influential disability activists saw social change as contingent on some form of internal emancipatory transformation. This finding is refreshing in the context of the influence of materialism, and a telling recognition of the hold of disablist prejudices on the global disabled community. The notion of internalised oppression first emerged in race theory, and – while regularly quoted – has received little real attention from disability studies.

The simple, definitive research question is: what is internalised by disabled people who suffer internalised oppression? The words of slain anti-apartheid activist and black consciousness writer Steve Biko (1978) are one place to begin. Interestingly, his understanding resonates closely with the words of Coleridge's (1993) respondents. He writes:

> At the heart of this kind of thinking is the realisation by blacks that the most potent weapon in the hands of the oppressor is the mind of the oppressed. If one is free at heart, no man-made chains can bind one to servitude, but if one's mind is so manipulated and controlled by the oppressor as to make the oppressed believe that he is a liability to the white man, then there will be nothing the oppressed can do to scare his powerful masters.
>
> (Biko, 1978, p. 92)

Clinical experience is, to me, replete with evidence of disabled people who consciously or unconsciously experience themselves as a liability to others. At work is a process in which denigrating social signals persist, re-awakening painful aspects of the life story. What this may create is a pattern of mutual, malignant confirmations between external and internal. The simple reality of being dependent on others for material access, against the backdrop of barrier-ridden societies, continually appeals to human worries about being burdensome or, in the words of French (1993b, p. 69), 'spoiling other people's fun'.

Fanon (1963, p. 203) characterised the colonial invasion of black minds by the worm of self-hatred as something which forced its victims to continually ask themselves the question 'In reality, who am I?' The creeping uncertainty described here regarding what is and is not me is evidence of projective identification, and familiar in the disability world. Consider, for example, the complex ambivalences of disabled group identification discussed earlier. To escape this, Fanon argued that political and inner liberation must go hand in hand – black people must wage war on personal and social levels, aware that these arenas are *in no way interdependent* (Fanon, 1952; Davids, 1996).

The central tenets of Fanon's (1952) argument are the following: through life under colonialism, black people internalise the black–white political relationship; it becomes part of the psychological world. But unconsciously black individuals identify strongly with whiteness, as overwhelming cultural signalling associates this with value. The 'black self' is thus rendered an unwanted outsider (Davids, 1996). Fanon (1952) expresses this bitter truth as follows:

> However painful it may be for me to accept this conclusion, I am obliged to state it: For the black man [sic.] there is only one destiny. And it is white.
>
> (Fanon, 1952, p. 12)

Disabled people are forged in a sea of messaging which continually values the whole, well, perfectly proportioned and functional body, to the shaming denigration of all else. No matter one's style of response, this de-legitimation tugs all towards the only method of partial salvation – a closer approximation of the shape and ways of the nondisabled. The incipient disabled self may grow in a world bathed in exclusion – an experience of being 'shut out', and wordlessly required to qualify to be 'let in'. From comic strip heroes to television personalities, sporting stars to film and fashion icons, virtually all figures of identification come with 'nondisabled-ness' as part of the package. What this may create, borrowing further from Fanon (1952), is a culturally internalised unconscious ideal which is not the embodied, disabled self, but a nondisabled 'prior' or 'truer' self (Kumari-Campbell, 2008). Pivotal here is the lack of validating experiences which mirror the embodied and existential self, opening the internal world and dislodging self-blame. Instead, all that is 'good', all that is aspired to in the labile process of self-formation – a game, a school, a social group, a sports team, a bodily ideal – exists at the opposite end of a closely guarded binary. In racism, these splits may be rigidified if colonised peoples are allowed some limited participation in the 'white world' (Davids, 1996). Black people who remain fully excluded are then denigrated as the bearers of 'real' inferiority in an intra-group fracture, where self-hatred is enacted as hatred of others. The reluctant identification and often painful in-group denigration we see in a proportion of the disabled community are called to mind here. Similar is the phenomenon of feeling complimented when others forget that one is impaired.

Deborah Marks (1999a) believes that developing the concept of internalised oppression will be a crucial part of understanding the relationship between discrimination and the psychological struggles of disability. Internalised devaluing of self, involving identification with a nondisabled ideal, can cause unconscious collusion with unequal relationships which allow material injustices to go unnoticed. It is not only hidden feelings about self and other which need conscious processing, but more importantly the life-traumas with which these originally became cemented. Traumatic assaults on identity which remain unconscious and unprocessed will tend to be repeated in self-sabotaging enactments.

Let us pause to imagine the distortions in relationship which may be present in the formative years of a congenitally disabled life: from the guilty or anxious emotional currents of families in distress to the controls and exclusions of rehabilitation; from the denigration of schoolmates to the pathologising imputations of well-meaning adults; from the perplexing exile of special schooling to the confusion of an unspoken, shared shame; from the anxiety of parents regarding one's finding a mate to the sinister institutional discourse of 'realistic expectations'. Again, our examination of disablist socialisation will not want for material. In this world, the splitting provoked by disability is everywhere, making it difficult to escape complicity. Finding buried contradictions in one's self-image is always an intricate and thorny business, but here ideological currents tugging one away from self are especially powerful.

Zola (1994, p. 85), with beautiful clarity, writes that oppression involves not only the loss of voice, but also of '*the tools to find it*' (my emphasis). Demonstrating this, Micheline Mason (1990) relates how she came to understand the impressions made on her sense of self by a discriminating world. She writes:

> A message clearly and firmly slipped into my unconscious saying that people would prefer it if I died … I am now 30 years old. Only now am I beginning to realise that I do not have to smile all the time, and that I can achieve mediocrity without feeling someone will come along and 'put me out of my misery'.
>
> (Rieser and Mason, 1990 in Sinason, 1992, p. 143)

An honest look at the aversive social worlds in which some disabled people grow up raises questions about the psychological defences needed for survival. Emotional trauma, and the harmful relationships which can cause it, tend to be repeated if we are not provided with the care needed to deal consciously with pain. For disabled people the repetition of hurtful prior relationships may take the form of dependency and compliance, self-pity or self-hatred, hostility and entitlement, colluding with social denialism, persistent blaming of the self or the world and much else. Trying to make sense of such feelings and behaviours need not reduce these to 'symptoms'. Our first port of call must be to see behaviour as coherent, communicative reactions to relationships and contexts. Further, the psychoanalytic principle of behaviour being *multiply* determined means that each response has both a conscious and unconscious meaning. So it is, recalling Chapter 3, that personal and political actions are always interwoven, but both remain legitimate. Limiting our understanding of disability to either will impoverish our ability to see and validate disabled lives.

Drawing on Marx, Charlton (1998) describes the internalisation of oppression as a twofold process. First, is 'hegemony', which is defined as the dominant class' instilling of its values in the broad population through methods such as 'double-speak', 'misdirection' (or victim-blaming), 'naturalised inferiority' and 'legitimated authority' (pp. 35–36). Second is the inflicting of psychological suffering, creating a stagnation of self-pity or self-annihilation, which makes awareness of oneself, one's peers and one's situation much more difficult. This is 'alienation' (ibid.). From my own point of view, it is this constriction of self-awareness, based in the rigid defences required to survive hurtful treatment, which is a fulcrum of the subordination of disabled people. The materialist view allows for one important sort of solidarity – that of the public, political domain – but tends to discourage a form which promotes candid self-exploration and communication, maintaining an estrangement from self.

In step with society's medicalising view, disabled people may unconsciously learn to project internal struggle into 'defective' parts of the body, or the imperfect body as a whole. To medical model logic it is the misshapen limbs, poorly functioning eyes, inarticulate speech centres, inert muscles and so on, which cause struggle and make an equitable life impossible. Biomedicine also trains us in dissection of the body into discrete Cartesian functional elements, clearly marking out those which are a nuisance to normalcy. Cultural messaging dovetails perfectly, confirming that 'of course', no-one would want a body with this 'broken' component. By consequence, 'damaged' body parts may increasingly become dissociated from the self, functioning as hold-all explanatory containers for conflicts of all sorts (Kumari-Campbell, 2008). Clinical experience shows family systems where significant impairments are never spoken of, as well as situations in which even a very minor impairment is constructed as the 'reason' for chronic, shared difficulties. The disidentification with one's body at work here shows a recruitment into cultural splitting, which must involve some rejection of self. Self-descriptions of being 'nondisabled inside' bear testament to the struggle of occupying a body which society, and from there the self, has come to hate. Michalko (2002) reflects on how he grew up experiencing his blindness not as a part of himself, but as a disruption of his true being (see also Wilson, 2003). Pervasive, inescapable images of disability as a difference to be prevented rather than lived in pull very hard against subjective wholeness. Of course, many other congenitally impaired people will grow into a clear, robust identification with their bodies, even in the face of social rejection, attempts at 'fixing' and the like (Parens, 2009).

Ussher (1989) presents a similar picture of gender ideology creating internal splits in growing women. The adolescent girl separates self from body, the pregnant woman splits sexuality from motherhood and archetypes of motherhood and menopausal redundancy may disparage the free expression of self. In both gender and disability, harsh dictates which derail individuation are all around us. Disabled people must somehow occupy a world of irreconcilable dissonance between ideals and experience. In lives of mistreatment, the resulting internalised persecutory objects are projected into the body, the self or the world, recreating oppressive relations. In the last case, the simple principle is that people who have undergone abuse, quite sensibly, expect more. This idea of projecting persecution onto the world is not a denial of social oppression. Instead, what is important is the internal sedimenting of relationships, laying a weighty, unconscious inertia on change. If different relationships are, at a deep level, not imaginable, there is little prospect of bringing these into being.

In the case of race, projecting feelings of shame into one's own black skin is not an efficient defence (Davids, 1996). Successful projection disowns the 'dirt' into another. The nondisabled cultural consensus, then, projects its disavowed parts into the disabled community, who may then re-project this material – now subjectively owned – into their own 'flawed' bodies. As with racism, there is no reciprocity in this picture. Disabled people are asked to 'swallow' the emotional jetsam of the dominant, redouble efforts at approximating their ideal and perhaps re-project shame and defect into those deemed 'more disabled'. The difficult choice for people interpolated into this harsh system is to either employ such frantic splits and deflections, or live with the pain of a deep wound to identity.

Mirroring

Winnicott (1974) traces our experience of self back to the gaze shared between mother and infant. It is in the mother's facial expression and responsivity that the baby begins to see, and feel, whom she or he is. For Winnicott, how the mother appears to the baby is a function of what she is seeing; the *good enough* mother validates the infant with her gaze, shoring up aliveness, integration and worth (Erskine, 1994). But if the mother's face shows distraction or distress the baby has a premature experience of the needs of the other, impinging on growing selfhood. In this interaction, affirmation begins to be replaced with self-consciousness (ibid.). The seeds of the shame of objectification are in that non-loving look, creating a template of being 'looked *at*' rather than 'looked *after*' (Erskine, 1994, p. 50, my emphasis; Wright, 1991). If this disjuncture is significant, the baby may unconsciously join forces with the mother's unspoken feelings, rejecting his or her growing self, which may become experienced as an unwanted, intruding other. The infant has assumed what Winnicott (1960) terms the *false self*, presenting to the mother an unreal pastiche of responses aimed at winning positive regard, while becoming alienated from the spontaneous expression of self.

To the infant the mother really is the world, creating both a template and a metaphor for later relating. And as with all psychological functioning, defences rooted in formative, perhaps difficult experiences lead to repetition. So it is that the dynamics outlined above generalise to adulthood, and to the collage of experiences of mirroring which shape and reshape who we are, and what we feel our place in the social world to be (Honneth, 1995). Moreover, Winnicott (1960; 1974) does not suggest discrete categories – all have aspects of selfhood which have been enlivened by acceptance and love, and other parts shrouded by rejection. In false self functioning the major portion of what is shown to the world is disconnected from authentic being. But all, by virtue of an imperfectly attuned world, carry some experience of the self being unworthy and unwanted.

Now, whatever pre-existing experiences of rejection may exist in disabled lives, these may be continually confirmed and re-aggravated by ongoing disablist social mirroring. The seeds of doubt regarding self-worth and entitlement are enlivened by a world which carelessly, unseeingly excludes and demeans. On top of material deprivation, thus, come personal meanings. These may recapitulate the hurtful messages of formative relationships, be these in medical, educational or institutional settings, or in the home and the community. It is not hard to see how the false self persona is evoked by lives of disentitlement, shaping disabled people as accommodating, silently smiling and self-deprecating. The constant confirming of one's most insecure parts batters the clear thought and self-regard so necessary for self--advocacy. All this may exist on top of the very real possibility of a complex early life, involving fear or distress in parents which calls the child to a premature appeasing role (Lussier, 1980; Watermeyer, 2002a). In Lussier's (1980, p. 182) words, 'one starts by loving oneself according to the love one has received in the pre-ego phase of life'; and, in parallel, one relates to one's body according to how it was responded to by influential figures (Raphael-Leff, 1994). The extent to which we are able to express the *true self* correlates to creativity – our ability to impress ourselves upon the world. Conversely, false self functioning understands the world as something to be 'fitted in' with (Hoggett, 1992, p. 10). In this picture, creativity is stifled, passivity fostered and injuries to identity re-infected by the projections and controls of the normate world.

Returning for a moment to Lacan (1977), we recall his view that the coherent identity we hold consciously is a flimsy, cosmetic deception, disguising the fragmentation below. Since coherent selfhood is an illusion, what we see in disablist mirroring is how impaired people are, through ideology, more exposed to the universal reality of the fragmented ego than others. In this sense the 'disabled identity', rather than being inferior, is in some way more human than the imperatives of modernity allow in mainstream life. According to Kernberg, what lies beneath the facade of the narcissistic personality is rage of the most paranoid-schizoid nature (Kernberg, 1970 in Frosh, 1991). This hidden, dissolving self may be what the mirror of the disabled body alerts the grandiose self to. Disabled people – harbingers of what lurks 'at the edge of the mirror' – may both evoke and serve as projective targets for the inner human truth of a vicious, vengeful human self.

As noted earlier, the fact that most disabled people live out their formative years and beyond surrounded only by nondisabled people must have strong implications for entitled selfhood (Wendell, 1996; Gill, 2001; Michalko, 2002). Living as a minority of one reduces the possibility of challenging prejudices, values, expectations and vocabulary (Ramlow, 2003) which carry meanings about impairment. The threats of isolation and typecasting are very real, as the spontaneous, creative and authentic self becomes weighed down by layers of internalised devaluing. Preece (1995) found a clear distinction between individuals impaired from birth or early childhood and those sustaining impairment later. The former showed less confidence, with special schooling being associated with lower levels of assertiveness and independent thought.

Michalko (2002) and Corker (1994) provide narratives of early life as, respectively, blind and deaf children, which have much in common. Both describe lives saturated with reminders of their status as 'unfortunates'; of being on the wrong side of a raft of social dichotomies. Corker (1994) tells of how she found refuge from hurtful imputations about her deafness in fantasy. She writes:

> I subsequently retreated into and gained solace from a fantasy world peopled by characters who were more companionable than those who occupied the real world. In this world, it did not matter what I lacked, because that could always be imagined and allowed to assume its proper place in the identity that was attempting to shape itself in spite of the wiles of the adult majority … I can remember feeling really confused, even angered by the dichotomy between the messages of the verbal and the more subtle communication of bodily language and facial expression, by the depth of a glance that could warm or freeze.
>
> (Corker, 1994, p. xv)

Corker describes how subtle, denigrating mirroring often occurs without awareness, and may be invisible to onlookers (ibid.). Deaf people growing up in this milieu may, with no alternative point of reference, *become* the hearing person's behaviour towards them – the essence of projective identification. In such circumstances, it is entirely understandable to unconsciously position all hearing persons as similarly prejudiced.

Research into communication patterns between nondisabled and disabled individuals reveals interactions which are abbreviated, and include: less eye contact, but more staring; less smiling, but more signs of anxiety; less information seeking, but more distancing speech patterns (Fox and Giles, 1996). Further, Emry and Wiseman (1987) found that nondisabled persons' expectations of disabled people included social introversion, emotional instability, depression and hypersensitivity – expectations reflected overtly or otherwise in patterns of mirroring. These responses are reminiscent of Winnicott's description of an anxious, distracted or depressed parent, reinforcing parts of the self where certainty and trust are scant and self-criticism is always nearby. The institutional discourses of tragedy, medicalisation and otherness in which disabled children are so often immersed, writes Priestley (1999, p. 92), are in turn 'reproduced through daily encounters with other children, with adults and with a variety of institutional contexts' (see also Todd, 2006). With moving clarity, Mutua (2001) describes the silent mirroring experienced by a physically impaired person in an inaccessible built environment. The account is of an unrelenting, wordless negation of one's experience, even existence. As the world goes about its business, inanimate structures whisper 'Why are you here?' Absence in the mirrored image of the world signifies omission of one's experience from what is assumed as commonly human.

One often unnamed (and to some unspeakable) area of denigrating mirroring is the 'discrimination of love' (Rossiter, 2001, p. 97). The body ideal, along with unconsciously driven aversions, may leave visibly impaired people framed as asexual and beyond consideration as potential love interests (ibid.; Shakespeare et al., 1996). Denying the culturally condensed prejudice at work, the mental pain of such rejection tends to settle on the individual, as a natural outcome of 'deformity'. We end this discussion with the words of a severely physically impaired man, which show up how cultural oppression and individual psychological narratives tend to be superimposed:

> My mother was also fearful that I might get hurt in pursuing romantic relationships. She was so fearful that she told me 'don't even think about women' … I was so angry inside I sort of forgot the girl's rejection and focused on my own mother's rejection.
>
> (Rossiter, 2001, p. 98)

Disability, psychology and development

Despite the broad influence of the social model, most international disability development policies reflect an individualistic welfare approach, with very little evidence of a human rights agenda (Albert, 2005). It remains to be seen whether the recent advent of the UN Convention on the Rights of Persons with Disabilities (2006) will alter this significantly. The problem of what, exactly, development *is* for disabled people rests on the question of 'needs', and who these are defined by. One basic principle is that any programme must involve disabled people centrally in design as well as implementation (Coleridge, 1993). 'Welfarism' is anachronistic, but the priorities of the social model are also lacking, in disregarding personal aspects of empowerment and growth. Quoting Lyotard, Fraser and Nicholson (1990) welcome the postmodern condition in development studies as an era in which we are no longer convinced by monolithic narratives of social truth, such as the enlightenment tale of progress, or the Marxian picture of proletarian revolution. Instead, development theory must straddle material and human worlds, welcoming individual subjectivity and embodiment, and the self-authoring of culture.

In an incisive, sobering critique of the cross-cultural application of models of disability empowerment, Grech (2009) questions a host of taken-for-granted assumptions about what disabled people around the world 'need'. A point of departure is that we know very little about any aspect of disability in the developing world. Set against the complex, uncertain implications of poverty and local culture, the simple exporting of social model or human rights discourse is highly problematic (ibid.). As we have seen, the need to create mass mobilisation always leads to the risk of over-simplification. In particular, advocating for human rights and equity legislation has little meaning in contexts where there are no resources for implementation or enforcement. Further, the social model's attempt to negate the meaning of impairment may have different implications in developing countries, where survival is more likely to depend on physical labour (ibid.). Grech (2009) concurs with Whyte and Ingstad (2007), who warn against promotion of a universal development discourse. They write:

> The basic approach is to start where people live, with their concerns and resources and the particular political ecology in which they are interacting. What is disabling for them there?
>
> (Whyte and Ingstad, 2007 in Grech, 2009, p. 775)

In developing contexts, the economic predicaments of disabled people often occur against the backdrop of mass unemployment, confounding questions of 'inclusion' (Grech, 2009). The need to build cooperative relationships across marginal identity groups towards a shared development agenda seems essential. Again, separatist politics must be questioned. In South African society, the reality of a catalogue of human rights which remain unenforceable to the vast majority of disabled people is painfully apparent. Disabled people's organisations (DPOs) show a strongly urban bias, and are often more accountable to donors or personal interest than their constituency (Coleridge, personal communication). Besides this, organisations forged under social model politics are prone to enforcing the orthodoxies to which this book objects. This is certainly the case in my country. Like myself, Grech (2009) emphasises the need to focus on social capital, building relational networks, mutual trust and personal integration.

In a progressive, illuminating social work text, Thompson (2003, p. 40) states bluntly that 'existential freedom is a prerequisite for political freedom', and that 'to deny the former is to foreclose the latter'. Jenny Morris (1993, p. 106) is equally unequivocal, stating that disabled peoples' liberation from prejudice will never succeed if viewed as 'solely a matter of changing others'. The simplicities of material 'emancipation' are attractive, and these priorities remain real. But in my view a new, different level of engagement is essential in directing the disability movement towards a phase of greater political maturity. Ever more, the idea of development occurring without devoting resources to individual transformation seems implausible. Honneth (1995, p. 164) sees political engagement and the fostering of personal entitlement to recognition as inseparable. One of Coleridge's (1993, p. 13) disability development activist respondents stated simply that 'if people feel good about themselves, they can begin to create change'. Courageously facing the reality of shared dynamics in unequal relationships, Coleridge (1993, p. 36) argues that 'discrimination and prejudice create the sense of being disabled that leads to further discrimination and prejudice'. Needless to say, we must beware of the stereotype that disabled people cause their own oppression. But Coleridge's (1993) respondents emphasise repeatedly that the self-regard of disabled individuals is at the core of transforming attitudes. Coleridge (1993) writes:

> The harsh reality is that if disabled people see themselves as victims, they will be treated as victims; if they are sunk in self-pity, they will be perceived as pathetic; if they are hostile towards non-disabled people, they will be shunned; but if they refuse to see themselves as victims, if they claim their own dignity, see themselves as positive and able to contribute, they will be seen as positive and able to contribute.
>
> (Coleridge, 1993, p. 36)

This is indeed a harsh reality, placing heavy, unfair demands on members of all oppressed groups. But all activists interviewed insisted that their work is primarily with disabled people themselves, believing that prejudiced sectors of society will not change unless the process is begun by the minority (ibid.). Coleridge (1993, p. 52) also gives his account of movement from a 'disempowered' stance to an 'empowered' one, describing the latter as:

> … open to change, assertive, pro-active, self-accountable, self-directed, uses feelings, learns from mistakes, confronts, lives in the present, realistic, thinks relatively, has high self-esteem.

By contrast, the person who has not yet moved to this 'empowered position' tends to be:

> … closed to change, aggressive, reactive, blames others, directed by others, overwhelmed by feelings, avoids, lives in the past or the future, unrealistic, thinks in absolutes, has low self-esteem.
>
> (Coleridge, 1993, p. 52)

It would be dreadfully wrong to assume that since it is the disabled individual's task to achieve empowerment, that the behaviours of disempowerment are unjustified or nonsensical. As we saw earlier, if we are willing to explore disabled subjectivity honestly, we will find coherent behavioural and emotional responses to unbalanced circumstances. Awareness of the scale of social suffering disabled people experience is essential as a point of departure. Coleridge (1993) is bold, facing the tough reality of lives in which there is no choice but to process one's own struggle. This is a massive challenge. Capitulation, embitterment and hostility may be quite natural and human responses to the madness of unjust circumstances.

Paolo Freire's (1970) model of empowerment through 'conscientisation' has great promise in the disability arena (Peters, 1999). Freire (1970) believed that political and personal emancipation could be achieved through a group-based process of critical reflection on everyday realities, exposing hidden mechanisms of oppression (Kalyanpur, 1996; Mercer, 2002). Through his 'dialogic method', individuals learn to 'perceive social, political and economic contradictions, and to take action against the oppressive elements of reality' (Freire, 1970, p. 19). Internal freeing from the self-blame and self-doubt engendered by subordination was, for Freire, as important as political mobilisation.

As I have alluded, it is important to not underestimate the gravity of this sort of personal reflection. Exploring one's losses, traumatic experiences and personal subjugation can be excruciating. It is for this reason that the unconscious need to manage such pain at times supports compliance with injustice. A combination of Freirian praxis with a critical psychoanalytic view of discrimination forms, I believe, a useful instrument set to begin integrating the psychological layer into disability equity strategy.

Disability and psychotherapy

If personal and social change are indeed closely related, the place of psychotherapy in the disability story must receive attention. To put it mildly, psychotherapy has a bad reputation with much of the materialist-dominated Western disability sector, due to its identification with biomedical discourse (Marks, 2002; Watermeyer, 2002b). Recalling the debate between Goodley and Lawthom (2005) and Forshaw (2007) in Chapter 2, the former contributors saw 'community psychology' as the only branch of the discipline worth considering. Clinical psychology, by contrast, was viewed as inevitably collaborating with disablism. Simi Linton (1998) agrees, believing that essential tenets of therapeutic psychology, as well as the discipline more broadly, run counter to an emancipatory view of disability in at least three ways. First, psychology is the basis for research conventions and constructs underpinning notions of normality, deviance and pathology – so influential in disabled lives. Second, psychology's empiricist bias and largely negative response to standpoint theory impede analyses of disability as a social construct. Last, the discipline tends to train professionals to intervene at the personal, intrapsychic level, obscuring contextual inequalities (ibid.). In my own experience as a trainer of graduate professionals, baseline awareness of disability as an axis of oppression is, indeed, minimal. Again, a fundamental question facing the disability movement here pits boycott politics against a policy of engagement with transformation. While there is certainly truth in the critique of Linton (1998) and Goodley and Lawthom (2005), there is also outdated stereotyping; the discipline of psychology continues to shift substantially. For example, Forshaw (2007) is correct in questioning the idea that psychology is resistant to standpoint approaches, noting the immense shift to qualitative methods in psychology over recent decades. Additionally, the assertion that quantitative methods necessarily silence or devalue disabled people is simply wrong (ibid.). The key issue is how these are applied. Resonant with other debates raised in this book, my own view is that the disability movement and disability studies cannot afford to dismiss psychology. Without the option of creating a new, ideologically pristine discipline to conceptualise its predicaments, it must engage; carefully, critically, fairly, continually.

Returning to the specific issue of psychotherapy, a basic question is whether disabled people need, or would benefit from it. Unsurprisingly, social modelist voices respond to the association of disability and psychotherapy with suspicion. Reeve (2004), notwithstanding her interest in psycho-emotional aspects of disability, asserts that a visit to a psychologist is likely to add to, rather than ameliorate, such difficulties. In this view, psychotherapy will always attribute emotional or behavioural responses to intra-psychic factors, neglecting context. Given the lack of critical disability theory in most psychotherapy training, Reeve's (2004) basic concern is well placed, but trashing psychotherapy to all of her disabled readers seems irresponsible. One will not change professional culture by stereotyping professionals. Instead, those with or without insight into disability issues will feel understandably alienated. This does not underplay the reality of how much change is required, both in disability awareness and demographic represention in mental health professions. Evidence is that disabled individuals' experience of psychotherapy has not, for the most part, been empowering. McKenzie (1992), for example, found that disabled people under psychological and psychiatric care saw practitioners as having little insight into life in a disablist society (in Oliver, 1995, p. 263). Besides this problem, part of the social modelist position involves eschewing psychological narratives altogether, positioning the choice to seek therapy as evidence of failure or, worse still, of collaboration with medical oppressors. The denigration of psychologists by Reeve (2004) and Thomas (1999a), while well intentioned, will only deepen these splits. Modalities of psychotherapy are immensely diverse, ranging from the narrowly 'medical' to the radically political. We will not deepen insight into the discipline's implications for disability with descriptions of a homogeneous monolith.

Of course, psychotherapists routinely fall into the trap of being so compelled by impairment as to underestimate contextual causes of distress, potentially reinforcing self-blaming (Abberley, 1993; Swain et al., 2006). Most mental health professionals have had little experience of disability work, limiting insight into discrimination as well as personal projections about impairment (Watermeyer, in press). Some social modelists respond to the excessive attribution of psychological difficulties to impairment by arguing that only disabling barriers, and never impairment, cause distress (Swain et al., 2006). The reasons for this position are clear, but these make it no less untrue.

Confirming social modelist misgivings, some rehabilitation-oriented models of disability psychotherapy aim to 'manage' emotional distress through, for example, cognitive-behavioural reformulation. Put very simply, the idea here is changing thought patterns in order to alter relationships with the world and the self. If uncritically applied, such methods certainly have the potential to sideline the social origins of struggle, instead problematising responses to lived realities. The difficulty with such work is analogous to the feminist critique of some models of psychotherapy (e.g. Hollway, 1998), where treatment is prescribed to modify 'maladaptive' responses to what are, in fact, intolerable circumstances. The error is often one of emphasis. Political awareness and action may be admitted, but more as an afterthought. The deeply socialised self-blaming of some disabled people may interact, creating a therapeutic discourse which is supportive, rather than subversive. For me, Vash and Crewe's (2004) influential volume, now in its second edition, shows up this problem of emphasis. They write:

> Contemporary understanding of disability, however, requires comparable recognition of the social dimensions of emotional distress.
>
> (Vash and Crewe, 2004, p. 269)

Here, the 'comparable' account of social factors is summoned in response to primary attributions to do with the body. As we have seen, psychological accounts of disability which begin with impairment typically become stuck in its compelling layers. Reeve (2000) is correct in observing that, while mental health practitioners are often aware of the need to reflect on racial or gender prejudices which they carry, little similar intent is visible regarding disability. In her experience some psychotherapists disbelieve the importance of environmental factors, probably leading to 'diagnoses' of 'denial' (ibid., p. 673). The influence of civil rights action and social theory surrounding race and gender are evident here in the minds of mental health practitioners. This is a challenge to the disability sector.

Perhaps the most well-read text from within disability studies on the relationship between disability and psychotherapy is Olkin's *What psychotherapists should know about disability* (1999). As it is influential, I will comment on the approach in some detail. Olkin (1999) strives to foreground contextual factors in approaching mental health problems among disabled people. But while her perspective is certainly critical, it also embodies a 'modernist' position, involving methods and models for 'managing' disability. These methods are, it must be said, probably very useful to many people. Perhaps the need for these is inevitable, but it is hard to present such strategies while holding a rigorous, irreverent critique of ideology at centre stage. An exacting encounter with difference requires the sort of thoroughgoing interpretation which leaves no stone of convention unturned, welcoming alternate ways of being even if – *especially* if – these provoke disquiet. An engagement which provides strategies for coping with life in a disablist society can foster perspectives and lifestyle choices which least disrupt broader cultural mores. The strength of critical psychoanalysis is again a contrast here, aiming not only to interrogate cultural accounts of disability, but also to reach 'underneath' to the psychic organisations which rely on the divisions of the status quo. Disability presents the opportunity for a mammoth critique of the 'ideology of the body'. This could not be expected of a work such as Olkin's, but it must be possible to create principles which are both therapeutic and steadfastly analytical, and consequently subversive.

Among much else, Olkin (1999) reviews research exploring factors associated with more positive disability attitudes. These include similarity of appearance to nondisabled people, lesser impairment severity, attractiveness, competence and good social skills (p. 67). Her intention is not to justify prejudiced attitudes, but there is also little problematising of these. Instead, a mood is created which begins with the cooperative attitudes shown by socially and occupationally successful disabled people, which offset prejudice. It will be clear that she concurs with Coleridge's (1993) activist respondents in this regard; but in the clinical setting these ideas carry a subtly different ideological valency. As we have seen, although responses to the social world may be maladaptive, even self-destructive, it is essential that we begin by viewing these as meaningful and communicative. At centre stage must be an inquiry into the hidden rationality at work in 'unhelpful' behaviours, which uncovers layers of experience and integrates meaning. Whether or not a response style is 'well adjusted', the sense and unconscious 'fit' of the behaviour with distorted socialisation is primary. We are reminded of Ray in Veck's (2002) work. Olkin's (1999) principles for dealing with the likely problems of disabled lives render a form of 'disability case management' which cannot help reconstructing subtle essentialist differences between disabled and nondisabled groups (see also Crisp, 2002). This is inadvertent, and a criticism equally applicable to a range of psychological interventions which cannot escape defining the 'ill' and their 'needs'. But subversive inquiry must be a constant companion to interventionism.

To be called subversive, psychotherapy must unpack social contradictions, harness entitlement and anger and lead to the giving back of unconsciously held imputations (Samuels, 1993; Marks, 2002). In Samuels' (1993, p. 55) words, there must be 'a modulation of feelings outward as well as inward'. Quoting Jean Laplanche, Frosh (2006) cautions against the tendency to view presence of a coherent life-narrative as evidence of 'health' or well-being. Psychoanalysis shows up our tendency to sculpt rational stories which actually obscure the reality of lives subject to the slings and arrows of a hostile, self-interested society. Psychotherapy which lacks an acute, critical edge may smooth over the inconsistencies of life, creating a narrative which dampens internal dissonance and relegates injustice to the shadows (ibid.). By contrast, a critical psychoanalytic view is curious about what we do not know. This may mean disrupting easy narratives borne of ideological sleight-of-hand. It is the fault-lines in the narrative which draw interest, as these may signal areas of trauma which cement unequal relationship. Efforts from within disability studies to oppose the tragedy narrative with an 'affirmative' view of disability (Swain and French, 2008), although commendable, may risk disguising important contradictions in internal life. Samuels (1993, p. 52) sees immense political potential in psychoanalytic enquiry, describing psychotherapy as 'a bridge between depth psychology and politics'. Active, educative engagement with the community of mental health professionals can, I believe, harness real emancipatory potential.

Samuels (1993) adds that political organisations would benefit greatly from applying resources to the psychological development of their members, for reasons of efficiency as well as humanitarianism. A model which combines curiosity about personal history with an awareness of the interpretive significance of political circumstances is the heart of subversive, socially responsive psychotherapy (Watermeyer, 2012).

Note

1 Interpellation here refers to how ideology recruits individuals into perpetuating its functions, largely without their awareness. We live steeped in discourses which provide limited, value laden and politically weighted views of reality. The impressions of ideology on the self are hard to recognise, and therefore hard to challenge.

7 Conceptualising the psychological predicaments of disablism

Disability, silence and trauma

Introduction

Theoretical ideas presented so far in this book have emerged from a new, psychoanalytically oriented synthesis of existing work in disability studies and related fields. This chapter is the first of three which aim to develop and enliven these ideas, along with some new ones. I do this with the help of fragments of experiential material gleaned from my group psychotherapy work with severely physically impaired adults. This is a relational phenomenology surrounding very visible, severe impairments such as quadriplegia, hemiplegia and global ataxia. Noting this, the dynamics described may appear somewhat exaggerated or situation-specific. Still, I believe the material offers useful grist to the mill for a more general discussion. Clinical accounts in these final three chapters are not intended to be read as data. This is a book of conceptual suggestions, not empirical claims. The intention is to give life to the ideas presented thus far, helping us assess whether these illuminate anything of disabled experience. I do not attribute generalisability to my formulations. But at the heart of this work is the conviction that people can be liberated from ideology through the naming of subtle mechanisms of othering. If we can trace the faint outline of hidden, oppressive relational dynamics, these become less constrictive. Psychoanalytic thinking provides us with tools to query what lies just beyond consciousness, in the places where socialisation has concealed contradictions in how we relate. Part of the experiment of this book, and especially these three chapters, concerns whether the ideas gathered here bring hidden experiences of the disabled reader into clearer relief. This is the work of trying to mirror subjective worlds that are obscured by ideology which, as we know, is good at covering its tracks. In this chapter I begin by considering the experiential reality of visible impairment in a world where bodily 'abnormality' tends to evoke anxiety in others. This leads into a discussion of how resultant dynamics can silence the voice of disabled experience. Finally, I offer an approach to the difficult issue of integrating personal experiences of trauma into a contextual view of disablist oppression.

Disability and anxiety

> **F**: … the difference is then how people manage that anxiety … There are some people who come and confront it by sort of revealing their anxiety, but

> I think they would probably be the smallest minority. And some people who … try and disarm it in some way … we feel a little bit like we're tiptoeing around something. And … then some which are far more rare for me … is a more confrontational way of dealing with it … where people come and … need to … understand why I'm disabled … the conversation moves to trying to find the blame for being disabled. And that, often times, either is God or the disabled person … and there's obviously the other which is just avoidance, when people try not to talk to you and try not to engage.

An axiom of this book is that anxiety is ubiquitous in relational spaces surrounding disability. Disabled people may feel encircled by a world of individuals who seem awkward, subtly hostile, embarrassed, at a loss or off-balance in the business of relating. As we noted earlier, Melanie Klein (1948) found the anxieties of young children to be largely rooted in aggressive impulses. Some of the anxiety we see, thus, probably stems from distancing, aversive urges. Freud's (1933) association of altruism with repressed sadism – though understandably seen by some as cynical – also brings some light to this issue. Quite simply, if and when people with impairments do carry our most shameful parts, momentary rageful responses at our worlds being intruded upon by these reminders should not surprise us (Watermeyer, 2006).

The implications of being a stimulus for anxiety are substantial, especially in relationships of little familiarity. Moving through the world as (in part) a cause of unease means confronting real obstacles to free, trusting, robust and authentic relating. There is messaging implicit in the mirroring experiences one encounters: from pity or subtle disgust, to the communication that one is unmanageable, un-containable or too much to bear. The self, in such circumstances, exists in the face of a current of unsettling imputations, being required to field the psychic 'excess' of others. Part of this relationship management involves constricting evidence of the psychic pain of which projections are composed.

Imperative to silence

> **J**: One thing that I have found, though, with my past peers … I get a very standard response. It's like, how are you doing, a standard response, and like, I'm fine. And when you say you're fine it's got absolutely nothing to do with how you're actually feeling. And, you know, conversation generally doesn't go past that … There's only one person that knows me the best, and that's myself. Every other person … gets a sliver, but they never get a big piece.

Through having to negotiate the uncertainties and insults of our development, shame is a universal aspect of human selfhood. The conflict between disclosure and disguise of parts of self we deem less admissible is an equally shared, ongoing feature of social life. Is what is inside us palatable, tolerable, lovable to others? These assessments determine our willingness to take risks in relationships. If we are able to risk, it improves the likelihood of experiences of being truly seen, which are so precious to psychological integration. This challenge of relating is, I believe, made much harder by cultural responses to impairment. As we saw in the previous chapter, Wendell (1997, p. 266) describes how 'coming into the world' as a disabled person provokes resistance to the 'mixing' of 'worlds', the 'normal' with the 'not normal'. For this reason, much of a disabled person's experience may go underground, through a lack of socially acceptable means of expression. The loss of control symbolised by bodily flux is 'despised, pitied, and above all, feared' (ibid., p. 267). Consequently, the urge to protect others from this danger, and oneself from others' responses, is difficult to resist. Impaired individuals may carry an unseen disability narrative made up of everyday experiences in which disability is salient. These experiences may have a positive or negative valency, but unite around disability-difference as the unsayable 'elephant in the room'.

Most inadmissible, though, are experiences such as discrimination, demeaning treatment, deprivation, impossible inconvenience, pain and fatigue and the like. Admission to mainstream social life may be felt as contingent on keeping this metanarrative hidden. But importantly, the material of this story is not qualitatively different from any other 'small talk'. It mirrors the daily events and tribulations of nondisabled life. The difference is that there is no place for it. Murphy (1987, p. 87) remarks simply on this code of silence, saying that no-one ever asked him 'what it is like' to live with quadriplegia. To do so, he continues, would 'violate all the rules of middle-class etiquette' (ibid.). Murphy (1987) is talking about regular restrictions on personal disclosure which are part of politeness; but for disabled people an extraordinarily large tract of experience falls into the 'impolite' category. Olkin (1999, p.77) regards the requirement that disabled people 'regulate affect' as commonplace in modern society. As will be recalled, Fanon saw this constraint as the first obstacle towards liberation to be overcome (Charlton, 1998). Fanon's 'mechanisms of concealment' alienated the colonised not only from one another, but from their own internal life (ibid., pp. 74–75).

Listening to someone else's experience is a demonstration of willingness and strength to tolerate what one imagines is 'inside' him or her, recalling Bion's (1962a; 1962b) construct of *containment*. In Bion's schema, the mother helps her infant to become more emotionally integrated through taking in his or her difficult feelings; that is, embodying an accepting state of 'reverie' (Rustin, 1996). This early picture is a template for emotional functioning which applies throughout the life course. We all need, provide and lack containment. In fact, Hinshelwood (1991) describes Bion's concept of 'container and contained' as a key mechanism through which projective identification takes place between groups (see also Young, 1994). What this boils down to is the question of who is willing to hear and accept the internal reality of the other. Or, conversely, who seeks to drive their unwanted internal material into the devalued other, denying the true experience to be found there. Are we able, for example, to simply accept the life stories of refugees in our country, or do we defend against the painful reality by adding our own distancing interpretations and attributions?

Rustin (1991) expresses what we need from others as an experience of being *thought about*; that is, feeling known in a manner which facilitates self-knowledge and self-acceptance. In modern society it appears that we are largely unable to think clearly about disabled experience. In part, the un-containment of such experience is demonstrated by society's failure to address the human needs of disabled persons. Experience must be thought about and validated if its realities are to come into relief and be addressed. But apparently, perceptions of that experience are so saturated with projections that thinking cannot take place.

The implication is not that disabled people are impossible to contain, but rather that unconscious evocations make an open, listening stance very difficult when impairment is visible. This hesitancy is probably so familiar to the congenitally impaired person as to go almost unnoticed – the 'second nature' of Winnicott's (1960) false self. In this picture, disabled people seldom have the experience of being emotionally held, as this relies on opportunities for self-expression. Instead, like Winnicott's parentified child, the disabled individual is likely to subtly take up a holding role. People continually receiving a tacit message that their inner worlds are somehow dangerous or toxic will, naturally, partially internalise that assessment. If, to echo Fanon, disability experience remains in the shadows, the reality of inequality will also remain somehow unreal.

In Bion's (1962a) terms, it is not *knowledge* carried by the listener – or the mother – which brings self-integration, but simply a stance which communicates acceptance and a readiness to be surprised (Frosh, 2006). Frosh (1991) attributes pervasive narcissism to disruption, in the modern world, of conditions allowing for experiences of containment. Modernity does little to facilitate the presence of a containing other, able to validate social distress. In fact, this sort of acceptance seems to fly in the face of what neoliberal, autonomous modernism is about, with disability appearing as the nemesis of its intentions. The perceived chaos of the narrative of bodily frailty is exceptionally hard for the Enlightenment mind to hear, reducing the teller to the ranks of those devoid of 'proper' stories, and hence of 'proper' lives (Frank, 1995, p. 97). In disabled lives, thus, the physical exclusion of built environments and inaccessible procedures – nowhere to be – is mirrored by a psychic experience of spilling over, of being too much. This is the experience of being emotional 'matter out of place' (Douglas, 1966), or rather, matter *without* a place. In my clinical experience, disabled people suffer an amplified version of the common human state of not having a place to put one's innards, the secretions of one's experience. Here, material unwelcome is mirrored in an existential homelessness.

Unfortunately, the social model leaves disabled people solely responsible for containing these aspects of life, through eschewing personal experience. To me, this exclusive emphasis on barriers seems, at times, connected to the protection of others from personal experiences of impairment. All humans need recognition; all need containment. In an ideological paradox, disabled people are expected to show impairment as something completely 'normal', as 'adjusted to' and unremarkable. This assessment may be true for many impaired persons, but is an oppressive misrepresentation for many others.

Trauma and its re-enlivening

> **L**: You know, I know these are pessimistic emotions that are not unique to people with disabilities, but I think they're probably magnified to a degree.

R: You lose out on the ability to recognise yourself as valuable, as worthy, yeah, and I think that was … a core part of that early [post-accident] process was figuring out a way of … almost like a lexicon, a language … that would allow me to recognise … again who I was. And … the only discourse available to you at that moment is … the survivor. You know, in the early days, the fact that you didn't die becomes … a great achievement [small laugh].

F: I think one other thing that has been my experience of being disabled is the … the huge amount of time you spend on the very mundane things. And just the huge amount of time I spend waiting for stuff to happen … kind of in limbo … and it means that … it's almost like there's an unhealthy amount of time to chew things over. When you're in, kind of, emotional turmoil, you really have the space to torture yourself. And not to go and do something which would take your mind off it for a while.

The term *trauma* has been used in more than one way in the social sciences. First, as a narrow, psychiatric concept describing emotional symptoms surrounding a life-threatening experience such as criminal violence or accident. The second, psychoanalytically oriented meaning is broader, referring to a hurtful intra-psychic or existential experience which, although relating to events in the relational world, may not involve physical danger. The trauma here is one of symbolic violence exercised on one's identity, sometimes through the re-evoking of prior annihilating experiences (e.g. Sinason, 1992). A traumatic experience may thus come in the form of an interaction, a realisation or the emergence of a memory. What defines the phenomenon is that it punctures the defences (A. Freud, 1967). Without questioning the material-world roots of social trauma, the focus here is on an emotional level in which chronic assaults on identity reinfect old wounds.

Part of the perennial splitting we see between experiential and materialist accounts arises from the fact that disability is associated with trauma. Life in a prejudiced world will visit trauma on those it shuns. Further, trauma is by definition difficult to think about (Bion, 1962b), as it confronts us with realities beyond our comforting expectations, beyond our defences. Awareness of trauma among the disabled community contributes, in my view, to a sort of 'performance anxiety' among disability theorists. Quite understandably, writers fear not doing justice to the gravity of human suffering (see Dalenberg, 2000). I certainly feel this in my own work. The evocativeness of disability and the diversity of impairment make it very difficult to commit any generalising description of 'disability trauma' to paper. Conversely, individual, autobiographical accounts have limited political potential. Evidence of how much is psychologically at stake in writing about disability shows up in the split discourse of 'acceptance and denial' (discussed later), which presents a hopelessly limited repertoire of being into which disabled people are discursively forced. In sum, the conflicting forces at work as one tries to write on this issue include a constrictive reverence for suffering (Dalenberg, 2000), the anti-phenomenological orthodoxy of the social model, the requirements of political correctness and expediency and the danger of supporting stereotypes of damage. Together, these are formidable challenges. But let us not be scared off any longer.

The word 'trauma' is drawn from a Greek root, meaning 'wound', denoting a piercing – here, of internal emotional safeguards. Davis (2002) describes how ideology maintains a silence around material trauma inflicted on disabled people, allowing us to reformulate systematic injustice as merely 'accidental'. He writes:

> One of the reasons why there is resistance to calling attacks against people with disabilities 'hate' crimes is because the general ideology toward people with disabilities rules out hate as a viable emotion. But the 'hate' toward people with disabilities is a much more subtle and ingrained hatred. It is a hatred of difference, or the fact that someone cannot see a clearly posted sign, cannot walk up unblocked stairs, needs special assistance above what other 'normal' citizens need. This kind of hatred is one that abhors the possibility that all bodies are not configured the same, that weakness and impairment are the legacy of a cult of perfection and able embodiment.
>
> (Davis, 2002, p. 156)

An emancipatory approach to disability trauma must avoid the victim-blaming of medical-psychological accounts, but also has to consider individual psychological development. We need an analysis which addresses the individual self, but locates this psychological reality within contextual factors. Thomas (1999b, p. 47) is at precisely this juncture as she considers the challenge of developing a psychology of 'personal identity formation' in disability, with a 'heavy sociological slant'. She offers no ideas regarding how this might be done without falling into an individualising logic.

The perspective I propose begins with the universal unconscious psychic wounds of development. As discussed, the subtle, ideologically propagated idea of some sort of qualitative difference in psychological experience between disabled and nondisabled people is a dangerous fallacy (Watermeyer, 2002a). All carry philogenetically equivalent, hidden scars of contextual misattunement; of shame, inadequacy, self-hatred and the like, with threads leading back to the templates of formative relationships. Where we begin to theorise 'disability difference' in the psychological realm is in the ways in which social positioning *selectively* enlivens and confirms malignant aspects of self in disabled individuals. What disablist culture produces is a sustained experience of perverse mirroring, re-evoking and aggravating the most vulnerable or self-attacking parts of the self-identity. I call this mirroring *perverse* because it is unconsciously motivated by precisely the sort of shame-ridden conflicts which its action speaks to in the inner worlds of those it targets. This is the essence of projective identification in the inter-group arena. Through this mechanism, distorted mirroring works to evoke, to realise the untold stories of the dominant.

As we saw earlier, Freud's (1914) view on disability, though ambiguous, framed impairment as a 'pretext' (p. 99) which may be used psychologically to live out what are, in fact, more basic, universal existential struggles. With reference to physical attractiveness as well as visible impairment, Freud (1914) pointed out that all carry neuroses, which may at times be ascribed to the nature of the body, but are in fact a combined product of constitutional psychological elements and cultural factors. Such factors may exist as differential, limited access to the material props which support our narcissism, or more overt, denigrating imputations. Young (1994, p. 139) explains how a trauma functions psychologically as a 'homing device' which 'ransacks … the history of the victim until it finds a congruent, early experience'. The new event then 'latches on' to split-off internal parts, further dividing the self (ibid.). Acute physical traumas leading to adventitious impairment are very relevant here. For a range of reasons relating to health provision and culture, individuals in these circumstances may have limited opportunities for processing psychological trauma. All forms of trauma are virtually inseparable from self-blame. The malignant, typically self-critical meanings assumed by such shadowy memories may set the tone for a subtle, unconscious collusion with prejudice. In other words, undigested trauma lends credence to cultural ascriptions of damage, which are directed at the body, but felt as the self. But even without acute trauma, the ongoing assault of aversive social responses will 'ransack' the inner world, seeking support in destabilising the self.

The crystallising picture, then, is one in which traumatic experiences are an ongoing part of impaired life in a disablist society. But beyond this drone, and especially for people with lifelong impairments, there is the probability of a history of more direct, hurtful assaults on selfhood. Consider the likelihood of difficulties in early attachment and separation, family relationships characterised by stress and uncertainty, rehabilitative imperatives to be 'more normal', personal meanings attached to special schooling or institutional care, the projections of peers and authority figures and many other influences on disabled lives which make it harder to grow a robust sense of self. A discriminatory world may then corroborate feelings of unworthiness, reopening old wounds. Internal battles to feel legitimate, entitled and whole may be a constant drain on emotional energy in the face of a world that 'disagrees' so consistently and in so many idioms.

Though not using a psychoanalytic framework, Paterson and Hughes' (1999) notion of the 'dys-appearing body' intersects well with these ideas. They write:

> When one is confronted by social and physical inaccessibility one is simultaneously confronted by oneself; the external and the internal collide in a moment of simultaneous recognition. When one encounters prejudice in behaviour or attitude, one's impaired body 'dys-appears'.
>
> (Paterson and Hughes, 1999, p. 603)

As one's body 'dys-appears', aspects of the body ego forged in early physical ministrations are selectively called forth by social experience. Simultaneously, impaired modes of being are de-legitimated by the 'carnal information' of cultural norms of embodiment (ibid., p. 604). Impairment, therefore, settles within experience as a blight on desirable embodiment, which leaves no space for alternative forms of physicality. In this way, the impaired body is excluded from contributing to shared 'carnal information' (ibid.), and from a psychological home in the social world. The potential disruption of access to a continuous, immediate stream of self (Winnicott, 1974) caused by bodily 'dys-appearances' must be a significant part of life with disablism.

In closing this discussion, Davids (1996) echoes my view on disablism by problematising Fanon's (1952; 1963) analysis of racism. Fanon, according to Davids (1996), fails to bring to life the unique, personal meanings of social mistreatment. Instead, the subject he presents is 'a passive, idealised child, the innocent victim of a malevolent split permeating down from the social' (ibid., p. 227). Fanon ignores what is – to Davids and myself – the crucial issue of the child's own awareness of colour, or disability. In each case, difference will be used psychologically as a means of making sense of the self and the world, by individuals who are, like all people, unique and complicated. The idea of mistreatment enlivening hurt aspects of the internal world brings disabled people into the picture as fallible, normal humans. These are not the uniform victims of oppression presented by the social model. The important paradox here is that it is in the personal meanings of oppression and impairment – the abjection these may evoke – that human universals are to be found. It is not, as the social model view would have us believe, that disabled people are 'like everyone else' in not being defined by damage, but rather that everyone else shares equally in the 'damage' of humanness which has become culturally signified by disability. This view begins to value the contribution which disabled experience stands to make to our appreciation of that humanness.

8 Disability and the distortion of personal and psychic boundaries

Introduction

Throughout my clinical experience of disability, a common denominator is relationships involving distorted personal and psychic boundaries. Understanding these dynamics is a key to mapping the psychological, relational circumstances of life with disablism. In one way or another, much of what I suggest in this book tracks back to shifting, permeable or unclear boundaries between bodies, groups or selves. The psychoanalytic critique of disablism in essence describes the movement of psychic material across boundaries separating individuals or groups, through processes such as projective identification. Of interest is the fact that norms of etiquette and privacy are routinely flouted when disability is involved. It is not easy to find a visibly impaired person who has not had the experience of being asked the question 'so ... what happened to you?' by a stranger (Slack, 1999, p. 33). The intimacy and shared history required to ask a similarly personal question of a nondisabled person would be considerable. There are clues here which point to the control and appropriation of the disabled figure that forms the core of the unconscious narrative of inequality. Clear boundaries would limit this appropriation, blocking the ascriptions required to create disabled people as the holders of shame and dependency. But what makes things impossibly complicated is that disabled people do often require assistance, muddying the waters at the confluence of need, projection and control.

Disability discrimination is, in its most important form, subtle and nebulous. Kindness and subordination may be very difficult to separate, allowing the latter to find a home in the self unnoticed. Inequality which is difficult to see is difficult to resist. Gill (2001, p. 366) observes how disabled people 'rarely encounter the clarity of contempt associated with racism and homophobia', as these sentiments are actively repressed around impairment. As we have seen, devaluing ideas about disability are not as clearly illogical as racist values, since impairment lends these not only a certain rationality, but also an admirable empathy. Gill (2001, p. 366) perceptively states that it is 'more difficult to refute a distortion of fact than an outright fiction'. Perhaps most importantly, it is very difficult to grasp the reality of one's subordinate status when it emanates not from 'prejudiced villains', but from persons with whom one may identify deeply (ibid.). Family members, friends and other 'good people' may, confoundingly, be the source of faint, but persistent inequality.

Boundary distortions and being 'an exception'

In a paper entitled *The exceptions*, Freud (1916) describes a style of psychological functioning which he associates with bodily difference. Patients with congenital impairments, or who had endured severe illness in early childhood, were found by Freud (1916) to be especially reluctant to accept his *reality principle.* Instead, they claimed the status of exceptions to the responsibility, independence and personal accountability of adult life. This special dispensation was justified with the idea of having 'suffered enough', and hence deserving to be spared the pain of taking responsibility for inner struggles, as well as material realities. In writing this, I do not imply that these perceptions of disabled people have any basis. But of interest is how disabled people have been constructed by theory, and why. Psychoanalytic work involves the very thing that 'the exceptions' eschew – delaying gratification, relinquishing defences and facing thorny realities. Freud found this group of patients extremely resistant to doing so. He writes:

> They say that they have renounced enough and suffered enough, and have a claim to be spared any further demands; they will submit no longer to any disagreeable necessity, for they are exceptions and, moreover, intend to remain so ... Their neuroses were connected with some experience or suffering to which they had been subjected in their earliest childhood, one in respect of which they knew themselves to be guiltless, and which they could look upon as an unjust disadvantage imposed on them.
>
> (Freud, 1916, pp. 312–13)

Freud (1916) animates his discussion with the character of Shakespeare's congenitally 'malformed' *Richard III.* Richard felt wronged by nature, through having been denied the physical beauty he believed necessary to win human love. So unjust was this fate that he felt entitled to reparation, and exempt from the moral imperative to treat others with respect or kindness. In Freud's (1916, p. 314) words, the logic at work here was 'I may do wrong myself, since wrong has been done to me'. As elsewhere in his remarks on disability, Freud (1916) then conflates psychological phenomena of bodily and cultural origin, by describing Richard's difficulties as an amplified version of what is, in fact, a universal human struggle. Quite reasonably, Freud (1916) suggests that at some pre-conscious level we all feel entitled to compensation for the ways we have been short-changed by nature, as well as historical chance. We have been left with imperfect bodies and minds, as well as dull material existences, while others live in a 'royal palace' (Freud, 1916, p. 314). The resulting wounds to our narcissism lead to the resentful conviction that 'it's not fair'. More controversially, Freud (1916) then relates disability to femininity, asserting that women are also prone to assuming the position of the 'exception', due to a subjective experience of bodily defect or lacking. An embitterment felt by some women towards their mothers, in his view, emanates in part from a reproach based on their having been born female rather than male. In the case of both disability and femininity, the key question is whether the value differential at play is of cultural or bodily origin.

Rosemarie Garland-Thomson (1997b, p. 37) slates Freud's (1916) musings as rank essentialism, understanding his position as one which sees 'deformities of character' as an inevitable, presocial consequence of impairment. Davis (2002), similarly, views Freud's formulations as a malignant reinforcement of stereotypes about disability, to do with malingering, passivity, profound damage and entitlements to special treatment. Resonant with this stereotyping is a familiar unease in conversations about integration, which reflects the idea that allowing one 'exception' will bring a tidal wave of others, leading to a fantasy of resources being inundated and chaos ensuing. Various psychoanalytic authors do, as we have seen, tacitly or otherwise assume an essentialist position. Jacobson (1959) endorses Freud's purported essentialism, writing of a number of psychoanalytic patients who claim the position of 'exceptions'. In this work women and disabled people are portrayed as likely to have weak super-egos – what may be loosely described as a lack of self-accountability. Hidden under these personality presentations, the argument continues, is unconscious self-hatred and a need to be punished (Jacobson, 1959). This self-hatred may be managed unconsciously through rebelling against laws to which others are subject, or disguised by sentimental beliefs such as the idea that one was chosen to suffer (ibid.).

Regardless of one's opinion on Freud's (1916) ideological stance, what is being described in *The exceptions* is a distortion of relational boundaries – in particular, the idea of being exempted from moral limits set on others. As we have seen, Freud's position on psychology and the body seems ambiguous, but it may be so by design. Freud (1916) starts by construing 'exceptionalism' as prominent with disabled people, but then repositions it as a universal artefact of human development, as something we all feel. Contrary to Garland-Thomson and Davis, I see it as unclear whether Freud (1916) denies the influence of social treatment on disabled peoples' experiences of self.

Returning to gender, the 'embitterment' at being born female mentioned above is part of Freud's notion of *penis envy*. This is an idea blasted by feminist critics, who see it as reflecting a simple sexist essentialism which positions women as 'envious' of men's inherently superior qualities. However, Juliet Mitchell (1974), herself working from a feminist stance, reinterprets Freud's intentions on this matter as virtually opposite to the essentialism of which he is accused. To Mitchell (1974) the 'penis' here was not an organ, but a symbol of patriarchal power in an unequal world. The envy at work – as, perhaps, the purported self-hatred – was a product of bodily differences being used psychologically by women to make sense of stark, bewildering political inequalities. In this reading, Freud positions himself as a critical social commentator, directing attention to how manifest gender inequality distorts relationships and identities. Thus, it was politics that imbued the female form with incompleteness, not female nature which informed social reality. In particular, we may elaborate Mitchell's (1974) argument by reinterpreting the 'exceptionalism' shown by some women as a response to the injustice – the unfairness – of patriarchy. In this picture a demand to be indulged was borne of two aspects. First, it emanated from an (initially) unconscious recognition of structural inequality. Second, sedimented sexist culture and socialisation may have created a field of spongy limits around the assumed frailty of women, involving a domesticating or patronising indulgence of needs, but also an implicit denigration of abilities. Now, if we apply this logic to Freud's (1916) reflections on disability, what we see is a picture of selves whose bodily difference has been imbued with psychological meaning through systematic distortions in treatment – the features of disablist socialisation. Where Davids (1996) above saw Fanon's (1952; 1963) account as lacking was in his disregard for how material and psychological struggles experienced by the black subject become projected into the skin. It is blackness which becomes the conscious, justifying 'reason' for inequality. Analogously, Mitchell's (1974) reading of Freud sees women as projecting socially engendered struggle into the myth of an inferior constitution. I add disabled people to this list. In each case, socialisation has led to the internalising of essentialist ideas, which save the self from the impossible dissonance of societal contradictions. As noted above, trauma and self-blame remain close companions.

Over the next sections we will consider distortions in personal and psychic boundaries (Watermeyer and Swartz, 2008), as an initial conceptualisation of how visible impairment shapes relationships. If, like Lussier's (1980) patient Peter, we inhabit our bodies 'as they are', rather than 'as they should be', this directs us to seeking connecting threads between 'exceptionalism' (if and where this pertains) and the nature of disablist socialisation. Psychoanalytic authors who embrace a presocial, essentialist view of the body ego must, if we look a little closer, also support the absurd idea that body image in general is not profoundly mediated by culture. Conversely, if we examine the ascriptions of lack, frailty and damage which disabled people are often subject to, a struggle to believe in one's ability to stand up to the limits of social rules is one perfectly plausible consequence. If the world says repeatedly that one is not capable, at times this will be hard to disbelieve. At a deeper level, if 'exceptionalism' reflects awareness of being wronged, the question of *how* and *by whom* remains. Perhaps, as in Mitchell's (1974) argument regarding gender, what we see consciously exists as counterpoint to an unseen awareness of trauma and injustice, reworked through ideology into self-blame and pathologisation. The self-hatred identified by Jacobson (1959) may also have a place, as one possible outcome of disabled people and women being constructed as inherently inferior and incomplete, leading to defensive narcissistic entitlements which barely cover the miserable introjections of a denigrating world. As noted, Jacobson (1959) describes 'exceptionalism' as being to do with the presence of a weak super-ego. At face value this makes sense; yet, my own clinical experience of disability is quite the contrary. Here, disabled individuals are regularly seen suffering under particularly punitive internal critics, presumably resulting from cultural messaging. If 'inappropriate' entitlements are seen, these often appear to be defensive responses to self-denigration, enacting suspicions that one is flawed, and thus can only live on charity. Deeply socialised links to disability altruism in its various forms re-enact these meanings, which may take up internal residence for lifetimes. Later we will explore how efforts to rid the self of imputations of 'exceptionalism' or the need for benevolence may lead to punitive, even harmful demands on the self.

If we apply Heinz Kohut's (1966; 1972) ideas on the nurturing of healthy narcissism to the 'exceptions', what we see in these individuals are the implications of inadequate formative relationships (Kohut, 1966; Greenberg and Mitchell, 1983; Frosh, 1991). While psychoanalytic ideas regarding attachment are strongly focused on early life, my use of 'formative' here applies to mirroring experiences throughout the life course. In Kohut's (1972) model, entitlements to special treatment are an outcome of rejection or disapproval by important mirroring figures. These hurtful experiences shape psychological strategies aimed at escape from the pain at the heart of the self, possibly showing as entitlement or prerogative. When a growing self receives insufficient affirming mirroring, his or her healthy narcissistic inclinations become repressed, instead of realistically modified (Frosh, 1991). The child has not received the means to trust his or her ability to stand up to the requirements and rules of social life – in other words, Freud's reality principle. Instead, he or she is left with a frightening sense of shame and inadequacy. Uncertainty about ability and worth, stemming from inadequate mirroring, results in a taut vacillation between inauthentic over-valuing of self, and painful feelings of inferiority (ibid.).

These ideas are, I believe, very helpful in making sense of the association between disability and 'exceptionalism'. As already discussed, socialisation in a segregated, disablist world may make it harder than usual for parents to have healthy, robust faith in their disabled child's capacity to develop and separate. This may easily present difficulties with nourishing a child's healthy narcissistic needs, with parents' worries leading to anxious or guilty permissiveness, or a controlled spartanism. I acknowledge that these reflections may appear to some as a pathologising of parents. I understand this view, but disagree. What I believe is that parenting a disabled child presents immense challenges from the internal as well as the external world. Real compassion allows for discussion to be opened, rather than foreclosed on political grounds.

The picture of disabled socialisation taking shape is one of a systematically, intersubjectively disadvantaged group, tending to have unreliable access to the narcissistic supports we all need. This is through the effect of unconscious evocations on a range of mirroring relationships. Beyond the closeness of family, as we shall see, is a world where unreal, enmeshed or patronising relating is commonplace, re-mirroring the message that one is different, requires 'special support' and thus has no place in the 'mainstream'. The crux of the issue is that these meanings are, to some extent, to be found everywhere – in intersubjective spaces, in cultural representations, in parents and families and in disabled persons themselves. As an important caveat to this entire discussion, we must take care to validate expressions of appropriate, entitled rage at disablist exclusion, as well as looking inside 'exceptionalism' to find the unconscious recognition of injustice. What is so fitting, so mystifying and confounding in disabled lives regarding the 'exceptionalist' logic of 'it's not fair' is that, in material reality, and often in the most brutal way, *it really isn't fair*. For all humans, the question of what one deserves, what one may ask from the world, has deeply embedded psychological connections and complex, often conflicting answers. In worlds inhabited by disabled persons the atmosphere remains thick with cross-cutting, contradictory and powerful assertions regarding one's entitlement, value and place. This din of confusing meanings spans the helpless pathos of the disabled figure in charity advertising, the imperatives to normalise of rehabilitation discourse, the stereotypes of bitterness and freeloading evident in popular culture, the call to greater independence heard everywhere, the quasi-spiritual or religious rhetoric of redemption and 'overcoming', and much else. If one is prone to guilt and uncertainty regarding entitlement – that is, if one is human – these circumstances are, to say the least, bewildering. This is life in a world of chronically and severely disrupted relational boundaries.

The relationship of psychic boundaries and anxiety

When psychological boundaries between individuals become indistinct and permeable, anxieties about emotional equilibrium arise. Not being able to 'see' the limits of one's emotional life, or the far reaches of fears reflected in another, brings anxiety about psychological dangers which may emerge without warning, or from hidden locations. The high emotional valency of disability promotes boundary-less relating involving the exchange of psychic material, leading to anxiety and the need for control. As a group therapist working with severely impaired persons, I see my own use of projective identification as I involuntarily live out part of myself through imagining the inner lives of those before me. Simultaneously, though, I feel a need to subdue and control what I 'see', in a fantasy of caring protection. It is, I believe, mostly myself who needs protecting.

'Healthy' relational boundaries, in psychoanalytic terms, are associated with what Klein (1948) termed the *depressive position* (Greenberg and Mitchell, 1983) – a type of psychological functioning where the ego 'can define the boundary between what is inside and what is outside, and can control the transactions between the one and the other' (Rice, 1965 in Palmer, 2002, p. 162). A key feature here is accepting ownership of one's internal struggles, rather than disowning and jettisoning these. Further, this way of being allows for nuance and ambiguity in self and other, rather than resorting to splits and projection. The heady unconscious emotional currents surrounding visible disability discourage this sort of relating.

I am speaking here of nondisabled responses to impairment, which may pull more towards *paranoid-schizoid* (splitting) than *depressive position* functioning. I do not imply that disabled people 'have poor boundaries'. But being immersed in a world in which others are repeatedly drawn into unbounded relating must impact on socialisation, as well as limit one's options in relationship. Anzieu (1989) introduces the concept of the 'skin-ego', an imagined membrane which separates inner mental contents from the outside world (Hinshelwood and Chiesa, 2002b). For all, the process of separation and development involves the coalescing of this membrane. Positive mirroring, involving influential others showing faith in one's capacity to mature beyond one's abilities, supports this growing demarcation of the self. Importantly, being around others who are able to hold clear relational boundaries shores up our own ability to do so. As we grow, what healthy boundaries provide for us is a reasonably confident sense of 'what is me', 'what is not me' and who delineates the difference. The relational disruptions described earlier can upset the development of clear boundaries, leaving, for example, congenitally impaired persons vulnerable – permeable – to the unwanted emotional material of others.

The 'freakishness' (Fiedler, 1978) of the impaired body threatens cultural boundaries of identity, through awakening split-off parts of self. The resulting anxiety is managed through the further boundary contraventions of projective identification, as the psyche struggles to regain the subjective control of 'clear separations'. Typically, these are separations of what is whole and healthy, 'me', from what is damaged and shameful, 'not me'. At an extreme, disabled people may be positioned in confusing social spaces, as parts of the self are inserted and extracted, appropriated and controlled, defined and claimed by an incessantly invested world.

Being real

> **L**: Yes, it's … authenticity. I mean, I think that's the heart of the problem … I feel like, if there is an answer to that … that would be the holy grail in terms of finding … a normal way of negotiating relationships … Spontaneous … I think spontaneity is the heart of it.

In accounts from my clinical work, it is especially unusual for severely physically impaired persons to be related to in a manner which is unambiguous, natural, spontaneous, robust and real – in a manner not significantly influenced by projections. It is a truism that when one party in an interaction slips into unreal, appeasing relating, the other participant will find it hard not to collude. Stubborn dynamics of a shared protectionism easily take root, stilting communication and contact. The silence around real or imagined disability experience takes many forms, and may also constrain more general personal disclosure. Nondisabled observers may pre-consciously imagine that what is unspoken is a dreadful reality which 'we all know about', and thus needs no discussion. This avoidance is often rationalised through the common, mistaken idea of 'protecting' disabled people from something they would not want to be reminded of. There is little opportunity for clear self-defining by the disabled individual in these circumstances, as he or she is, in turn, drawn into silently protecting observers from their own fears. Awareness of the need to reassure, to contain something unspoken, discourages the showing of experience, as this will lead – in the words of one respondent – to 'having to do more looking after'. Such a turn in the interaction would leave the disabled individual feeling even more unseen, as energy and attention shift towards the observer, and his or her subtly visible fears. The predicament leaves one between a rock and a hard place. Either one placates and protects, colluding with unrealness and remaining invisible, or risks showing authentic experience, possibly evoking splits, reparative impulses, withdrawal or prejudice. The common denominator is that the disabled self remains largely unseen.

While disabled people report that the need to placate others creates disconnect between public persona and private self, research suggests that most choose to tolerate this rather than continually face confrontation (Gill, 2001). Frosh (1991) describes how parents who are self-absorbed may foster false self-functioning in children (Winnicott, 1960), due to the relational space being dominated by parents' needs. Adult interactions around visible impairment may, analogously, be dominated by observer needs. Conformity, inauthenticity and barriers to intimacy are one possible result. My clinical work also concurs with research showing that young children tend, refreshingly, to relate to impaired adults in a quite robust, real way (Coleman, 1997). Children do not typically reject or ignore difference, often expressing interest and curiosity without stigmatisation (ibid.). In order to read the attitudes of others, Hahn (1997) found that visibly disabled people developed particular proficiency in discerning non-verbal cues. Correspondingly, Braithwaite (1990) found signs of discomfort in nondisabled people confronted with impairment, including fidgeting, minimal eye contact, staring, physical distancing, expressions of sympathy, avoidance of the individual and acting as though the impairment does not exist. In response to this affected treatment, disabled people employed various strategies to promote acceptance, such as making conversation about 'normal' things, sensitively managing curious questions and 'taking control of helping behaviours in ways that signal their full personhood' (Gill, 2001, p. 361). Similarly, Fox and Giles (1996) summarise research assessing nondisabled non-verbal interaction in the presence of visible disability. Features include shorter interactions that end prematurely, increased physical proximity, less smiling and heightened galvanic skin response. In verbal behaviours, nondisabled people often expressed opinions dissimilar to their own, but more aligned to those of the disabled participant, or used lower verbal immediacy (a measure of psychological distance indicated by word choice) (ibid.; see also Hordon, 1994). In Sinason's (1992, p. 139) clinical experience, 'fake cheerfulness' is the most common way intellectually impaired people deal with the exclusions of everyday interaction – a strategy 'often encouraged and rewarded as a sign of genuine good humour'. Disturbingly, abused and disabled children are the only two groups who show statistically significant exaggerated smiles on their drawings (ibid.). This shows relational defences extending into inner life, based in worlds offering little containment (Bion, 1962a). Importantly, such lack makes it especially hard to maintain contact with traumatic aspects of experience and history.

> **R**: Yes, … because I'd cultured my own behaviour in a way … pretty much whatever the nondisabled students I was around felt like doing, I'd sort of modify my behaviour so that it gels with what's going on … we are the minority, and so we just sort of gel in. It's not something that I question, really, it's something I've done all my life.

Resonating with these words, Murray (2006, p. 39) characterises the 'deep pain' of disablism as 'the denial of access to "ordinary" relationships'. Murphy (1987, p. 121), likewise, writes of a 'forced artificiality', involving 'joviality', the 'pretense of humour' and 'effusive friendliness', limiting the engagement which brings a greater, shared realisation of self. The 'de-realising' of subjectivity implied by disablist relational dynamics is an immense obstacle to a clear, articulate voice of disabled experience. Because dynamics are shared, change is difficult. Consider the following:

> **F**: … kind of hyper-managing your relationships like this means that you create the room to have … 'normal' … relationships, but only up until a certain point, and then … people … realise that they don't have access to parts of you that they would with other people … I feel it creates a certain … glass ceiling to relationships. Yeah, you hit … a line in the sand.

In Coleridge's (1993, p. 39) words, in order to 'break the spell' of disability projections, it is 'robust friendships' which are needed, not 'kid gloves'. Simi Linton (2006), with a visceral clarity, describes her need for realness in the following anecdote. Soon after an accident in which she suffered a spinal cord injury an old friend telephoned her, anxious to hear what had happened and how she was. 'I'm OK', she said, to which her friend loudly objected, '*You're fucking paralysed!*' (p. 17). After everyone else had 'been so nice', this friend's straightforward honesty was a powerful signal of inclusion, of normalcy. In the following excerpt a quadriplegic man expresses a similar sentiment after an incident in a disability awareness seminar which he chaired:

> **R**: Then one guy put up his hand, and he says, 'I avoided you last year because I'm terrified, not just scared, I'm terrified of what you represent'; and that was refreshing, so I could just take it from there. That was real. I said 'great, this is the kind of response I want. You're expressing what you, and probably what a lot of other people feel'.

Over-politeness signifies difference as much as outright discrimination, asking for collusion around an illusion of intrinsic difference. 'Stifling pity' can, indeed, be 'murderous' to the 'very nature' of the objectified individual (Sullivan, 1923 in Byrom, 1999, p. 159).

Being seen

> **F**: For me it would be quite a simple thing for a person to do … you know, take a functional limb, say, if you're right handed, tie it behind your back. Spend a day with it like that … just one day … Get some kind of idea of, you know, the life that I've been forced to lead … You wouldn't even have to have an impaired leg like me, or be treated weirdly by people. But just for a day, and you know, what's the big issue … in twelve and a half years I haven't got one person to try.

As a disabled person, French (1999) describes the continual experience of having to 're-present' oneself in a manageable form, while rarely having one's experience seen. Not being seen is the constant corollary to not feeling allowed to be real. Symbolic messaging confirms both principles, as in Wendell's (1997) experience:

> Much of the world is also structured as though everyone is physically strong, as though all bodies are 'ideally shaped', as though everyone can walk, hear and see well, as though everyone can work and play at a pace that is not compatible with any kind of illness or pain, as though no one is ever dizzy or incontinent or simply needs to sit or lie down.
>
> (Wendell, 1997, p. 266)

One key theme of this book is that disablism threatens not only material needs, but emotional ones as well. In terms which are deeply cultural, but felt as instinctual, it is simply 'not OK' to not be fully able to see, hear, speak, walk or otherwise function (Watermeyer and Swartz, 2008). The illegitimacy of impaired embodiment combines material and social worlds in a failure of containment which reverberates across physical, relational and intra-psychic levels. Against this backdrop, the daunting human challenge of gathering up one's experience into some sort of wholeness of being seems especially tricky in disabled lives. Put bluntly, it is hard to find one's way to feeling whole if one's life has been steeped in signs that one simply is not, and cannot, be so.

Axel Honneth (1995, p. 174) views 'freedom' or 'lack of coercion' as more than the absence of aversive structural forces – again contrasting with a materialist analysis. The key signifier of being free, instead, is the absence of 'inner barriers' and 'psychological inhibitions'. Most interestingly, Honneth construes these aspects as 'a form of trust directed inward', which lends confidence in the articulation of needs and the exercise of abilities (ibid.). This 'confidence', or, as he puts it, 'these unanxious ways of feeling with oneself', can only grow through experiences of recognition (ibid.). As should be clear, these concepts harmonise well with psychoanalytic ideas of containment, mirroring and integration. Being seen brings the ability for self-recognition, and consequently self-definition. What denotes prejudice is definition from the outside, which then recruits individuals into its realities. In short, we need to be seen in order to see ourselves more clearly, so that we may make ourselves more seen.

We understand the political reasons for social model resistance to engaging with the personal, but what of more subtle motivations? Here is a simple interpretation. There is ample reason to believe that disclosures of culturally 'unpalatable' subjective material will not be easily accepted by the majority, instead possibly leading to heightened stigmatisation. One wonders, then, whether the social modelist position reflects something of the emotional oppression of disablism, where shame and self-concealment are elemental. Does the social modelist moratorium rest, in part, on the knowledge that the already precarious belonging of disabled people depends on the continued protection of others from the messy, complicated vicissitudes of impaired life? Perhaps some political strategists see a value in constructing the world as less complicated to reassure dominant social groups. Perhaps this is a necessary stage in gaining political rights before the possibility of being known, and authentically belonging, becomes more feasible.

Manic defence

In the quotation below a physically impaired man compares his experience to that of an acquaintance who, like him, suffered a spinal injury. The writer's injury led to quadriplegia, whereas that of the acquaintance proved over time to be minor, causing no lasting impairment.

> **R**: … so he was fixed, and I can't be fixed. And I think that's a big thing for people; and I think sometimes there's a collective feeling in society that … it's a failure, because we couldn't fix you. And we're sorry, and because we couldn't fix you we don't know what to do with you …

Anxious fantasies surrounding disability often evoke reactions which may be understood as *manic defence* (Watermeyer and Swartz, 2008; Watermeyer, 2009). A manic defensive response involves warding off a diffuse but frightening feeling of lack or emptiness with a 'corrective' action. It is a 'doing' defence. Familiar to all is the scenario of a visibly impaired person being gently coerced into receiving, even appreciating, unwanted assistance with everyday tasks, such as crossing the road or pouring tea. This gentle coercion may be driven by the helper's fantasies to do with shameful inability, or a need which must be filled. The action which keeps the feeling at bay transgresses both physical and psychological boundaries. There has been little negotiation of actual needs; instead, both the nature of experience and what is required to remedy it are assumed. As already acknowledged, the need for assistance is fundamental in the lives of a vast population of impaired persons. This discussion does not problematise this. At issue though, is how the reality of needing assistance creates opportunities for unconscious, defensive enactments, confounding relating in a manner which tends to obscure the inner lives of disabled people.

Clinical accounts connect reluctance to disclose disabled experience to expectations of a manic, 'fixing' response. Sharing an experience of exclusion or functional limitation evokes helplessness, which leads to unsolicited 'helping'. If helping is not feasible, or the defence it offers is insufficient, subtle blaming, withdrawal or other modes of distancing may result, as the unmanageable feeling is 'given back'. Seemingly, it is difficult for people to see disability without intervening – to alter, remedy or obscure it. Through the course of this exchange, the experience which was originally disclosed is, in all likelihood, lost.

To exemplify dynamics surrounding this 'flight into action', I provide the following anecdote from my teaching on a postgraduate university programme in clinical psychology (see Watermeyer and Swartz, 2008):

C, a sensitive and thoughtful student, described to the class her difficulties with managing the transport needs of Z, her partially sighted housemate. C had her own car, while Z was not eligible for a driver's licence due to her impairment. C noted that her friend was always polite regarding her need for lifts, but wondered whether Z felt angry or resentful behind her courtesies. A further feature was C's stated difficulty with being 'real' in her responses to the situation. It was hard to say no, and at times she, too, felt unexpressed resentment at what was asked of her. In a familiar twist neither of C's other two housemates had their own transportation and both regularly called on her for lifts. Yet the emotional valency of these favours felt, by comparison, innocuous.

Present here are the key features of a 'doing defence'; that is, actions to address a material need which occur, in part, to the exclusion of communication. Addressing the need – even against C's own wishes – in effect foreclosed a discussion of what, for both Z and herself, lies underneath the engagement. For example, we do not have the opportunity to learn what it is like for Z to constantly occupy a position of courteous, unassuming 'asking' for access to an essential resource, over which she has no control. Of course, the main reason for this difficulty is the failure to provide accessible public transportation to South Africa's disabled population. But in a world where material inequality is everywhere, examining its impact on power and silence in relationships is important. It should be clear that in my view C is not to blame here. She is tangled in dynamics of unreal, partial relating in which all participate. One in C's position is certainly structurally conferred with power, but how that power may be wielded, shared or guiltily disowned is a complex question. The heart of what I wish to demonstrate is how structural factors, unconscious discrimination, interpersonal dynamics and intra-psychic identity factors combine in leaving Z's story of her world and herself untold. We don't know what it is like to be in her predicament, and probably do not want to hear. A key to more authentic relating, to seeing one another more clearly, involves being able to discuss disability experience without, as a first port of call, needing to do something about it; that is, to listen and speak while holding clear boundaries. This is the heart of containment, of Rustin's (1991) idea of our need to be *thought about.* Being able to freely compare experiences would render a more solid, respectful platform for later decisions regarding assistance, while – most importantly – debunking faint, pre-conscious feelings of inherent difference. The latter issue is elemental, since it lays the groundwork for real relationship which is unfettered by guilt, repressed resentment, fantasies of vulnerability or whatever else may be at play.

It appears that allowing the injustice of disability-related deprivation to be real in the interpersonal space feels unbearable. In response to a spectre of lack, a common fantasy reformulates problems as soluble, and the world as fair. This anxiety-driven wish – what I term the *fantasy of filled needs* – is a familiar cultural phenomenon composed of vague, illusory, yet firmly held beliefs to do with 'special' services and provisions 'out there' in society for those 'in need'. One consequence is that the layer of disabled experience for which no solutions are available is rendered invisible, papered over by the notion of a just world. This experience must go underground.

At the core of the broader community's inability to cease acting or resisting, and begin listening, are two sets of factors. The first is the complex of projected fantasies about what impaired experience is like – anxieties to do with damage, adequacy and shame. The other intolerable knowledge set is the appalling reality of deprivations suffered at the hands of cruelly unconscious societies. This knowledge lurks preconsciously, threatening to bring on a rush of guilty implications to do with privilege, and even complicity. With this picture as a point of departure, it is not difficult to make sense of a range of responses to disability-related disadvantage, be these quizzical, victim-blaming, confused, impatient or patronising. There are parallels between discourses of assimilation and normalisation (at times present in rehabilitation), and the manic defences visible in everyday disability-related interactions. Each proffers resources to the business of 'making normal'; needing, at an unconscious level, to fill an imagined void. But in doing so both may silence the lived reality of being different, or the simple experience of being who one is.

Solutions, entitlement and passivity

> **L**: You know, the reality I see is that I pose some … opposition, to these solutions, because, it feels like this person doesn't know what it's like to … spend a day in my shoes.
>
> **F**: … a lot of the way that people who really care about me interact with me is to offer those [solutions] … a way of showing that you care is to provide answers. Which, of course, ends up in this strange cycle of … needing to thank people for caring, and for providing the answers, and explaining why you … don't or can't make that choice … it becomes more work if people try and provide you with answers than if they didn't.
>
> **J**: … you get the problem-solvers. Well, some of them have valid points. But often you see people listening, and they're trying to say 'well, what about this?', and as you talk they're trying to work out how to overcome it [laughs]. And so I've had this conversation with people, and they go 'Yeah, but, but, but', and I go 'Yeah, but, but, but', and they say 'well what about … ', and then at the end of the day they sort of go 'Yeah, OK', [sighs]. And they're kind of … deflated.

The simple proposition of this section is the following: people chronically deprived of resources readily available to others may internalise material inequalities, making it harder to feel deserving. In the case of disability, socialisation to do with deserving – what one is and is not entitled to – is likely to have been distorted. Ongoing experiences of exclusion, guilt or permissiveness in formative relationships, and awareness of the stereotype of the entitled disabled person, buffet the growing self and confuse perceptions of fairness. Given this, it is not surprising that we see conditioned distortions of deserving among disabled people, including self-denial, spartanism and acquiescence to marginal lives, and the stereotype of passivity and entitlement (as in Freud's 'exceptions'). Entitlement may at times be based on reaction formation, responding, in fact, to feelings of undeserving. Of course, at other times it may be a simple, appropriate anger at injustice. The resilient stereotype of the passive victim seems a simple consequence of the fact that vast numbers of disabled people live lives of continuous deprivation with little prospect of change. Clinical accounts characterise this experience as an 'insane' distinction between 'haves' and 'have nots', somehow casual and arbitrary, yet brutally policed. An example is the distinction between those who may go to a restaurant or bar, onto a beach, to the home of a friend, to a theatre or cinema, to a party, wedding or other celebration, to an antenatal class, a library, a gallery, onto several forms of public transport – and those who, due to the nature of the built environment, simply cannot. These examples all appear in my clinical work with physically impaired people, but similar silent exclusions are easily identifiable with a range of impairments. The core experience described by respondents was of a numbing, senseless expulsion from sharing in that most basic resource – human contact. As with any trauma, it is unlikely that such experiences would be integrated in a value-free, sterile way; instead, unconscious meanings are attached relating to personal history and worth.

According to Marks (1999a), passivity and acquiescence may be a defence against rage at repeated exclusion. But also demonstrated in the quotations which opened this section is a dynamic relationship between manic needs to repair, and the withdrawal of disabled people into a passive, possibly angry position. In disabled lives a familiar experience is of 'solutions' to practical difficulties being mooted by nondisabled others. 'Why don't you try this?' or 'what about doing it this way?', and 'haven't you thought of that?' are common, mild confrontations. Such questions apparently assume that the disabled person concerned does not, as a rule, explore options or resources in facilitating functionality. Meanwhile, unseen to the querying observer, life may be filled with a daily onslaught of intractable dilemmas, exclusions and discomforts. Against this backdrop, the hopeful or cheery suggestions of the observer may feel patronising and defensive, attending more to projected fears than practical realities. The stream of 'solutions' may appear as an exhausting sign of the chronic un-recognition of the realities faced in such lives. Further, while some 'solutions' might be feasible, observers are probably oblivious to the fact that the careful organisation and planning required is simply impossible in light of the time-consuming, physically demanding, unpredictable and complicated nature of impaired life in a barrier-ridden world. The psychological crux of the *solutions discourse* is control, demanded of individuals in the absence of real knowledge of their circumstances. One quadriplegic man compared his feelings about 'solutions' to the response of black consciousness to white liberalism; he commented:

> **F**: You know, the notion of black consciousness, the attack on white liberalism … It's like 'you guys, I know that you're trying, but you … reaffirm everything that the harsh oppressor says about us by trying to be positive … but [small laugh] in this deeply patronising way'. It's a … deeply disabling experience. Like of somebody coming to the townships and explaining to you how to … solve your problems.

The unconscious psychological flipside of these energetic imperatives is, I believe, a basic human fear of 'deathly inertia', of giving in to depression. This is the ominous, yet also inviting part of us which – true to Freud's (1920) *death drive* – feels like 'lying down and giving up'. Winnicott (1963) describes a dynamic in early attachment relationships in which the gratifying of needs, such as through feeding, actually embodies a *silencing* of the infant's experience. This seems analogous, in adult relating, to a focus on material needs displacing recognition of emotional realities. For disabled people the putting forward of 'solutions' may momentarily sever contact between inner and social worlds, as the expression of experience is inundated and repelled inward by the weight of resolution.

Burlingham (1961), in her work with congenitally blind children, found that subtle signs of guilt and withdrawal in mothers rendered a passivity in infants 'far beyond' (p. 122) what she could ascribe to impairment. She also identified a relationship between physical dependency, such as that caused by sight impairment, and the concealment of rage (ibid.). Exclusion from participation, anger or confusion at being unseen and passive withdrawal thus seem closely entwined. Passivity may hide what is, in fact, a hostile giving over of control, which enacts the unseen reality of a constant symbolic disenfranchisement. Importantly, anger expressed in one locale may have been evoked in a range of others – what Olkin (1999, p. 77) refers to as 'decontextualised rage' – leading to disabled individuals being branded irrational or maladjusted. Consider accounts of institutionalised persons with cerebral palsy. In these stories, episodes of rage were thought to result from organic causes. Sinason (1992) reinterprets these emotions as rational responses to the control, guilt-ridden permissiveness, over-protection and abuse which were routinely part of institutional life. Passivity, here, is a sensible defence against repercussions which an honest expression of rage may evoke from a milieu unable to see 'impaired behaviour' as coherent.

The reality of limited choices

> **M**: But, I think, in terms of disability and managing being disabled in society, there are very stark prices to be paid no matter which fork of any road you take. You make a choice, but it's kind of … between evils. Most of the time you're on … the losing side, and the choice is just … what form of losing you're going to be doing. It's constant compromise … although often times I recognise what the choices are in terms of being in those relationships.

A reality which sets the tone for all the relational distortions described here is the lack of accessible environments, resources and services. Inequality places disabled people in chronically compromising positions, as access to essential resources may hinge on the way relationships are managed. Murphy (1987) makes the following comments on his experience of transport-related dependency:

> In all this, they [people with mobility impairments] are passive recipients, waiting for the world to come to them – in its own time, if at all.
>
> (Murphy, 1987, p. 77)

Later, and in more general terms, he describes the distorting effect of physical dependency on relationships:

> [dependency is] … a condition that warps all one's … social ties and further contaminates the identity of the dependent … [dependence] … assails and tests even some bonds that we hope are impermeable, such as those of marriage.
>
> (Murphy, 1987, p. 199)

The simple need for assistance may place disabled individuals in the role of managing multiple relationships. In particular, they may be challenged with monitoring, understanding and preventing the control and enmeshment so prevalent around disability. Assistance often affords a degree of preconscious, gratifying control to the helper – what Marks (1999a, p. 22) terms a 'psychic pay-off'. If compromising relationships are not deliberately altered, dynamics quickly become entrenched, making realignment a thorny, difficult task (see Shaw, 2001). It may seem sensible here to give the disabled individual responsibility for defining boundaries, and blame him or her for relationship problems. But this ignores the reality of limited material choices faced by disabled people in an inaccessible world. Individuals may be forced to collude with ways of relating which feel wrong, for the sake of survival. If Z, in the example above, lived in a society with accessible transportation, her ability to understand and manage her relationship with C would be greatly enhanced, through operating from a position of equal power. But most engagements between disabled and nondisabled people occur across an array of inequalities, clouding the possibility of bounded, self-assertive relating (Eberhardt and Mayberry, 1995).

No-one would question that relationships can be baffling at the best of times. But in an uncertain, disablist world requiring hard work and creativity for simple survival, it is unrealistic to expect individuals to possess the energy and insight required to unpick these largely unconscious transactions. The model which emerges is one of interlocking relational and material forces, drawing disabled people away from internal experience, and undermining the power and legitimacy needed for authentic relating. Because of requiring assistance from friends, family members, health practitioners or care workers, disabled people have a specific need for the skills of managing relationships in a clear, bounded and assertive manner. Ironically and painfully though, such individuals may have undergone socialisation which directly contradicts these needs, instead fostering placation and accommodation. In light of these ideas, it is not difficult to see how the stereotype of the manipulative disabled person has come into view. In a depriving world, disabled people may be forced into relating in terms of pragmatic trade-offs where, for example, controlling or intrusive relationships are tolerated in order to retain access to a vital resource. Such trade-offs may be conscious and deliberate or unconscious products of layered socialisation, where boundaries have been contravened and resources are out of reach. Morris (1993, p. 102), as a disabled person, describes feeling enraged or undermined without clearly understanding why. Unequal relating may be so embedded that strong emotional responses may appear unreasonable, even to the self (ibid.).

Collusion and complicity

While unequal access to material resources creates distorted relationships, their unconscious perpetuation is always a reciprocal matter. Further, making sense of the hidden, tangled dynamics of relationships shaped by disability is as confusing, if not more so, for nondisabled persons than their counterparts. There is reflection and debunking to be done on all sides. A theme of this book is that to construct disabled people as passive recipients of a unidirectional force called 'oppression' is to mystify and re-bury the workings of inequality. Temperley (1984) describes feeling unease at a similarly reductionist view of gender oppression:

> It seems to me fatally easy for a group that has been disadvantaged or exploited to idealise itself and to believe that, once the privileges of the oppressors are removed, the hated qualities associated with those oppressors will cease to be the social problems they were before.
>
> (Temperley, 1984, p. 25)

If we fail to theorise the role played by disabled people in unequal relationships we, in effect, support the illusion of essential difference between disabled and nondisabled people. Again, we are confronted with an inviting but misleading split. It is a split which, in my view, demeans disabled people by constructing them as victims, while maintaining that social trauma has not made impressions on styles of relating. This is misguided nonsense. If oppressive relations involving any identity were not bi-directional and dynamic, society would long since have achieved unseen levels of equality. Interpellation into unconsciously supporting power relations is a fundamental reality. And, together with this, projective identification is at the psychological heart of social oppression. Shame-ridden parts are elicited in the other, which are then exaggerated, preparing the way for further projections. The object of projection then experiences these as his or her own (Young, 1994). The uncertainty expressed by Morris (1993) about the reasons for her emotional responses fits well here – uncertainty about ownership of feelings and characteristics often signals the presence of projective identification. Projected materials have found a home inside the recipient, intermingling with the range of feelings which life in a barrier-ridden world will evoke: anger, shame, hurt, guilt and much else. If we honestly consider this painful picture, complicity is an unavoidable reality, albeit a political taboo. Exploring the ambivalence and uncertainty rooted in lives of trauma is a first step to diminishing the power of projective identification. The social model's materialist focus has simplified the disabled subject. Getting to grips with the experience of disabled people will involve hearing internal conflict, ambivalence, collusion, confusion. Self-knowledge is the crux of de-colonisation.

The discourse of independence

> **L**: … I think it's also a psychological … fear that we all have, that we're … less than … we want to be. It [dependency] speaks to that basic insecurity … And I would term my disability … hyper-dependent … that hyper-dependence I think becomes like the high water mark of our insecurities … you really are stripped back to an infantile state, and so … everything that gives you value in society is stripped away … in a moment … but I think it also speaks to a very deep fear we have … that we've … failed in a very profound way … that we've failed full stop.
>
> **R**: … after a lot of work I manage to transfer myself onto my bed and then back onto my chair, which is an incredibly difficult process for me … it took me … about six months to get that right. Well the problem is when you're getting out of bed into your chair, and by the time you get into your chair you feel like getting back into bed. And I realised that actually … it's not where I really need to put my energy every day.
>
> **T**: And so as part of my rehab as well I had to learn to take off and put on my shoes, but I obviously don't have any hands and so I had to use my mouth. I had to use my teeth to undo my shoes, to put them on again. It was just insane, I was literally completely exhausted after doing that.

It is commonly assumed that disabled people desire and strive for independence (French, 1993c). Whatever the position, what is clear is that dependency is a highly contested cultural idea. The reasons for avoiding it have complex socio-political as well as psychological roots. As should be evident from the discussion so far, one reason why a disabled individual may seek independence is to avoid the relational entanglements which accompany assistance. Cheerful gratitude, the repression of anger and the sidelining of emotional and physical needs are familiar to all. But beyond this, disabled people may be socialised into an experience of self as dependent on benevolence, through material deprivation and disablist discourse. The idea of the 'independent subject' is a culturally specific one, mobilised by the discourse of neoliberal autonomy, some strands of feminism and the tradition of humanistic psychology (Treacher, 1989). Dependency, in this thought environment, is viewed as toxic and destructive to the human spirit. In a world where the shame and relational distortions of need are a consequence of ostensibly just modes of exchange, dependency also represents failure in accumulating the trappings of the autonomous citizen. Underscoring the cultural specificity of this picture, noted social anthropologist Clifford Geertz writes:

> The Western conception of the person as a bounded, unique, more or less integrated motivational and cognitive universe, a dynamic centre of awareness, emotion, judgment and action organised into a distinctive whole and set contrastively both against other such wholes and against its social and natural background, is, however incorrigible it may seem to us, a rather peculiar idea within the context of the world's cultures.
>
> (Geertz, 1993 cited in Hughes, 2001, p. 25)

Echoing the respondents above, disability studies carries many accounts of the 'normalising' drive of rehabilitation involving excessive strivings for independence in everyday tasks. Critical here is that medical discourse may draw practitioners and clients towards an ideal of material independence which easily marginalises psychological needs. French (1993c) cites examples quite similar to those above. In one case, for a severely physically impaired man the basic task of removing socks became a rehabilitative goal consuming enormous physical and emotional energy, to the detriment of more rewarding activities. Corbett (1989) presents the picture as follows:

> The basics of self-help, which are second nature to the able bodied, might be an intolerable chore to some people with disabilities. Why should they bother with them? A narrow focus upon basic skills impedes the quality of life and inhibits self-expression.
>
> (Corbett, 1989 cited in French, 1993c, p. 44)

Whose psychological needs are being filled by securing fragments of independence? Discourses of rehabilitation tend to orient all towards physical adjustment, while seldom posing questions about the cultural imperatives at work (Phillips, 1985; Ingstad and White, 1995). Culturally informed anxieties about difference shape health care practices which view alternative lifestyles as, at best, a final port of call; at worst, as failure. It must be reiterated, though, that these motivations are most often shared by all – practitioners, patients and families. The devaluing of life possibilities characterised by difference, in these circumstances, seems inevitable.

Social model thinkers view dependency as a context-specific outcome of unequal resource distribution (Oliver, 1993b). Extending this position is the idea that 'independence' is a relative concept rather than a categorical one, as society is built on universal inter-dependence (Lonsdale, 1990). This perspective sees non-disabled independence as a myth. Against a backdrop of universal dependency, the 'dependencies' of disabled people are singled out and disallowed by a culture which abhors difference. As a partially sighted person in an occupational setting, it became evident to French (1993c) that all employees – disabled and not – had limitations, and needed help and support from one another. But the legitimacy of these needs was unequal. She writes:

> … able-bodied people's problems are regarded as normal and acceptable, and thus they can ask assistance of each other without feeling guilty or inferior. Disabled people can ask for help too as long as they steer clear of any problems directly associated with disability … thus disabled people are often expected to cope with their limitations in a way not expected of other people.
>
> (French, 1993c, p. 46)

Asch (2001) comments wryly that all in modern societies depend on service providers to perform tasks which are beyond us – from car mechanics to computer technicians, plumbers to lawyers. But the normative status of these needs neutralises evidence of dependency, while qualitatively indistinguishable assistance in, say, dressing and washing, is a signal of failure. This discussion applies where essential services are provided. Across most of the world this is not the case, leaving physically impaired people reliant on the voluntarism of family and friends. Of course, we must recognise disabled individuals' desire for independent living, advocating for appropriate services, universal design and client-driven rehabilitation. But careful reflection by all is needed to make sense of why independence seems so irresistibly attractive. Interlocking material and psychological forces are at work. These are mutually constitutive and very difficult to disrupt.

Shakespeare (2006), ever watchful about accepted wisdom, views the reasoning that all are dependent as rather disingenuous, even trite. Conventional dependency is, in his assessment, 'very different' to the extreme needs for care of, say, severely physically impaired people (p. 146). With Shakespeare (2006), I believe that the disability movement's largely deconstructionist position on this issue risks sidestepping the real, thorny experience of acute dependence. A part of this is the inescapable, complex problem of inequalities in the giving and receiving of physical care. This does not contradict earlier thoughts on the positioning of disabled people as emotional carers, silently taking responsibility for managing relationships. The picture, instead, is one where these issues support and compound one another, as silence around the taboo of physical need translates into a compensatory holding of the emotional needs of carers, including needs for projection. Clinical accounts of severely physically impaired persons show the exhausting complexity of negotiating relationships with employed care workers or family members, with the nagging idea of dependency as shame continually draining emotional energy. Dependency as a human universal is philosophically undeniable. But this position risks foreclosing an examination of lifelong relationships of potentially acute dependency which are integral to disabled socialisation. The idea that adequately resourced social services will make these complexities 'go away' is both naïve and disrespectful, ignoring the very real influence of unconscious transactions.

Frosh (1991) sees the glittering veneer of narcissistic society as primarily a means to disguise a fear and hatred of being dependent on others. Acknowledging need exposes the individual to a possible repetition of the primary rejection which is at the heart of narcissistic functioning. In Klein's (1957) framework, destructive envy – so evident in late modern, consumerist society – is intimately connected to the hatred of dependency. The hatefulness of envy lies in impulses to destroy that which is valued simply because it cannot be controlled, and is thus evidence of dependency – of need. In Hoggett's (1992) words, envy embodies 'both a desperate attempt to deny this sense of lack and an attack upon the things which prompt it' (p. 23). Attacks on the 'dependencies' of disabled people may, thus, reflect a complex of shame-ridden dissociation from need, and hatred emanating from envy for an illusory, idealised dependent state. This latter aspect is a projection of the fantasy of a perfectly attuned caring relationship, in which all needs are admissible and attended to. Earlier we explored the possible connection of this fantasy to disability hate crime.

Control

> **L**: It's … predictability … there's just a higher level of predictability about your place in the world and your interaction with the world when you're not disabled.
>
> **F**: The thought of never being secure … and maybe I'm generalising here a bit, but that is one of the characteristics of what it feels like to be disabled. It's never having absolute security … and so to live your life having experienced, you know, complete security, probably means you now fill … quite a different space.
>
> **T**: Something I'm trying to learn at the moment is how to … how to balance the life I'm wanting to live with … the life my body is able to accommodate. Just trying to find that balance, and it's an ongoing thing for me.

Clinical experience of people with a range of impairments reveals the painful work of endlessly having to relinquish control. As an adjunct, living according to the schedules of others, and often having to wait, is ubiquitous. Reasons at play here are a mix of material barriers, the complexity of helping relationships, and the realities of impairment-based limitation. But the common denominator is enduring a continuing lack of feelings of control, needed by most people to enhance security and positive self-identity. It is far harder to find one's secure, self-accepting inner foundations when alienated from choice. Showing oneself – 'being' oneself – occurs here despite circumstances, rather than because of the comfort and safety one would choose. Further, prejudiced, barrier-ridden environments bring daily unpredictability, creating lives in which improvisation, disappointment, 'making do', realigning expectations and enduring discomfort are the norm. Managing the emotional experience of un-control here requires its own energy, draining resources needed for material action. Oliver (1995) concluded that it was this lack of control over physical and social worlds, rather than the experience of impairment, which was at the root of emotional difficulties among disabled people. Again, we see the ideologically driven logic of 'one or the other'. My own clinical experience is more mixed. Welcoming embodiment means foregoing convenient distinctions; and we can do so without losing sight of the cruel inequality which is the cornerstone of life with impairment.

Clinical material shows subjective control to be bound up with the unconscious pacts of assistive relationships, set against functional limitation. The risks of claiming control are based on assessment of the unconscious investments of carers regarding dependency, altruistic roles, anxieties about separation and much else. It has become clear to me that few severely functionally impaired persons are not aware of the tender, even precious unconscious investments in the caring role which form the unspoken backdrop to assistance. The awkward, at times excruciating difficulty of transforming the sedimented helping culture of some charity organisations presents the same picture. Taking back control is hard when this means subverting the hidden identity needs of the other. But as noted, it may be as difficult for the disabled 'patient' to see through these layered investments. The key is identifying boundary distortions, and how these are created and maintained. The co-occurrence of a physical and relational world which denies control with a culture demanding autonomy, leaves the disabled person to wrestle with an impossible incongruity. 'This', says the world, 'is how you must be', but simultaneously 'this, too, is how you cannot be'.

At the heart of control of one's environment is the expression of identity. Personal lifestyle options, spontaneous choices about one's day, preferences in personal contact – being able to realise inner currents in these actions is an expression of self. These possibilities may often be overwhelmed by limited choices and pragmatic requirements for survival. Murphy (1987) describes the deadening of self-expression in his life:

> This loss of spontaneity invaded my entire assessment of time ... It rigidified my short-range perspectives and introduced a calculating quality into an existence that formerly had been pleasantly disordered ...
>
> (Murphy, 1987, p. 76)

Echoing clinical accounts, Murphy (1987) mentions such everyday activities as going outside for fresh air, getting a snack, going shopping or to visit a friend. All such activities came to require planning, substantial effort and, most of all, the cooperation of others. This is a life-world very far removed from the autonomous control of the modernist vision, and the trappings of narcissism which bolster it. The view of disabled people being unconsciously appropriated as public bearers of the human struggles denied by others again seems convincing. Assessing the inequality in access to 'materials of narcissism', one notes the common expectation that disabled people show gratitude for virtually any level of inclusion. In a dramatic contrast, products, technologies and living spaces are meticulously designed and redesigned to satisfy not only the needs, but the wants of the majority. Fitting interestingly with these ideas on narcissism, Hunt (1998) remarks that disabled people have a 'special insight' to offer the human world, through living the 'passive aspect that is one half of the human reality' (p. 11). He writes:

> Those who lead active lives are perhaps especially inclined to ignore man's [sic.] need to accept passivity in relation to so many forces beyond his control. They may need reminding sometimes of our finiteness, our feminine [sic.] side in the hands of fate or providence.
>
> (Hunt, 1998, p. 11)

Depression

> **M**: ... and I think there's something there as well in terms of us developing an alternative, collective voice. You know, it's the same reason ... why the long awaited for [racial/class] revolution never happened, that that level of passivity becomes expressed in ... the least destructive form of self-hatred you can find ... whatever that expression might be ... I don't think that disabled

> people are even that enabled, I don't think we've even been able to express in material ways ... or. ... through beating people up ... There's no ... literally no lower power person to take it out on.

In the quotation above a severely physically impaired man compares his psycho-social circumstances to those of dislocated, racially oppressed communities in South Africa. He paints a picture of suffering engendered by both disablism and impairment, with little or no outlet – adaptive or otherwise – for its expression. The rageful, violent acting out prevalent in disadvantaged communities seems out of reach, as he observes that there is 'no lower person to take it out on'. His intentions are not at all violent; these observations are abstract, and to me reflect a highly sophisticated analysis of where the severely physically impaired identity fits into society's hierarchies. The crux of his message was of feeling and enduring so much, but being positioned in a way which stifles expression or resistance, as well as opportunities for sublimation.[1] The effect is silently living or swallowing the internal consequences of a denigrated identity, and feeling domesticated into the binary lies upon which modernity rests. My own clinical experience often relates depression in disability to the pain of a lack of authentic relating from others, in conjunction with experiences of hurtful mirroring – both from the human world and barrier-ridden environments.

> **F**: I think my own journey is particularly lonely because ... I feel I see the dynamics that other people ... don't, and often times choose not to. It's the Pandora's box kind of moment, of kind of recognising ... the real unhappiness of what's going on, rather than the surface unhappiness of it all.

F reflects here on how relational spaces around him have become distorted since he became impaired, leaving him feeling starved of direct, honest contact. Living in the face of a current of projections requires constant re-girding of self, especially with little access to the material distractions of consumerist life. One severely impaired woman associated her bouts of depression with the constant need to be 'nice', while managing feelings of rage and loss at relentless exclusion. It was the personal meanings of exclusion, as well as the material deprivation, which at times brought despair. Exclusions destabilised self-worth, as hurtful mirroring reinforced self-criticism. This self-attack relegated her to an old, familiar confusion about the 'real' meaning of impairment; whether it did indeed (as in common prejudices) imply that she was of intrinsically less worth.

As we have seen, material aspects of disablism are very difficult to separate from psychological meanings which, in turn, are in part informed by socialisation in a prejudiced world. The meaning of impairment is contested daily in disabled lives, at manifest and invisible levels. This is a continuous battle to overcome cultural imputations of abjection. Coleridge (1993, p. 37) views impairment-based rejection as carrying 'catastrophic' results. Dismissal or disgust from the social world 'provokes despair and retreat, which in turn widens the gap and produce[s] further rejection and stereotyping' (ibid.). In clinical experience I am mostly amazed at the robustness of self shown by disabled individuals in the face of discrimination. But often, it seems, it is the *consistency* of exclusion – the presence of ongoing trauma – which exhausts emotional resources. At issue is the difficulty of waging a battle on two fronts; that is, in inner and outer worlds. Internally, the re-aggravation of old wounds to identity is a constant source of destabilisation.

With particular reference to disability, Charlton (1998, p. 77) views nihilism as a central aspect of oppression, describing this as 'alienation in its most desperate stage'. Social manifestations of nihilism include suicide, crime, domestic violence and substance abuse – the sorts of 'acting out' which M above regards as largely out of the disabled community's reach. Besides the physical, material nature of marginal living spaces, self-blame may be a key reason for this. Suicidality is the exception and, as we have seen, carries specific relevance in bioethics debates around disability. With characteristic vehemence, Adrienne Asch (2001) places such struggle firmly at the door of an abandoning society. She argues that the desirability of dying to some disabled people is a consequence of how 'there is so little medical or social assistance in living' (p. 315).

Disabled super-ego

> **L**: But that doesn't change the fact that you've got a conditioned mind. You know, you say something, and all of a sudden, you're hearing yourself, and starting to judge yourself … it's like, you're just not good enough, you don't deserve to have good experiences.
>
> **R**: I've got a mind that likes to try and solve problems. I think up problems just to solve them … And then I find myself confronted with my disability, and trying to work out, how can I actually solve the problem, and I would just beat my head again and again against the wall, because there was no logic … It's like … a conundrum.
>
> **J**: I don't want to just be an equal human being or a … good disabled person … For a disabled person being exceptional, not just because they're disabled, but because they're exceptional, is kind of read as … a larger feat. But it means that the things I ask of myself are that much more intense, the road I walk is that much more … steep. There's very little room there for … fallibility.
>
> **F**: But you see, where I'm coming from … I always feel I have to achieve, achieve and achieve, and I'm never happy with who I am … The disability makes it worse. I feel like … I'm never good enough. And that I have to not have ataxia in order to be good enough … That's how I feel, but I'm trying to change it.

The approach that this book takes is to be curious about all constructions of disability, be these theoretical or colloquial, politically correct or ideologically ignorant. I believe that psychoanalytic exploration can tie contradictory ideas together, connecting all as differing responses to a shared unconscious narrative that disability brings. As already described, the traditional psychoanalytic reading of Freud's (1916) essay *The exceptions* views impairment as leading to a weak super-ego, where rules of fairness and morality are seen as inapplicable (Jacobson, 1959). My own impression from clinical experience is the converse. Social control, communicated in many forms, is a core element of life with disablism. It should not surprise us that this at times translates into strict internal self-evaluations. Imperatives to normalise, change and overcome are literally everywhere, and appeal to the most stringent, self-critical parts. The language of solutions points to what is wrong or should be done differently, reiterating why subjective struggle is essentially the fault of the individual. Media representations revere those who, instead of 'making excuses', choose to 'see adversity as challenge'. This messaging may haunt individuals with doubt, blaming the self for going about things the wrong way, not planning adequately, neglecting relationships, not being assertive enough, being too negative; and so the list continues. In the midst of ongoing, traumatic assaults on identity, it is very difficult to find the thought space to separate one's own views from prejudiced demands. Instead, one may fulfil the dance of projective identification by actively focusing on *disproving* what is ascribed. As will be clear, I do not view the punitive super-ego as a 'pathology' of impaired people, but as a consequence of ideological control – one which makes self-compassion more difficult to find. But let us return to Freud (1916) and the 'exceptions'. Of interest is how two such contradictory ideas about disability could emerge. On one hand is the view that disabled people tend to be dependent and shirk accountability, claiming 'exceptional' status. On the other, disabled people seem prone to overly harsh, self-imposed standards. How can this be? There is, I believe, more in common between these positions than it may seem.

Both reflect the effects, in disabled and nondisabled actors alike, of boundary distortion. As noted earlier, the question of 'what I deserve' is a human fundamental. Disabled lives are filled with a culturally and unconsciously informed clamour of disagreement about this. The chaotic, contradictory limits of material deprivation, spartan institutional life, permissive charity culture, 'special needs' services, anxious or ambiguous familial relationships and much else compose a chequered world of messaging about what is fair. Over this past week I have heard many people say that Oscar Pistorius' omission from South Africa's team for the 4 × 100m men's final at the World Athletics Championships was 'unfair' and 'a shame'. Others say 'well, he wasn't fast enough'. Still others say 'his place is in paralympic, not mainstream sport'. Some paralympic commentators believe that his category qualification for paralympic competition was a mistake, and that he has an unfair advantage (Howe, 2011 – personal communication). This example shows the diverse cultural commodification of disabled stories. The fact is that all observers are invested, all have strong feelings about who one is and what one deserves (Swartz and Watermeyer, 2008). Burkett et al. (2011) express Pistorius' public phantasm as follows:

> Oscar Pistorius might be viewed as: an athlete attempting to achieve his potential at the 100m sprint; a vanguard figure, challenging the deficit model

> of disability; someone whose performative self challenges the borders of human identity and technology; a sub-elite athlete attempting to break into the lucrative world of elite commercialised sports via technological assistance; or an athlete using unfair means to compete at the Olympics. These options are not exclusive.
>
> (Burkett et al., 2011, p. 645)

Such are the life-worlds of visibly impaired persons. Confused narratives of entitlement seem a predictable consequence. Cultural responses to the disabled body are nothing if not ambivalent. Further, a psychoanalytic view would see entitlement and self-deprivation as closely related for any population. The so-called entitlements of 'exceptionalism' are associated with both political recognition of inequality, and unconscious struggles with deserving. Jacobson's (1959) identifying of self-punishing fantasies fits with this, but with the huge proviso that no recognition of social injustice was considered. According to Davids (1996, p. 231), projected 'psychic dirt' most often contains psychotic fragments, far too hazardous to readily 'welcome back' – the fervent cultural, emotional and political commodification of disability stories is testimony to this. If change is to happen it will involve 'great pain, anguish and upheaval', through the re-owning of chaotic, traumatising aspects of inner life (ibid.). Also coming into view are the punitive demands of narcissistic culture, applying to all. In response to authoritarian requirements to measure up, disablist culture turns on incipient failures, as a proportion of any population will do when fighting attacks on identity. In a culture which subverts containment of its humanity, it is inevitable that someone be found to carry the humiliation of the collective.

Note

1 Sublimation is a defence mechanism involving the managing of difficult unconscious feelings through useful activities. These actions give some symbolic expression to the unseen emotion, such as using competitive sport to healthily channel aggression, or the creative arts to express conflicts to do with identity or intimacy.

9 Disability and loss

Introduction

The questions of whether disability involves loss, what the nature of this may be, and what it results from remain emotive and politically charged. As we shall see, ascriptions of loss to disabled life are everywhere. In this chapter I critically examine the discourse of loss as it pertains to disability, exploring how political and cultural contestation of the disabled figure can combine in silencing authentic expression of life with disablism. The disability movement's understandable drive to provide counter-narratives to the view of disability as pathology may place disabled people in invidious circumstances in relation to their own inner lives. The debate around loss is a useful demonstration.

Medical and rehabilitation discourse invariably associates disability with loss (e.g. Vash and Crewe, 2004). Similarly, artistic and media representations that characterise disabled life as material and emotional loss are ubiquitous. The bereavement model of some psychological approaches to disability revolves around loss – its denial, acceptance and implications (Oliver, 1995; Olkin, 1999; Gill, 2001; Watermeyer, 2009). 'Acceptance' here implies submission to the essentialist reality of impairment (Lenny, 1993). Disabled people live in the teeth of a gale of projections to do with loss (Watermeyer, 2009). The misery of loss presents less here as a human consequence of impairment than as its intrinsic, self-evident nature. Understandably, the idea of 'disability loss' has been rejected in strong terms by social model authors (e.g. Morris, 1989; Lonsdale, 1990; Oliver, 1990; Abberley, 1993; Finkelstein and French, 1993). At the centre of the loss discourse are the sentimental disability images exploited by some charity organisations. Rituals of conspicuous benevolence such as the telethon rely on constructions of disability as loss, in order to provoke giving (Garland-Thomson, 1997b; Longmore, 1997; Michalko, 2002).

Social model rejection of ideas of loss relates to the construction of disabled people as incomplete, justifying segregation and other forms of control. Media representations miss the opportunity to reflect disabled people going about the business of life, full as it is of the universal ups and downs of muddling through. Instead, tragedy, dependency, redemption and every other companion to the spectre of loss are ever-present. The disabled imago epitomises loss in modern society, crying out for intervention, benevolence or consolation (Watermeyer, 2006). My intention here is to critique the selecting out of disabled people as the primary custodians of the layer of humanness, but also – perhaps more controversially – to question the politically motivated dissociation of disabled lives from loss. To be alive, to grow and develop, to hope and relate means to experience loss. At issue is the way in which disablist discourse distorts access to, and representation of, that part of inner life in disabled people.

The loss discourse

> **R**: It's like with old friends of mine I used to know, and they'll see me at a party or something, and they can't relate. To them it's … the whole tragedy. And so they ask me how are you doing and how's your work and stuff, and they want reassurance from me that I'm OK, which I'll duly tell them, and that's kind of that.
>
> **F**: Oh, yeah, people pray for you. I've been prayed for so many times it's a miracle I can't walk. And people can be … incredibly rude and invasive about it.
>
> **G**: I think, in my case, if I could move my arms, I could be seen to be doing something, but what I can do, people just don't see … they have no idea what I'm capable of or not capable of. All they see is me being fed and watered … not … doing anything else. Like a big … baby … I guess that's how they see it.

The work of Thomas and Siller (1999) is a useful example of psychology's approach to 'disability loss', drawing explicitly on Freud's *Mourning and melancholia* (1917). They write that emotional responses to disablement 'frequently' follow 'identical lines' to those of bereavement, including 'shock, expectation of recovery, mourning, defence … and adjustment' (p. 186). But more than two decades of research has failed to validate stagewise models such as theirs (Gill, 2001). Instead, disabled people have been found to follow unique, personal styles of managing life situations (Oliver, 1995). Most psychological support for people who have become disabled almost certainly remains rooted in a grief model, setting impairment up as the only real problem. Mental state or quality of relationships here is viewed as a function of adjustment to impairment. Trouble in these areas may attract the label of 'denial'.

Deliberately countering the discourse, disability studies research presents evidence that many disabled people do not identify the onset of disability as a loss (e.g. Campling, 1981; Morris, 1989; Finkelstein and French, 1993; Lenny, 1993); Disability, it seems, may be experienced as enriching, through stimulating a process of questioning assumptions about human life and the nature of society. As we have seen, a range of writers see disabled subjectivity as having much to contribute to the creation of a more humane, caring and critical society (Davis, 2002; Michalko, 2002). A core proposition of this book is that disablism, like other forms of oppression, is based on a denial of the right to define one's experience.

The symbolic violence which accompanies disability makes self-definition very difficult. While there is no reason to question the experiences of disability in the studies just mentioned, of interest is their position as counterpoints to stereotype. An important question is whether these stories involve an exclusion of parts of disability experience which *do* carry loss, resulting from whatever combination of contextual and bodily factors. It seems to me that deliberately excluding loss means colluding with a false binary, re-enacting a silence cast on real lives. The heavily criticised sentimentality of some phenomenological research may fall into the same binary, but in the alternate position. The path to an articulate, measured and authentic voice of disabled subjectivity is not the reactionary emphasising of the positive in response to a damning negative. Instead, the discourse which underpins both accounts must be overturned. Quoting Arthur Kleinman and colleagues, Michalko (2002) contemplates where the truth of social suffering lies. In other words, asking whether it is possible to escape suffering while steeped in cultural messaging which attaches it to the essence of the self. Kleinman et al. (1997) write:

> Social suffering is a feature of cultural representation both as spectacle and as a presentation of the real … how we 'picture' social suffering becomes that experience, for the observers and even for the sufferers' perpetrators. What we represent and how we represent it prefigure what we will, or will not, do to intervene. What is not pictured is not real. Much of routinised misery is invisible; much that is made visible is not ordinary or routine. The very act of picturing distorts social experience in the popular media. … even personal 'witnessing' is compromised. We are living through a great historical transformation in the imaging, and therefore perhaps also in the experience, of social adversity.
>
> (Kleinman et al., 1997, pp. xii–xiii)

Applying this to the disability arena, we see how the grief model creates specific spaces for the imagining of disabled subjectivity which inform social responses. The more we imagine, the less we hear. The discourse of loss functions culturally as a means of mastery over disability's frightening unknowns (Watermeyer, 2009). At the heart of the observer's control is the illusion that what has been lost can be clearly seen from the outside. Ideas about 'overcoming denial' relate almost exclusively to impairment; discrimination is seldom named as loss. Consequently, many in the disabled community experience the idea of losses to be dealt with as an affront, seeing these as existing in the minds and defences of the observer. Loss is in all, and as we have seen, the disabled body is a lightning rod for split-off, painful projections from the social world. Disabled people's rejection of this ascribed loss, based on recognition that 'this is not mine', provides neat evidence of denial. But simultaneously, the disabled individual is aware that any acknowledgment of loss will usher in a pre-existing, highly elaborated stereotype of tragedy, which will cover him or her completely.

Acceptance and denial

> **M**: And I think because … there's that desperate search for meaning … everybody around you [is] … desperately trying to find that same thing. Like, 'where's the silver lining here?' … so there's this … sense of desperation to the whole conversation …
>
> **L**: I think before, there was this whole thing of we need to accept it. And then, saying I'd accepted it, when I knew I hadn't accepted it, and fighting with myself to accept something that I know I can't accept, because I can't accept it. Are there too many 'accepts' in that sentence?

The grief model requires attaining an imagined place of 'acceptance'. If difficult feelings or 'poor adjustment' persists, this is attributed to ongoing 'denial'. But in fact the discourse of acceptance and denial is a dynamic phenomenon, fluctuating in the intersubjective space, and serving the emotional needs of the observer. In a very moving account of her family life as a partially sighted child, French (1993b, p. 69) describes being surrounded by 'anxious relatives who were trying to get me to see things'. She presents a picture of adults struggling to digest the unthinkable knowledge that their beautiful niece or granddaughter could not see a rainbow, a hillside, a pretty bird. They would position her carefully, a gentle hand tilting her head to exactly the right angle, before pointing; 'look … look, there it is … there!' Even as a toddler French was acutely aware of the anxiety which would be evoked if she could not see what was being pointed out. Quite quickly she learned that the best option for everyone was for her to simply say 'yes', perhaps pretend to be excited and allow the unease to pass. In this way she was taught to deny her disability for the benefit of those around her. These familial experiences are certainly not uncommon, positioning such 'denial' as entirely rational. It is easy to see how such pressures extrapolate to every social context, leading to disguise. In French's (1993b) narrative, even adults not close to her elicited denials, through disbelieving her, or viewing her 'not seeing' as manipulation or mischief. The pressure to deny continued throughout adulthood; interestingly, however, it became more subtle. She writes:

> Disabled adults frequently evoke anxiety and embarrassment in others simply by their presence. Although they become very skilful at dealing with this, it is often achieved at great cost to themselves by denying their disabilities and needs. It is not unusual for disabled people to endure boredom or distress to safeguard the feelings of others … In situations like these reassuring phrases like 'I'm all right' or 'don't worry about me' become almost automatic.
>
> (French, 1993b, p. 74)

Bowlby (1979) describes a family dynamic in which parents subtly require their children to shut off from painful information, in the wish that the events or knowledge concerned had been kept from them. The silence is for everyone's protection. In the picture French (1993b) describes, adults may be operating from a dim fantasy of protecting the child from loss, failure or misconduct. Familial hierarchies are disrupted by such protectionism, as children learn to act as containers for grown-ups. According to Bowlby (1979), children in these circumstances may grow up struggling to trust their own senses, to trust others easily and to freely exercise curiosity. The subtle sense of danger present in adults' anxieties remains. In essence, Bowlby is talking about perceiving one reality and being told that another is true. In light of all we have seen, this experience of having one's subjective life contradicted is probably very pervasive in the lives of visibly impaired people. This supports the picture of a systemic withholding of containment; a moratorium on what one is allowed to feel.

Clinical accounts of the sudden onset of severe impairment show a picture of entire social systems shaken by trauma. As all struggle to integrate the traumatic change, dynamics of projection, protection, lack of containment and silence are clearly in evidence. The following excerpt is representative:

> **R**: Yeah, like this guy came in and said 'you're never going to walk again', and it just didn't sink in at all. He said 'you won't be able to move your arms again'; yeah, right. You can't comprehend that. It's impossible, it doesn't make sense … it just doesn't gel. And then, also the reaction of other people is very strange. And suddenly you're this [horrified sound] tragic figure and people you've known all your life are coming in and walking out crying and you think 'what's going on?' It's very odd. And there you are comforting them … [It's] very paradoxical. One of my best buddies came, he stayed a bit. And he kind of said I want to come and talk to you, I'm battling with this. And I remember being in hospital, my head kind of still in traction, and I'm like 'don't worry D, I'm strong, I'll be fine'. And he's cracking up by my bedside … but … you lose a lot of people you're involved with because they can't handle the situation.

From the first moments of regaining consciousness in his new life as a quadriplegic man, R was aware of pressure to contain others, as familiar faces above his bed crumpled and turned away. In the midst of the raw, overwhelming feelings reverberating through human networks after a traumatic event, he was required to safeguard contacts by reassuring. In time, though, much of this care proved ineffective, as many social contacts withdrew – a common experience in the traumatic onset of impairment (Braithwaite, 1990). Against this backdrop of an entire system struggling with chaotic feelings, the individualising demands of the 'acceptance discourse' show up as an almost ludicrous miscarriage. Further, the marginalising of R's own feelings about what is, in fact, his predicament alone, is painfully evident.

What relational signs have communicated to these disabled people is that their inner experience – in some sense, their nature – is not tolerable to others. It is on this marshy relational ground that the self must somehow find a way to validate experience, building the legitimacy so important for the growth of personal power.

The 'maladjustment' of behaviour labelled as denial may, in fact, be the tangled manifestation of the titrated losses of entire tracts of culture, channelled through the bodies and minds of disabled persons. Far from being solipsistic, these meanings are deeply social, pragmatic and political mechanisms supporting the social and psychological order.

On being 'un-disabled'

> **L**: The problem with this idea of heroes … there's pressures put upon you to be Superman, like 'you're amazing', or like 'I'm your biggest fan', and we've never even met before. And so you do so much, and there's just not a balance. You can't be just a regular guy trying to get on with your life … they elevate it to that status … And that gets in the way of just … being.
>
> **G**: And so … you work harder to be seen that you can do it. Or you try to. And even in yourself, it's like, 'am I wasting my time, am I not?'; 'am I tired, how tired am I?' You can get quite confused about it.
>
> **J**: … it's almost a case of if you can't join them you try and beat them … 'if an able-bodied person can climb Kilimanjaro, then so can we'. I think it has … a psychological flavour of 'we're going to do things you recognise', but, because we're doing them everyone recognises that it's fundamentally different … And I think that's a process of trying to find … a positive way of being different.

In *Moby Dick*, Herman Melville's Captain Ahab lives a life based on resisting categorisation, seeking to infinitely re-prove that he has not become what the world expects him to be (Kriegel, 1987). As a disabled man, Ahab is deeply aware of cultural assumptions portraying him as damaged and defeated. His life is an endless project of overturning this prejudice. Quite similarly, polio survivor F. D. Roosevelt knew that successfully leading the United States would require presenting a convincingly vigorous, nondisabled image to the American people (Finger, 2006). He countered the common attributions of tragedy and shame with a story of triumph over adversity, presenting a man who had been galvanised, not weakened, by disability (ibid.). Strategically, he went to great lengths to ensure that photographic images depicting his impairment were tracked down and excised from public view. What we see in Ahab and Roosevelt are disabled people feeling responsible for undoing both perceived and real implications of impairment. In a culture which celebrates the 'supercrip' (Marks, 1999a, p. 75), the need to disprove projections easily draws one away from what is internally real. Modern culture is replete with moral dictates about what one should *not be*. A consequence of this is efforts at disowning parts of experience or self which hint at stereotype. All of this tugs against self-empathy, restricting candid and compassionate recognition of what one's struggles mean.

'Anti-stereotyping behaviour' provides evidence of efforts to avoid being seen as caricatures of prejudice (Watermeyer and Swartz, 2008). These stories, familiar in popular media, deal with 'fiercely independent' disabled people undertaking fantastic physical challenges, in defiance of assumptions about their capabilities. Viewers' hearts are warmed by the reassuring knowledge that, despite their 'challenges', disabled people have the courage and character to overcome. At work here is an amplified version of an everyday predicament presented by disablism. It involves being stuck in an absurdly limited, split repertoire of identity ascriptions; the conquering hero(ine) or the useless invalid. The heroism of superhuman feats responds to assumptions about vulnerability. In managing these, the individual publicly repudiates every last fragment of fallibility. But ironically, this reassuring probably serves to confirm rather than overturn the stereotype, through identifying hopeful exceptions to it (ibid.). It is entirely wrong to generalise these interpretations to all disabled people attempting difficult achievements. This is not my intention at all. No matter the motivations at work in particular instances, my point is to do with the high cultural salience of such feats, and hence the pressures at work in individual lives.

The organising feature of psychological life with disablism is, in my view, being forced to define oneself *in opposition* (Watermeyer, 2009). Disproving negative imputations often has to take precedence over expressing selfhood. But selves chronically unseen by the social world may not only aim to overturn expectations of, say, dependency, but also wish to ensure that no shred of evidence could connect such a shame to their lives (Watermeyer and Swartz, 2008; Watermeyer, 2009). But it's often impossible for disabled people to successfully conceal evidence of disability stereotypes. Inhabiting a world of barriers to inclusion makes this so. What comes into view is a paradoxical picture in which disabled people are precluded from showing universal aspects of emotional life, such as loss. In a deep but resonant irony, people forced to occupy worlds of deprivation are also disallowed from articulating – even consciously experiencing – the emotional implications of their circumstances. But is this not what oppression is all about?

Wherever an identity is demeaned and splits are created, some negotiate the world by capitulating to stereotype – that is, effectively obscuring individual uniqueness, and 'performing' according to cultural expectation. For disabled people adopting this position there may be some acknowledgment of self buried between the disablist assumptions that surround them. That is, fragments of real, human struggle may be validated, as if by coincidence, through the ascribing of a 'suffering identity'. Or perhaps internalised oppression has led disabled people to experience themselves as nothing more or less than that dictated by stereotype. At work here is the same socialisation that may underpin the opposite, 'anti-stereotyping' behaviour described above. What is consistent is the destructive splitting of the subject. At an extreme, the latter strategy may aim to excise demeaning assumptions about impairment from one's own mind, as well as the minds of prejudiced observers. It is inevitable that battles for social justice be played out on the intra-psychic as well as the material terrain.

Therefore, in a key respect identity may operate in a manner inverse to the norm in the disability realm. Instead of carrying points of identification along with elements of othering, identity here is mainly concerned with rejecting ascribed difference – it is about 'what I'm not' rather than 'what I am'. One critical view of stereotype-busting would see it as *mimesis* (Taussig, 1993) – an attempt to fulfil the prescriptions of the adaptation narrative. Mime, though, only underlines difference, re-emphasising inequality. Pointing to this does not mean a pathologising of disabled lifestyle choices. It is not material actions which require our attention, but the drone of ideological forces which confer meaning. Disabled people have every right to climb mountains, swim oceans or engage in whatever other activity takes their fancy, but let us examine the systematically different mechanisms of social identity formation in which these choices function. Culture will refract the identity-meanings of such activities in profoundly different ways for those with unusual bodies. Normalising culture calls all to constantly remake the body – the self – as ideal, as able. In Murphy's (1987, p. 20) powerful words, the 'first commandment' of infirmity is "*get well*"' (my emphasis).

Disability, entitlement and loss

> **M**: … what I think … is that if I was more accepted in society, that I wouldn't be feeling the loss as much as I do … because … I would have a lot more support around me. As a community, that would be helping me get through this, but as it is it's just like 'this is your problem, now cope with it'. The best thing would be if I could just like say to some guy, 'you know I really wish I could move today, it's really crap that I can't move at the moment'. And to turn to anybody and be able to say that. To say this is how I feel.
>
> **R**: … I don't know if I would use the word acceptance. I'd use the word … adapting … Yeah, and saying, well, this is what I have to deal with and I make no excuses, I have to do this now. And I'm going to do it.
>
> **J**: [on the disabled community] … there's … so much trauma … And it confirms in my own mind a suspicion … that … great people are really forged out of fire, it's really when you're going through those amazingly trying periods in your life … where those people who are phenomenal people because they are forced to make difficult decisions about who they are, and who they want to be. And they become very conscious about that journey. But on the other hand they are broken people, they are scarred people. You know, that's kind of the price you pay for the knowledge you get, you pay the price.

Psychotherapy work with severely physically impaired people, in my experience, presents loss as a continual reality. But the loss at work here is complex – a layered amalgam of social ascriptions and material exclusion, in mutually constituting relationships with impairment. Pathologising cultural attributions may create a complicated, ambivalent relationship with all loss, disrupting clear, self-empathic articulating of struggle. At the best of times acknowledging loss is a painful business, but it is more hazardous when it risks deepening prejudice, leaving one even more unseen.

Like all humans, disabled people do carry loss, but typically not the losses attributed to them. Some losses relate directly to disability, some do not. Often disability and impairment are interwoven with identity and experience in a complex narrative which makes separating out 'disability losses' meaningless. What is clear is that the psychological commodification of 'disability loss' in disablist discourse puts disabled people at risk of banishing aspects of subjective life. In the Kleinian view of personality, fulfilling relationships depend on the ability to allow one another to feel and communicate loss (Frosh, 1991). This sort of relating fosters integration, nurturing a healthy entitlement based on compassionate self-understanding. Hindering us in bringing loss to consciousness is the conditioned shame which is our universal human legacy. These struggles confront all, but at issue is the especially strict sanctioning of expressions of loss imposed on disabled people. Here, prescriptions of what is permissible are heightened; loss is imagined, denied, concealed, suspected and silently attributed. In my experience, lives of visibly disabled people are replete with unspoken psychological transactions involving the negotiation of loss for all participants. The disabled figure, in this sense, is a cultural commodity appropriated for navigation of the wild terrain of human loss.

In disclosing our losses, all face the uncertainty of whether our identity will be contaminated in the view of the listener, or whether we will remain the same. Courage to disclose involves trusting another to know that 'this is not all that I am'. In disabled lives these risks are much greater, because identity is so mediated by fantasy. A range of self-fulfilling prophecies await confirmation; the common, entrenched view of the disabled figure whose internal life is nothing but loss, is never far away. Consciously and unconsciously therefore, disabled people may have to defend against welling negative ascriptions, as a sort of relational default. Such persons may thus be left in a paradoxical, invisible borderland, carrying attributions of losses which are not theirs, and living with the concealment of losses which are real. One imagines that obscuring can only continue to breathe life into the defensive myth of essential difference. The social space disabled people may be forced to occupy is a hesitant and ambiguous one, not truly 'being', yet searching for authenticity, while anticipating rather than relating. This is a place of inherent relational compromises. Finding clarity in the midst of the cross-cutting, deeply conditioned assumptions of disablist culture is, to say the least, challenging. Internalised uncertainties about justice and entitlement are as much an obstacle to self-expression as anticipated othering. The two issues are mutually constitutive, and present as continuous. Finding solid internal ground in the midst of this gallery of past and present voices is the difficult work of an internal reclaiming of self.

Rather than denying loss, empowerment involves its deliberate and thoughtful claiming (Watermeyer, 2009). The intention is to disrupt stereotyped splits between stoic strength and misery, by turning, carefully, to internal referents rather than external constraints. This means weaving an increasingly overt narrative in which losses and hopes are intermingled. The identity of 'disabled' here has varying salience, relating closely to some losses and less or not at all to others. The enforced attachment or dissociation of loss from disability is rejected. Instead, loss is decolonised and welcomed back, claimed as precious and described in one's own words. Through this sort of reclamation, disabled subjectivity assumes its rightful place in the continuous stream of the human condition, showing up valuable truths about the nature of society and relationship along the way. Because subjectivity is always layered, it is both naïve and unfair to assume that disabled people simply 'know' what is wrong with the (disability) world, what it means to individuals, and what ought to be done. There is much that we do know, but there is also much that we all need to find out for ourselves. Allowing an understanding of personal meanings of loss must form one crucial arena of this work.

10 Concluding reflections

> **G**: ...well, I think it's a process of grappling with meaning, you know ultimately that becomes my way of finding control. It's understanding ... the nature of the dynamics which lead to ... the way things happen. In many ways it allows me to normalise my life. Because ... if you don't understand these dynamics as having these kinds of root causes, you end up being ... sucked that much more into them, and ... in many ways ... I end up feeling more disabled when I don't feel like ... I get it. That's been an over-arching experience from the initial injury ... initially the ways a lot of people reacted to me just didn't make sense at all. But then slowly, over time, you start to understand the patterns.
>
> The basic social institution is the individual human heart. It is the source of the energy from which all social action derives its power and its purpose.
>
> (Dass and Gorman, 1985, pp. 164–65)

What G describes is a subtle layer of relational distortions which form part of his unequal social positioning. These are to do with projections, avoidance, boundary contraventions, inauthenticity and much else – a host of factors militating against clear, bounded and equitable relating. This psychological predicament is not separate from material exclusion, but co-constituted with it. A central argument of this book is that a drive for change which acts only at the material level will miss an important layer of how oppression operates. In worlds where individuals live in close parallel, but with starkly unequal privileges and power, the idea that relationships and psychological experience may not be implicated or affected is absurd.

In my own disabled reality, psychological, interpersonal and material levels are all important. To differing degrees, all have social, ideological origins. The many layers of meaning I attach to my impairment are embedded in culture, in family history, in an unprepared material world and in many other arenas. Emancipatory politics always involves a rejection of ascribed characteristics, be these to do with race, gender, disability or any other aspect of identity. It is about saying what we are *not*, which is in opposition to a social world which affirms its own identity through othering. Early phases of political movements centre on a forceful rebuttal of prejudiced assumptions. Disability politics, in this sense, has taken a course of helping us identify what we are not, but is limited in the work to follow. This is the question of what we are.

The critique of separatist identity politics reflected in this book sees it as a necessary stage in the evolution of a more equal society, but one with limited relevance. The clamour of conflicting needs for redress in societies full of inequality must be transmuted into a politics which builds relationships across identities. Separatism requires difference to justify its cause. But there is an intrinsic contradiction in opposing inequality based on ascribed difference by affirming that very difference. It is inevitable, if difference is what we rely upon, that the rejected dictates of a prejudiced society will, to some extent, be displaced by intra-group orthodoxies. Part of rejecting stereotypes involves consenting to constraints on what we are able to be, or how we are able to feel. Ironically, difference also has its comforts; adversarial relationships can be familiar, safe ground to occupy.

The vision of a more caring society based on foregrounding commonality is not, to me, a naïve political ideal. As a South African the predicaments of members of various marginal groups in my society show all too much in common. The politics I suggest is not one which denies difference. In this work I make it clear that impairment is real, bodies are different and this difference needs to be talked about. In South Africa we understand too well the dangerous illusions of a politics which denies colour, and hence denies history. Race remains, it shapes lives in different ways, and holds firm to its position as primary cultural symbol. But if we are caught together in this racist predicament, the question then becomes what we share in terms of common, universally human responses to social adversity. What is it about us that some are protected from, and others exposed to? What do we all fear, and how do we use culture and history to escape it? How has an illusion of inherent difference become a defence for all against the hope, and fear, of change? Thus far, the reluctance of some segments of the disability movement to forge public bonds with other minorities is a missed opportunity. I am curious about the extent to which the long history of impairment-based separatism in disability social service organisations has left its mark on the disabled community. If we feel we have something to lose by becoming part of a larger movement, then let us begin by thinking carefully about what that may be.

Many writers in disability studies have reservations, even suspicions, about the idea of a universalist ontology – the position reflected in this book. This perspective holds that disability struggle is no more or less than human struggle. Taking this position does not question that disabled people are subject to systemic disadvantage. Disabled people suffer an increased risk of exposure to painful parts of the human condition through material deprivation, heightened experience of prejudices to do with the body, functional limitation, pain and fatigue and so forth. One fear some authors have expressed is that disability-related suffering will be subsumed under a trite idea that 'all suffer', or 'all are oppressed'. This need not be the case. It is possible, in fact essential, that we combine a clear analysis of the material deprivation of disablism with a recognition that disabled people are people like anyone else, who are caught in harmful and unjust circumstances. What is familiar about disability is what makes it hard to think about; but its familiarity and closeness to home also represent the only possible bridge to unity. The idea of a united movement for citizenship rights may spark fears of being left out or forgotten – *again*. These fears are not at all baseless, but the result of very real and relentless exclusion. Nevertheless, many times I have witnessed how an expectation of exclusion has played a part in sabotaging organisational engagements for change in the disability sector in my country. The expectation, as I have said, is not unwarranted. But it is also poorly understood, and hence plays a part in ongoing relational splits which require careful attention.

It will be clear that I view it as fundamental that the disability movement invest resources in human development. In other words, undertaking real initiatives which facilitate empowerment based on reflection, on mutual validation, and an honest recognition of history. The idea of 'internalised oppression' is heard often enough in disability studies circles, but is seldom described, let alone responded to. There is an ambivalent silence around the idea that people have been hurt or damaged by lives of deprivation and prejudice. We must get over this. The disability movement's aversion to psychology and mental health care has missed an opportunity for educating professionals, allowing individuals to acknowledge struggle where this exists, and recreating therapeutic services as vehicles of empowerment. But even more significantly, a fear of the pathologising of medicine or psychiatry has led to an inability to converse honestly with one another about lives which regularly include trauma. The vacuum in disability studies where the psychological realm ought to be is testimony to this. If, as this book suggests, imagined or real disabled experience is difficult to think about in the dominant culture, it is that much more important that it be thought about inside the disabled community. Splitting is part of the very fabric of disablist socialisation. We must work to understand and uproot the ways in which it has infiltrated ourselves, creating an alienation from personal truth. Group-based programmes of empowerment drawing on the Freirian model hold much promise. In my own work as a group psychotherapist, one lasting impression was of how inadmissible disability-related experiences were in everyday interaction. In a world unready to hear, we must begin by hearing ourselves as clearly as we can. To disabled people quoted in this book, much of the inequality embedded in everyday interaction would have remained invisible unless specific examination had begun. This call to reflection is not a signal to stop fighting for inclusion and material equity. Not at all. What I advocate is an addition to the movement's intentions, as well as a careful stocktaking of orthodoxy, organisational character and strategy.

The idea that any politics brings inherent limitations and silences is an important point of departure. Psychoanalysis teaches that any paradigm functions partly as a defence – every position we take will illuminate some parts of the world, and obscure others. Social model politics has, I believe, obscured from ourselves some of what makes us marginal. If disablist socialisation is the most influential force in inequality, as I believe it is, we must understand it as thoroughly as we can, both individually and collectively. None of the work I propose is easy. Much of it may feel awkward or frightening, and represents a break from the safety of familiar binaries and political correctness. But if impairment does have a misleading mystique, it seems clear that these familiar paradigms can only deepen this illusion, in the minds of observers as well as disabled people themselves. At the heart of internalised oppression is the projection of feelings of damage or inadequacy into one's body. In order to understand and dislodge this, a candid conversation about what impairment *is* must be allowed. My own response to the social model's original implication that, for the purposes of understanding inequality, impairment is 'nothing' is this: Impairment is definitely not nothing, but it is also almost certainly not what you think it is. I address these words mainly to the nondisabled majority, but also acknowledge that to me impairment remains, in part, mysterious. The bewilderingly complex conceptualisation of embodiment – some of which is recounted here – would not be necessary if the topic was a simple one.

What much of the above amounts to is the idea of disabled people being less likely than others to find experiences of containment; in relationships, institutions, the workplace, the state. The containment of a mother's acceptance of her infant's distress, and the responsivity of a cultural world which validates and welcomes one's experience are, to me entirely analogous. Impaired life in an excluding, prejudiced society means constant experiences of misattunement and invisibility, demonstrating that one was not, and is not, thought about. For all, not having someone who is willing and able to think about and accept one's experience will limit the ability for self-compassion. Being shown that one's inner life feels unknowable to others will tend to make it seem less knowable, less tolerable, to the self. These are not emotional dilemmas peculiar to disabled people, but broadly human ones. Again, disabled people may be strongly confronted with this sort of adversity. As humans, finding self-compassion is not one of our strong points. But attending to this need is particularly important in lives where trauma is a reality, and cultural signalling silences inner experience.

In his description of an infant's perception of non-acceptance by a parent, Winnicott (1974) contrasts feeling looked *after* and looked *at.* In both literal and ephemeral terms, the latter experience is very real in the lives of visibly impaired people. While others are parented by a state which responds to its needs, and a culture which mirrors its experience, the disabled figure is looked 'at' in a way which objectifies, invalidates and alienates. The act of looking at is infused with difference, with distance. This mirroring must appeal to psychological parts where self-worth is doubted – places where needs for acceptance and care were not sufficiently met. To suggest this in the lives of disabled people does not single out mothers of impaired infants as inadequate in their ability to hold. Instead, the picture is one of the universal reality of imperfectly met infantile dependency needs. This is explained in Winnicott's (1960; 1971) idea of 'good enough' mothering, involving the reality that perfectly attuned care is impossible, and would in fact be an impediment to development and separation. So all carry unconscious parts of self where containment has been inadequate; in disabled lives this experience is recapitulated and re-enlivened through both a material and psychological abandonment by the human world and the state. We all carry memories or fears of not being truly 'thought about', which are systemically re-realised in impaired lives by disablism.

Modernity, meanwhile, continues its work of developing living spaces, technologies and services which are ever more attuned to the entitled demands of its consumers. Both the body and the self of the disabled figure must adjust to the material world – influence very seldom flows in the opposite direction. Like the infant with a depressed mother, he or she is drawn into attuning to cues about how to be, how to justify being there, how to compensate.

In this book I have begun a project of conceptualising psychological aspects of disablist discrimination and impairment, exploring the usefulness of psychoanalytic ideas. The intention, at every point, is to connect the psychological predicaments of disabled people to the ways in which disablism distorts relationships and socialisation. These predicaments involve what it is like, as a self, to live in a social world which systemically ignores some of one's material needs, and much of one's experience. Invisibility has both a tangible and psychological face, and is at the heart of oppression. Disabled people are materially isolated from the production of culture, but the phenomenology of disabled life is also muffled by a world that avoids hearing what it fears. The world fears its own fantasies about disabled life, as well as its own subtle awareness of being part of a society shot through with injustice.

All humans need to be seen, to be heard, in order to flourish into a fuller experience of self. Ironically, much of what we see around us in narcissistic society is itself a defensive response to the experience of having felt profoundly unseen. Through the trappings and lifestyles of capitalist culture the consumer is able to purchase escape from these feelings, which are passed onto those designated as the truly, appropriately 'forgotten'. Disabled people, in this picture, are left alone with their humanity, as well as the disavowed shames of others. Finding a voice for this predicament is the first step to change.

> If we had a keen vision and feeling of all ordinary human life, it would be like hearing the grass grow and the squirrel's heart beat, and we should die of that roar which lies on the other side of silence.
>
> (*Middlemarch* – George Eliot)

I was drawn to the quotation from *Middlemarch* which opened the book by its resonance with the fear of complexity that underlies revolutionary politics. The justification of needing to work in binaries for political ends is real enough, but also obscures other resistances to engaging with what is hidden in ordinary lives. The psychological layer of disablism is as ordinary as it is powerful. It deserves our attention.

References

Abberley, P. (1987). 'The concept of oppression and the development of a social theory of disability'. *Disability, Handicap and Society*, 2, 5–19.

——(1993). 'Disabled people and "normality"'. In J. Swain, V. Finkelstein, S. French and M. Oliver (eds), *Disabling barriers – enabling environments* (pp. 107–15). London: Sage.

——(1996). 'Work, utopia and impairment'. In L. Barton (ed.), *Disability and society: Emerging issues and insights* (pp. 61–79). New York: Addison Wesley Longman.

——(1998). 'The spectre at the feast: Disabled people and social theory'. In T. Shakespeare (ed.), *The disability reader: Social science perspectives* (pp. 79–93). London: Cassell.

——(2002). 'Work, disability, disabled people and European social theory'. In C. Barnes, M. Oliver and L. Barton (eds), *Disability studies today* (pp. 120–38). Cambridge: Polity Press.

Abelow Hedley, L. (2006). 'The seduction of the surgical fix'. In E. Parens (ed.), *Surgically shaping children: Technology, ethics, and the pursuit of normality* (pp. 43–48). Baltimore, MD: Johns Hopkins University Press.

Adorno, T. W. (1951/2005). *Minima moralia: Reflections on a damaged life*. London: Verso.

Albert, B. (2005). 'Finally included on the development agenda? A review of official disability and development policies'. In C. Barnes and G. Mercer (eds), *The social model of disability: Europe and the majority world* (pp. 131–47). Leeds: Disability Press.

Albrecht, G. and Bury, M. (2001). 'The political economy of the disability marketplace'. In G. Albrecht, K. Seelman and M. Bury (eds), *Handbook of disability studies* (pp. 585–609). Thousand Oaks, CA: Sage.

Albrecht, G., Seelman, K. and Bury, M. (2001). 'The formation of disability studies'. In G. Albrecht, K. Seelman and M. Bury (eds), *Handbook of disability studies* (pp. 1–9). Thousand Oaks, CA: Sage.

Altman, B. (2001). 'Disability definitions, models, classification schemes, and applications'. In G. Albrecht, K. Seelman and M. Bury (eds), *Handbook of disability studies* (pp. 97–122). Thousand Oaks, CA: Sage.

Anzieu, D. (1989). *The skin ego: A psychoanalytic approach to the self*. New Haven, CT: Yale University Press.

Archer, M. (1995). *Realist social theory: The morphogenetic approach*. Cambridge: Cambridge University Press.

Armstrong, F. (2005). 'Pupil or "patient": Difference, disability and education in France'. In C. Barnes and G. Mercer (eds), *The social model of disability: Europe and the majority world* (pp. 49–64). Leeds: Disability Press.

Asch, A. (1984). 'The experience of disability: A challenge for psychology'. *American Psychologist*, 39(5), 529–36.

——(2001). 'Disability, bioethics, and human rights'. In G. Albrecht, K. Seelman and M. Bury (eds), *Handbook of disability studies* (pp. 297–326). Thousand Oaks, CA: Sage.

——(2006). 'Appearance-altering surgery, children's sense of self, and parental love'. In E. Parens (ed.), *Surgically shaping children: Technology, ethics, and the pursuit of normality* (pp. 227–49). Baltimore, MD: Johns Hopkins University Press.

Asch, A. and Fine, M. (1988). 'Introduction: Beyond pedestals'. In A. Asch and M. Fine (eds), *Women with disabilities: Essays in psychology, culture and politics* (pp. 1–38). Philadelphia, PA: Temple University Press.

——(1997). 'Nurturance, sexuality and women with disabilities: The example of women and literature'. In L. Davis (ed.), *The disability studies reader* (pp. 241–59). New York: Routledge.

Asch, A. and Rousso, H. (1985). 'Therapists with disabilities: Theoretical and clinical issues'. *Psychiatry*, 48, 1–12.

Asch, A. and Stubblefield, A. (2010). 'Growth attenuation: Good intentions, bad decision'. *The American Journal of Bioethics*, 10(1), 46–48.

Aspinall, C. (2006). 'Do I make you uncomfortable? Reflections on using surgery to reduce the distress of others'. In E. Parens (ed.), *Surgically shaping children: Technology, ethics, and the pursuit of normality* (pp. 13–28). Baltimore, MD: Johns Hopkins University Press.

Atkinson, P. (1997). 'Narrative turn or blind alley?' *Qualitative Health Research*, 7(3), 325–44.

Avery, D. (1999). 'Talking "tragedy": Identity issues in the parental story of disability'. In M. Corker and S. French (eds), *Disability discourse* (pp. 116–26). Philadelphia, PA: Open University Press.

Bach, J. R. and Tilton, M. C. (1994). 'Life satisfaction and well-being measures in ventilator assisted individuals with traumatic tetraplegia'. *Archives of Physical Medicine and Rehabilitation*, 75, 626–32.

Badinter, E. (1981). *The myth of motherhood: A historical view of the maternal instinct*. London: Souvenir Press.

Bakhtin, M. (1981). *The dialogic imagination: Four essays*. (C. Emerson and M. Holquist, Trans.). Austin: University of Texas Press.

Balikov, H. (1960). 'Functional impairment of the sensorium as a result of normal adaptive processes'. *Psychoanalytic Study of the Child*, 15, 235–42.

Barnes, C. (1990). *'Cabbage Syndrome': The social construction of dependence*. London: Falmer Press.

——(1998). 'The social model of disability: A sociological phenomenon ignored by sociologists'. In T. Shakespeare (ed.), *The disability reader: Social science perspectives* (pp. 65–78). London: Cassell.

Barnes, C. and Mercer, G. (2001). 'Disability culture: Assimilation or inclusion'. In G. Albrecht, K. Seelman and M. Bury (eds), *Handbook of disability studies* (pp. 515–34). Thousand Oaks, CA: Sage.

Barnes, C. and Mercer, G. (eds). (2005a). *The social model of disability: Europe and the majority world*. Leeds: Disability Press.

Barnes, C. and Mercer, G. (2005b). 'Understanding impairment and disability: Towards an international perspective'. In C. Barnes and G. Mercer (eds), *The social model of disability: Europe and the majority world* (pp. 1–16). Leeds: Disability Press.

Barnes, C., Oliver, M. and Barton, L. (2002a). 'Introduction'. In C. Barnes, M. Oliver and L. Barton (eds), *Disability studies today* (pp. 1–17). Cambridge: Polity Press.

——(2002b). 'Disability, the academy and the inclusive society'. In C. Barnes, M. Oliver and L. Barton (eds), *Disability studies today* (pp. 250–60). Cambridge: Polity Press.

Bartky, S. (1990). *Femininity and domination: Studies in the phenomenology of oppression*. London: Routledge.

Barton, L. and Armstrong, F. (2001). 'Disability, education, and inclusion: Cross-cultural issues and dilemmas'. In G. Albrecht, K. Seelman and M. Bury (eds), *Handbook of disability studies* (pp. 693–710). Thousand Oaks, CA: Sage.

Basnett, I. (2001). 'Health care professionals and their attitudes toward and decisions affecting disabled people'. In G. Albrecht, K. Seelman and M. Bury (eds), *Handbook of disability studies* (pp. 450–67). Thousand Oaks, CA: Sage.

Begum, N., Hill, M. and Stevens, A. (eds). (1994). *Reflections: The views of black disabled people on their lives and community care*. London: CCETSW.

Berger, P. and Luckmann, T. (1966). *The social construction of reality: A treatise in the sociology of knowledge*. New York: Anchor.

Bickenbach, J. (1998). 'Disability and life-ending decisions'. In M. Battin, R. Rhodes and A. Silvers (eds), *Physician assisted suicide: Expanding the debate* (pp. 123–32). New York: Routledge.

——(2001). 'Disability human rights, law, and policy'. In G. Albrecht, K. Seelman and M. Bury (eds), *Handbook of disability studies* (pp. 565–84). Thousand Oaks, CA: Sage.

——(2011). 'The world report on disability'. *Disability and Society*, 26(5), 655–58.

Bickenbach, J., Chatterji, S., Badley, E. and Ustun, T. (1999). 'Models of disablement, universalism and the international classification of impairments, disabilities and handicaps'. *Social Science and Medicine*, 48, 1173–87.

Biko, S. (1978). *I write what I like*. London: The Bowerdean Press.

Biley, A. (1994). 'A handicap of negative attitudes and lack of choice: Caring for inpatients with disabilities'. *Professional nurse*, 9(12), 786–88.

Bion, W. (1957). 'The differentiation of the psychotic from the non-psychotic personalities'. *International Journal of Psycho-Analysis*, 38, 266–75.

——(1961). *Experiences in groups and other papers*. London: Tavistock Publications Limited.

——(1962a). *Learning from experience*. London: Maresfield.

——(1962b). 'The psycho-analytic study of thinking'. *International Journal of Psycho-Analysis*, 43, 306–10.

——(1967). *Second thoughts*. New York: Jason Aronson.

——(1970). *Attention and Interpretation*. London: Tavistock Publications Limited.

Blank, H. R. (1957). 'Psychoanalysis and blindness'. *Psychoanalytic Quarterly*, 26, 1–24.

Bliss, S. (1994). 'Perfection or preconception – some thoughts on reactions to disability in the therapist'. *British Journal of Psychotherapy*, 11, 115–19.

Bogdan, R. (1988). *Freak show: Presenting human oddities for amusement and profit*. Chicago: University of Chicago Press.

Bollas, C. (1987). *The shadow of the object: Psychoanalysis of the unthought known*. New York: Columbia University Press.

Bordo, S. (1993). *Unbearable weight: Feminism, western culture, and the body*. Berkeley and Los Angeles: University of California Press.

Bornstein, M. (1977). 'Analysis of a congenitally blind musician'. *Psychoanalytic Quarterly*, 46, 23–47.

Borsay, A. (2002). 'History, power and identity'. In C. Barnes, M. Oliver and L. Barton (eds), *Disability studies today* (pp. 98–119). Cambridge: Polity Press.

Bosch, X. (1998). '"Voluntary" sterilisation in Spain clarified in new legislation'. *The Lancet*, 352, 24.

Bowlby, J. (1979). 'On knowing what you are not supposed to know and feeling what you are not supposed to feel'. *Canadian Journal of Psychiatry*, 24, 403–8.

Braddock, D. and Parish, S. (2001). 'An institutional history of disability'. In G. Albrecht, K. Seelman and M. Bury (eds), *Handbook of disability studies* (pp. 11–68). Thousand Oaks, CA: Sage.

Braithwaite, D. O. (1990). 'From majority to minority: An analysis of cultural change from able-bodied to disabled'. *International Journal of Intercultural Relations*, 14(4), 465–83.

Bronfenbrenner, U. (1977). 'Toward an experimental ecology of human development'. *American Psychologist*, 32, 513–30.

Burke, P. (2008). *Disability and impairment.* London: Jessica Kingsley.

Burkett, B., McNamee, M. and Potthast, W. (2011). 'Shifting boundaries in sports technology and disability: Equal rights or unfair advantage in the case of Oscar Pistorius?' *Disability and Society*, 26(5), 643–54.

Burlingham, D. (1961). 'Some notes on the development of the blind'. *Psychoanalytic Study of the Child*, 16, 121–45.

Burman, E. (1996). 'The spec(tac)ular economy of difference'. In S. Wilkinson and C. Kitzinger (eds), *Representing the other: A feminism and psychology reader* (pp. 138–40). London: Sage.

Bury, M. (2000). 'A comment on the ICIDH2'. *Disability and Society*, 15, 1073–77.

Byrom, B. (1999). 'Joseph F. Sullivan and the discourse of "crippledom" in progressive America'. In M. Corker and S. French (eds), *Disability discourse* (pp. 157–63). Philadelphia, PA: Open University Press.

Calton, C. (2010). 'The obscuring of class in memoirs of parents of children with disabilities'. *Disability and Society*, 25(7), 849–60.

Campling, J. (1981). *Images of ourselves: Women with disabilities talking.* London: Routledge and Kegan Paul.

Castelnuovo-Tedesco, P. (1981). 'Psychological consequences of physical defects: A psychoanalytic perspective'. *International Review of Psychoanalysis*, 8, 145–54.

Chapman, E. (1978). *Visually handicapped children and young people.* London: Routledge and Kegan Paul.

Charlton, J. (1998). *Nothing about us without us: Disability oppression and empowerment.* Berkeley: University of California Press.

Cixous, H. and Clement, C. (1975/86). *The newly born woman.* Minneapolis: University of Minnesota Press.

Clegg, J. (2006). 'Understanding intellectually disabled clients in clinical psychology'. In D. Goodley and R. Lawthom (eds), *Disability and psychology: Critical introductions and reflections* (pp. 123–40). Basingstoke: Palgrave Macmillan.

Coleman, L. (1997). 'Stigma: An enigma demystified'. In L. Davis (ed.), *The disability studies reader* (pp. 216–30). New York: Routledge.

Coleridge, P. (1993). *Disability, liberation, and development.* Oxford: Oxfam.

Colker, R. (2005). *The disability pendulum: The first decade of the Americans with Disabilities Act.* New York: New York University Press.

Conroy, C. (2008). 'Active differences: disability and identity beyond Postmodernism'. *Contemporary Theatre Review*, 18(3), 341–54.

Conwell, Y. and Caine, E. D. (1991). 'Rational suicide and the right to die: reality and myth'. *The New England Journal of Medicine*, 325(15), 1100–101.

Cooper, A. and Treacher, A. (1995). 'Free associations, truth, morality and engagement'. *Free Associations*, 5(1), 1–9.

Cordner, S. and Ettershank, K. (1997). 'Australia's illegal sterilisations revealed'. *The Lancet*, 349, 1231.

Corker, M. (1994). *Counselling – the deaf challenge.* London: Jessica Kingsley.

Corker, M. and Shakespeare, T. (2002). 'Mapping the terrain'. In M. Corker and T. Shakespeare (eds), *Disability/postmodernity* (pp.1–17). London: Continuum.

Crisp, R. (2002). 'A counselling framework for understanding individual experiences of socially constructed disability'. *Disability Studies Quarterly*, 22(3), 20–32.

Crow, L. (1992). 'Renewing the social model of disability'. *Coalition*, July, 5–9.
——(1996). 'Including all our lives: Renewing the social model of disability'. In J. Morris (ed.), *Encounters with strangers: Feminism and disability*. London: The Women's Press.
Crowther, N. (2007). 'Nothing without us or nothing about us?' *Disability and Society*, 22(7), 791–94.
Dalenberg, C. J. (2000). *Countertransference and the treatment of trauma*. Washington, DC: American Psychological Association.
Darke, P. (1998). 'Understanding cinematic representations of disability'. In T. Shakespeare (ed.), *The disability reader: Social science perspectives* (pp. 181–96). London: Cassell.
Dass, R. and Gorman, P. (1985). *How can I help? Stories and reflections on service*. New York: Alfred Knopf.
Davids, M. F. (1996). 'Frantz Fanon: The struggle for inner freedom'. *Free Associations*, 6 (38), 205–34.
Davidson, M. (2003). 'Phantom limbs: Film noir and the disabled body'. In R. McRuer and A. Wilkerson (eds), *Desiring disability: Queer theory meets disability studies*. Special issue, *Gay and Lesbian Quarterly*, 9(1–2), 57–77.
Davis, L. J. (1995). *Enforcing normalcy: Disability, deafness, and the body*. New York: Verso.
——(1997a). 'Constructing normalcy: The bell curve, the novel, and the invention of the disabled body in the nineteenth century'. In L. Davis (ed.), *The disability studies reader* (pp. 9–28). New York: Routledge.
——(1997b). 'Introduction: The need for disability studies'. In L. Davis (ed.), *The disability studies reader* (pp. 1–6). New York: Routledge.
——(1997c). 'Nude venuses, medusa's body and phantom limbs: Disability and visuality'. In D. T. Mitchell and S. L. Snyder (eds), *The body and physical difference: Discourses of disability* (pp. 51–70). Detroit: University of Michigan Press.
——(2001). 'Identity politics, disability, and culture'. In G. Albrecht, K. Seelman and M. Bury (eds), *Handbook of disability studies* (pp. 535–45). Thousand Oaks, CA: Sage.
——(2002). *Bending over backwards: Disability, dismodernism and other difficult positions*. New York: New York University Press.
Diekema, D. S. and Fost, N. (2010). 'Ashley revisited: A response to the peer commentaries'. *The American Journal of Bioethics*, 10(1), W4–W6.
Disability Discrimination Act 1995. London: HMSO.
Dodd, J., Saggers, S. and Wildy, H. (2009). 'Constructing the "ideal" family for family-centred practice: Challenges for delivery'. *Disability and Society*, 24(2), 173–86.
Douglas, M. (1966). *Purity and danger: An analysis of concepts of pollution and taboo*. London: Routledge.
Drake, R. F. (2001). 'Welfare states and disabled people'. In G. Albrecht, K. Seelman and M. Bury (eds), *Handbook of disability studies* (pp. 412–29). Thousand Oaks, CA: Sage.
Dreger, A. D. (2006). 'What to expect when you have the child you weren't expecting'. In E. Parens (ed.), *Surgically shaping children: Technology, ethics, and the pursuit of normality* (pp. 253–65). Baltimore, MD: Johns Hopkins University Press.
Drotar, D., Baskiewicz, A., Irvin, N., Kennell, J. and Klaus, M. (1975). 'The adaptation of parents to a birth of an infant with a congenital malformation: A hypothetical model'. *Pediatrics*, 56(5), 710–17.
Eberhardt, K. and Mayberry, W. (1995). 'Factors influencing entry-level occupational therapists' attitudes toward persons with disabilities'. *American Journal of Occupational Therapy*, 49(7), 629–35.
Eliot, G. (1871/2003). *Middlemarch*. Basingstoke: Michael Faber.
Emry, R. and Wiseman, R. L. (1987). 'An intercultural understanding of able-bodied and disabled persons' communication'. *International Journal of Intercultural Relations*, 11, 2–27.

Engel, D. M. (1993). 'Original myths: Narratives of authority, resistance, disability, and law'. *Law and Society Review*, 27(4), 785–824.
Engel, G. (1977). 'The need for a new medical model'. *Science*, 196, 129–36.
Erskine, A. (1994). 'The initial contact: Assessment for counselling in the medical context'. In A. Erskine and D. Judd (eds), *The imaginative body: Psychodynamic therapy in health care* (pp. 43–58). London: Jason Aronson.
Erskine, A. and Judd, D. (1994). 'Introduction'. In A. Erskine and D. Judd (eds), *The imaginative body: Psychodynamic therapy in health care* (pp. 1–10). London: Jason Aronson.
Fanon, F. (1952/1986). *Black skin, white masks*. London: Pluto Press.
——(1963/2004). *The wretched of the earth*. (R. Philcox, Trans.). New York: Grove Press.
Fenichel, O. (1946). *The psychoanalytic theory of neurosis*. London: Routledge and Kegan Paul.
Ferguson, P. M. (2001). 'Mapping the family: Disability studies and the exploration of parental response to disability'. In G. Albrecht, K. Seelman and M. Bury (eds), *Handbook of disability studies* (pp. 373–95). Thousand Oaks, CA: Sage.
Ferguson, P. M. and Asch, A. (1989). 'Lessons from life: Personal and parental perspectives on school, childhood and disability'. In D. Biklen, D. Ferguson and A. Ford (eds), *Schooling and disability* (pp. 108–40). Chicago: University of Chicago Press.
Fiedler, L. (1978). *Freaks: Myths and images of the secret self*. New York: Simon and Schuster.
Figlio, K. and Richards, B. (2002). 'Psychoanalysis in the public sphere: Some recent British developments in psychoanalytic social psychology'. In R. Hinshelwood and M. Chiesa (eds), *Organisations, anxieties, and defences: Towards a psychoanalytic social psychology* (pp. 183–203). Philadelphia, PA: Whurr Publishers.
Finger, A. (2006). *Elegy for a disease: A personal and cultural history of polio*. New York: St. Martin's Press.
Finkelstein, V. (1980). *Attitudes and disabled people: Issues for discussion*. New York: World Rehabilitation Fund.
——(1996). 'Outside, inside out'. *Coalition*, April, 30–36.
——(1998). 'Emancipating disability studies'. In T. Shakespeare (ed.), *The disability reader: Social science perspectives* (pp. 28–49). London: Cassell.
Finkelstein, V. and French, S. (1993). 'Towards a psychology of disability'. In J. Swain, V. Finkelstein, S. French and M. Oliver (eds), *Disabling barriers – enabling environments* (pp. 26–33). London: Sage.
Fisman, S. and Wolf, L. (1991). 'The handicapped child: Psychological effects of parental, marital, and sibling relationships'. *Psychiatric Clinics of North America*, 14(1), 199–217.
Flood, T. (2005). '"Food" or "thought"? The social model and the majority world'. In C. Barnes and G. Mercer (eds), *The social model of disability: Europe and the majority world* (pp. 180–92). Leeds: Disability Press.
Forshaw, M. (2007). 'In defence of psychology: A reply to Goodley and Lawthom (2005)'. *Disability and Society*, 22(6), 655–58.
Forster, E. M. (1921). *Howards End*. New York: Vintage.
Foster, A. (2001). 'The duty to care and the need to split'. *Journal of Social Work Practice*, 15 (1), 81–90.
Foucault, M. (1976). *Birth of the clinic: An archaeology of medical perception*. London: Tavistock
——(1979). *Discipline and punish: The birth of the prison*. (A. Sheridan, Trans.). New York: Vintage Books.
——(1995). *Madness and civilization: A history of insanity in the age of reason*. London: Routledge.
Fougeyrollas, P. and Beauregard, L. (2001). 'Disability: An interactive person-environment social creation'. In G. Albrecht, K. Seelman and M. Bury (eds), *Handbook of disability studies* (pp. 171–94). Thousand Oaks, CA: Sage.

Fox, S. A. and Giles, H. (1996). 'Interability communication: Evaluating patronising encounters'. *Journal of Language and Social Psychology*, 15(3), 265–90.

Frank, A. (1995). *The wounded storyteller: Body, illness and ethics.* Chicago: University of Chicago Press.

——(1998). 'From dysappearance to hyperappearance: Sliding boundaries of illness and bodies'. In J. Henderikns (ed.), *The body and psychology* (pp. 205–32). London: Sage.

——(2006). 'Emily's scars: Surgical shapings, technoluxe, and bioethics'. In E. Parens (ed.), *Surgically shaping children: Technology, ethics, and the pursuit of normality* (pp. 68–88). Baltimore, MD: Johns Hopkins University Press.

Frank, A. W. (2000). 'The standpoint of storyteller'. *Qualitative Health Research*, 10, 354–65.

Frank, G. (1988). 'Beyond stigma: Visibility and self-empowerment of persons with congenital limb deficiencies'. *Journal of Social Issues*, 44(1), 95–115.

Fraser, N. (1989). *Unruly practices: Power, discourse and gender in contemporary social theory.* Minneapolis: University of Minnesota Press.

——(1995). 'From redistribution to recognition? Dilemmas of justice in a "post-socialist" age'. *New Left Review*, 212, 68–92.

——(2000). 'Rethinking recognition'. *New Left Review*, 3, 107–20.

Fraser, N. and Nicholson, L. J. (1990). 'Social criticism without philosophy: An encounter between feminism and postmodernism'. In L. J. Nicholson (ed.), *Feminism/postmodernism* (pp. 19–38). New York: Routledge.

Freire, P. (1970). *Pedagogy of the oppressed.* New York: Continuum.

French, S. (1988). 'Experiences of disabled health and caring professionals'. *Sociology of Health and Illness*, 10, 170–88.

——(1993a). 'Disability, impairment or something in between?' In J. Swain, V. Finkelstein, S. French and M. Oliver (eds), *Disabling barriers – enabling environments* (pp. 17–25). London: Sage.

——(1993b). '"Can you see the rainbow?" The roots of denial'. In J. Swain, V. Finkelstein, S. French and M. Oliver (eds), *Disabling barriers – enabling environments* (pp. 69–77). London: Sage.

——(1993c). 'What's so great about independence?' In J. Swain, V. Finkelstein, S. French and M. Oliver (eds), *Disabling barriers – enabling environments* (pp. 44–48). London: Sage.

——(1994a). 'Disabled people and professional practice'. In S. French (ed.), *On equal terms: Working with disabled people* (pp. 103–18). Boston: Butterworth-Heinemann.

——(1994b). 'Attitudes of health professionals towards disabled people: A discussion and review of the literature'. *Physiotherapy*, 80(10), 687–93.

——(1999). 'The wind gets in my way'. In M. Corker and S. French (eds), *Disability discourse* (pp. 21–27). Philadelphia, PA: Open University Press.

French, S. and Swain, J. (2001). 'The relationship between disabled people and health and welfare professionals'. In G. Albrecht, K. Seelman and M. Bury (eds), *Handbook of disability studies* (pp. 734–53). Thousand Oaks, CA: Sage.

——(2006). 'Telling stories for a politics of hope'. *Disability and Society*, 21(5), 383–96.

Freud, A. (1952). 'The role of bodily illness in the mental life of children'. *Psychoanalytic Study of the Child*, 7, 69–81.

——(1967). 'Comments on trauma'. In S. S. Furst (ed.), *Psychic trauma* (p. 236). New York: Basic Books.

Freud, S. (1912). *A note on the unconscious in psycho-analysis. The Standard Edition of the Complete Psychological Works of Sigmund Freud, Volume XII (1911–13): The Case of Schreber, Papers on Technique and Other Works*, 255–66.

——(1914). *On narcissism: an introduction. The Standard Edition of the Complete Psychological Works of Sigmund Freud, Volume XIV (1914–16): On the History of the Psycho-Analytic Movement, Papers on Metapsychology and Other Works*, 67–102.

——(1916). *Some character-types met with in psycho-analytic work: The exceptions. The Standard Edition of the Complete Psychological Works of Sigmund Freud, Volume XIV (1914–16): On the History of the Psycho-Analytic Movement, Papers on Metapsychology and Other Works*, 309–33.

——(1917). *Mourning and melancholia. The Standard Edition of the Complete Psychological Works of Sigmund Freud, Volume XIV (1914–16): On the History of the Psycho-Analytic Movement, Papers on Metapsychology and Other Works*, 237–58.

——(1919). *The 'uncanny'. The Standard Edition of the Complete Psychological Works of Sigmund Freud, Volume XVII (1917–19): An Infantile Neurosis and Other Works*, 217–56.

——(1920). *Beyond the pleasure principle. The Standard Edition of the Complete Psychological Works of Sigmund Freud, Volume XVIII (1920–22): Beyond the Pleasure Principle, Group Psychology and Other Works*, 1–64.

——(1923). *The ego and the id. The Standard Edition of the Complete Psychological Works of Sigmund Freud, Volume XIX (1923–25): The Ego and the Id and Other Works*, 1–66.

——(1930). *Civilization and its discontents. The Standard Edition of the Complete Psychological Works of Sigmund Freud, Volume XXI (1927–31): The Future of an Illusion, Civilization and its Discontents, and Other Works*, 57–146.

——(1933). *New introductory lectures on psycho-analysis. The Standard Edition of the Complete Psychological Works of Sigmund Freud, Volume XXII (1932–36): New Introductory Lectures on Psycho-Analysis and Other Works*, 1–182.

Friedrich, W. N. and Boriskin, J. A. (1976). 'The role of the child in abuse: A review of the literature'. *American Journal of Orthopsychiatry*, 46(4), 580–89.

Frosh, S. (1989). 'Psychoanalysis and racism'. In B. Richards (ed.), *Crises of the self: Further essays on psychoanalysis and politics* (pp. 229–44). London: Free Association Books.

——(1991). *Identity crisis: Modernity, psychoanalysis and the self.* London: Macmillan.

——(2006). *For and against psychoanalysis* (2nd edn). New York: Routledge.

Fujiura, G. T. and Rutkowski-Kmitta, V. (2001). 'Counting disability'. In G. Albrecht, K. Seelman and M. Bury (eds), *Handbook of disability studies* (pp. 69–96). Thousand Oaks, CA: Sage.

Garland-Thomson, R. (1995). 'Ann Petry's Mrs. Hedges and the evil, one-eyed girl: A feminist exploration of the physically disabled female subject'. *Women's Studies*, 24, 599–614.

——(1997a). 'Feminist theory, the body, and the disabled figure'. In L. Davis (ed.), *The disability studies reader* (pp. 279–92). New York: Routledge.

——(1997b). *Extraordinary bodies: Figuring physical disability in American culture and literature.* New York: Columbia University Press.

——(2009). *Staring: How we look.* New York: Oxford University Press.

Gergen, K. J. (1985). 'The social constructionist movement in modern psychology'. *American Psychologist*, 266–75.

Gill, C. J. (2001). 'Divided understandings: The social experience of disability'. In G. Albrecht, K. Seelman and M. Bury (eds), *Handbook of disability studies* (pp. 351–72). Thousand Oaks, CA: Sage.

——(2004). 'Depression in the context of disability and the "right to die"'. *Theoretical Medicine*, 25, 171–198.

——(2010). 'No, we don't think our doctors are out to get us: Responding to the straw man distortions of disability rights arguments against assisted suicide'. *Disability and Health Journal*, 3, 31 38.

Gliedman, J. and Roth, W. (1980). *The unexpected minority: Handicapped children in America.* New York: Harcourt Brace Jovanovich.

Glover, J. (2006). *Choosing children: The ethical dilemmas of genetic intervention.* Oxford: Oxford University Press.

Goffman, E. (1963). *Stigma: Notes on the management of spoiled identity.* Englewood Cliffs, NJ: Prentice-Hall.

Golden, C. S. and Scheer, J. (1995). 'Murphy's contribution to disability studies: An inquiry into ourselves'. *Social Science and Medicine*, 40(11), 1443–45.

Goodley, D. (2011a). 'Social psychoanalytic disability studies'. *Disability and Society*, 26(6), 715–28.

——(2011b). *Disability studies: An interdisciplinary introduction.* London: Sage.

Goodley, D. and Lawthom, R. (2005). 'Epistemological journeys in participatory action research: Alliances between community psychology and disability studies'. *Disability and Society*, 20(2), 135–51.

Goodley, D. and Lawthom, R. (eds). (2006). *Disability and psychology: Critical introductions and reflections.* Basingstoke: Palgrave Macmillan.

Goodley, D. and Runswick-Cole, K. (2010). 'Emancipating play: Dis/abled children, development and deconstruction'. *Disability and Society*, 25(4), 499–512.

Gordon, P. (1995). 'Private practice, public life: Is a psychoanalytic politics possible?' *Free Associations*, 35, 275–88.

Grech, S. (2009). 'Disability, poverty and development: Critical reflections on the majority world debate'. *Disability and Society*, 24(6), 771–84.

Greenberg, J. and Mitchell, S. (1983). *Object relations in psychoanalytic theory.* Cambridge, MA: Harvard University Press.

Gunther, D. F. and Diekema, D. S. (2006). 'Attenuating growth in children with profound developmental disability: A new approach to an old dilemma'. *Archives of Pediatric Adolescent Medicine*, 160, 1013–17.

Hacking, I. (1999). *The social construction of what?* Cambridge, MA: Harvard University Press.

Hagrass, H. (2005). 'Definitions of disability and disability policy in Egypt'. In C. Barnes and G. Mercer (eds), *The social model of disability: Europe and the majority world* (pp. 148–62). Leeds: Disability Press.

Hahn, H. (1997). 'An agenda for citizens with disabilities: Pursuing identity and empowerment'. *Journal of Vocational Rehabilitation*, 9, 31–37.

——(2001). 'Adjudication or empowerment: Contrasting experiences with a social model of disability'. In L. Barton (ed.), *Disability, politics, and the struggle for change* (pp. 59–78). London: David Fulton.

——(2002). 'Academic debates and political advocacy: The US disability movement'. In C. Barnes, M. Oliver and L. Barton (eds), *Disability Studies Today* (pp. 162–89). Cambridge: Polity Press.

Handley, P. (2000). 'Trouble in paradise – a disabled person's right to the satisfaction of a self-defined need: Some conceptual and practical problems'. *Disability and Society*, 16(2), 313–25.

Harris, A. and Wideman, D. (1988). 'The construction of gender and disability in early attachment'. In M. Fine and A. Asch (eds), *Women with disabilities: Essays in psychology, culture and politics* (pp. 115–38). Philadelphia, PA: Temple University Press.

Heifetz, L. J. (1980). 'From consumer to middleman: Emerging roles for parents in the network of services for retarded children'. In R. Abidin (ed.), *Parent education and intervention handbook* (pp. 349–84). Springfield, IL: Charles C. Thomas.

Herr, S. S., Bostrom, B. A. and Barton, R. S. (1992). 'No place to go: Refusal of life-sustaining treatment by competent persons with physical disabilities'. *Issues in Law and Medicine*, 8(1), 3–34.

Hevey, D. (1992). *The creatures time forgot: Photography and disability imagery*. London: Routledge.

——(1997). 'The enfreakment of photography'. In L. Davis (ed.), *The disability studies reader* (pp. 332–47). New York: Routledge.

Hinshelwood, R. D. (1987). *What happens in groups: Psychoanalysis, the individual and the community*. London: Free Association Books.

——(1991). *A dictionary of Kleinian psychoanalysis*. Northvale, NJ: Aronson.

Hinshelwood, R. D. and Chiesa, M. (2002a). 'General introduction'. In R. Hinshelwood and M. Chiesa (eds), *Organisations, anxieties, and defences: Towards a psychoanalytic social psychology* (pp. 1–11). Philadelphia, PA: Whurr Publishers.

——(2002b). 'A conceptual overview of international contributions'. In R. Hinshelwood and M. Chiesa (eds), *Organisations, anxieties, and defences: Towards a psychoanalytic social psychology* (pp. 15–34). Philadelphia, PA: Whurr Publishers.

Hoggett, P. (1992). *Partisans in an uncertain world: The psychoanalysis of engagement*. London: Free Association Books.

Holden, C. and Beresford, P. (2002). 'Globalisation and disability'. In C. Barnes, M. Oliver and L. Barton (eds), *Disability studies today* (pp. 190–209). Cambridge: Polity Press.

Hollway, W. (1998). 'Gender difference and the production of subjectivity'. In J. Henriques, W. Hollway, C. Urwin, C. Venn and V. Walkerdine (eds), *Changing the subject: Psychology, social regulation and subjectivity* (pp. 223–61). New York: Routledge.

Holmes, J. (1996). 'Attachment theory: A secure base for policy?' In S. Kraemer and J. Roberts (eds), *The politics of attachment: Towards a secure society* (pp. 27–42). London: Free Association Books.

Honneth, A. (1995). *The struggle for recognition: The moral grammar of social conflicts*. Cambridge: Polity Press.

Hordon, L. D. (1994). 'Attitudes of medical students to disabled people'. *British Journal of Rheumatology*, 33, 203–4.

Hubbard, R. (1997). 'Abortion and disability: Who should and who should not inhabit the world?' In L. Davis (ed.), *The disability studies reader* (pp. 187–200). New York: Routledge.

Hughes, B. (2001). 'Disability and the constitution of dependency'. In L. Barton (ed.), *Disability, politics, and the struggle for change* (pp. 24–33). London: David Fulton.

——(2002a). 'Disability and the body'. In C. Barnes, M. Oliver and L. Barton (eds), *Disability studies today* (pp. 58–76). Cambridge: Polity Press.

——(2002b). 'Bauman's strangers: Impairment and the invalidation of disabled people in modern and post-modern cultures'. *Disability and Society*, 17(5), 571–84.

——(2009). 'Wounded/monstrous/abject: A critique of the disabled body in the sociological imaginary'. *Disability and Society*, 24(4), 399–410.

Hughes, B. and Paterson, K. (1997). 'The social model of disability and the disappearing body: Towards a sociology of impairment'. *Disability and Society*, 12(3), 325–40.

Hunt, P. (1998). 'A critical condition'. In T. Shakespeare (ed.), *The disability reader: Social science perspectives* (pp. 7–19). London: Cassell.

Hurst, R. (2005). 'Disabled Peoples' International: Europe and the social model of disability'. In C. Barnes and G. Mercer (eds), *The social model of disability: Europe and the majority world* (pp. 65–79). Leeds: Disability Press.

Imrie, R. (1996). *Disability and the city: International perspectives*. London: Paul Chapman.

Ingstad, B. (2001). 'Disability and the developing world'. In G. Albrecht, K. Seelman and M. Bury (eds), *Handbook of disability studies* (pp. 772–92). Thousand Oaks, CA: Sage.

Ingstad, B. and White, S. (1995). 'An overview'. In B. Ingstad and S. White (eds), *Disability and culture* (pp. 3–32). Los Angeles: University of California Press.

Jack, R. (1995). 'Empowerment in community care'. In R. Jack (ed.), *Empowerment in community care* (pp. 11–39). London: Chapman and Hall.

Jackson, J. (1994). 'Chronic pain and the tension between the body as subject and object'. In T. J. Csordas (ed.), *Embodiment and experience: The existential ground of culture and self* (pp. 201–28). Cambridge: Cambridge University Press.

Jacobson, E. (1959). 'The "exceptions": An elaboration of Freud's character study'. *Psychoanalytic Study of the Child*, 14, 135–54.

James, P. and Thomas, M. (1996). 'Deconstructing a disabling environment in social work education'. *Social Work Education*, 15(1), 34–45.

Johnson, R. (1993). '"Attitudes don't just hang in the air ... ": Disabled people's perceptions of physiotherapists'. *Physiotherapy*, 79(9), 619–26.

Kalyanpur, M. (1996). 'The influence of Western special education on community-based services in India'. *Disability and Society*, 11(2), 249–70.

Kelly, M. P. (2001). 'Disability and community: A sociological approach'. In G. Albrecht, K. Seelman and M. Bury (eds), *Handbook of disability studies* (pp. 396–411). Thousand Oaks, CA: Sage.

Kermit, P. (2009). 'Cochlear implants, linguistic rights and "open future" arguments'. In K. Kristiansen, S. Vehmas and T. Shakespeare (eds), *Arguing about disability: Philosophical perspectives* (pp. 137–53). London: Routledge.

Kittay, E. F. (2006). 'Thoughts on the desire for normality'. In E. Parens (ed.), *Surgically shaping children: Technology, ethics, and the pursuit of normality* (pp. 90–108). Baltimore, MD: Johns Hopkins University Press.

Klein, M. (1946). 'Notes on some schizoid mechanisms'. *International Journal of Psychoanalysis*, 27, 99–110.

——(1948). 'A contribution to the theory of anxiety and guilt'. *International Journal of Psychoanalysis*, 29, 114–23.

——(1952). 'The origins of transference'. *International Journal of Psychoanalysis*, 33, 433–38.

——(1957/1975). 'Envy and gratitude'. In *Envy and gratitude and other works: 1946–1963* (pp. 176–235). New York: Dell.

——(1959). 'Our adult world and its roots in infancy'. *Human Relations*, 12, 291–303.

——(1960). 'On mental health'. *British Journal of Medical Psychology*, 33, 237–41.

Kleinman, A. (1986). 'Illness meanings and illness behaviour'. In S. McHugh and T. M. Vallis (eds), *Illness behaviour: A multidisciplinary model* (pp. 149–60). New York: Plenum Press.

——(1987). 'Anthropology and psychiatry: The role of culture and cross-cultural research on illness'. *British Journal of Psychiatry*, 151, 447–54.

——(1988). *The illness narratives: Suffering, healing and the human condition.* New York: Basic Books.

Kleinman, A., Das, V. and Lock, M. (1997). *Social suffering.* Berkeley: University of California Press.

Kohut, H. (1966). 'Forms and transformations of narcissism'. In A. Morrison (ed.), *Essential papers on narcissism* (pp. 61–88). New York: New York University Press.

——(1972). 'Thoughts on narcissism and narcissistic rage'. *Psychoanalytic Study of the Child*, 27, 360–400.

Kraemer, S. and Roberts, J. (1996). 'Introduction: Holding the thread'. In S. Kraemer and J. Roberts (eds), *The politics of attachment: Towards a secure society* (pp. 1–20). London: Free Association Books.

Kriegel, L. (1987). 'The cripple in literature'. In A. Gartner and T. Joe (eds), *Images of the disabled, disabling images* (pp. 31–46). New York: Praeger.

Kristeva, J. (1982). *Powers of horror: An essay on abjection.* (L. S. Roudiez, Trans.). New York: Columbia University Press.

Kumari-Campbell, F. A. (2008). 'Exploring internalized ableism using critical race theory'. *Disability and Society*, 23(2), 151–62.

Lacan, J. (1977). *Ecrits: A selection.* (A. Sheridan, Trans.). New York: Routledge. (Original work published 1948).

Lane, H. (1992). *The mask of benevolence: Disabling the deaf community*. New York: Alfred A. Knopf.

Lasch, C. (1978). *The culture of narcissism: American life in an age of diminishing expectations*. New York: W. W. Norton.

——(1984). *The minimal self: Psychical survival in troubled times*. London: W. W. Norton.

Lawson, A. and Matthews, B. (2005). 'Dismantling barriers to transport by law: The European journey'. In C. Barnes and G. Mercer (eds), *The social model of disability: Europe and the majority world* (pp. 80–97). Leeds: Disability Press.

Lawthom, R. and Goodley, D. (2006). 'Conclusions: Making enabling alliances between disability studies and psychology'. In D. Goodley and R. Lawthom (eds), *Disability and psychology: Critical introductions and reflections* (pp. 187–204). Basingstoke: Palgrave Macmillan.

Lee, P. (2002). 'Shooting for the moon: Politics and disability at the beginning of the twenty-first century'. In C. Barnes, M. Oliver and L. Barton (eds), *Disability studies today* (pp. 139–61). Cambridge: Polity Press.

Lenny, J. (1993). 'Do disabled people need counselling?' In J. Swain, V. Finkelstein, S. French and M. Oliver (eds), *Disabling barriers – enabling environments* (pp. 233–40). London: Sage.

Levinson, F. and Parritt, S. (2006). 'Against stereotypes: Experiences of disabled psychologists'. In D. Goodley and R. Lawthom (eds), *Disability and psychology: Critical introductions and reflections* (pp. 111–22). Basingstoke: Palgrave Macmillan.

Linton, S. (1998). *Claiming disability: Knowledge and identity*. New York: New York University Press.

——(2006). *My body politic: A memoir.* Detroit: University of Michigan Press.

Lollar, D. J. (2001). 'Public health trends in disability: Past, present, and future'. In G. Albrecht, K. Seelman and M. Bury (eds), *Handbook of disability studies* (pp. 754–71). Thousand Oaks, CA: Sage.

Longmore, P. K. (1997). 'Conspicuous contribution and American cultural dilemmas: Telethon rituals of cleansing and renewal'. In D. T. Mitchell and S. L. Snyder (eds), *The body and physical difference: Discourses of disability* (pp. 134–53). Detroit: University of Michigan Press.

Lonsdale, S. (1990). *Women and disability: The experience of physical disability among women.* London: Macmillan.

Low, J. (1996). 'Negotiating identities, negotiating environments: An interpretation of the experiences of students with disabilities'. *Disability and Society*, 11, 235–48.

Lunt, N. and Thornton, P. (1994). 'Disability and employment: Towards an understanding of discourse and policy'. *Disability and Society*, 9, 223–35.

Lussier, A. (1960). 'The analysis of a boy with a congenital deformity'. *Psychoanalytic Study of the Child*, 50, 430–53.

——(1980). 'The physical handicap and the body ego'. *International Journal of Psycho-Analysis*, 61, 179–85.

MacKeith, R. (1973). 'Parental reactions and responses to a handicapped child'. In F. Richardson (ed.), *Brain and Intelligence* (pp. 131–41). Hyattsville, MD: National Education Consultants.

Main, T. (1989). *The ailment and other psychoanalytic essays.* London: Free Association Books.

Marks, D. (1999a). *Disability: Controversial debates and psychosocial perspectives*. London: Routledge.

——(1999b). 'Dimensions of oppression: Theorising the embodied subject'. *Disability and Society*, 14(5), 611–26.

——(2002). 'Introduction: Counselling, therapy and emancipatory praxis'. *Disability Studies Quarterly*, 22(3), 1–5.

Marsh, J. L. (2006). 'To cut or not to cut? A surgeon's perspective on surgically shaping children'. In E. Parens (ed.), *Surgically shaping children: Technology, ethics, and the pursuit of normality* (pp. 113–24). Baltimore, MD: Johns Hopkins University Press.

McDonough, P. A. (1997). 'The social patterning of work disability among women in Canada'. *Journal of Disability Policy Studies*, 8(1–2), 75–98.

McLaughlin, J. (2003). 'Screening networks: Shared agendas in feminist and disability movement challenges to antenatal screening and abortion'. *Disability and Society*, 18, 3, 297–310.

McLaughlin, J. and Goodley, D. (2008). 'Seeking and rejecting certainty: Exposing the sophisticated lifeworlds of parents of disabled babies'. *Sociology*, 42(2), 317–35.

McRuer, R. (2006). *Crip theory: Cultural signs of queerness and disability*. New York: New York University Press.

McRuer, R. and Wilkerson, A. (2003). 'Cripping the (queer) nation'. In R. McRuer and A. Wilkerson (eds), *Desiring disability: Queer theory meets disability studies*. Special issue, *Gay and Lesbian Quarterly*, 9 (1–2), 1–17.

McWilliams, N. (1994). *Psychoanalytic diagnosis*. New York: Guilford Press.

Menzies-Lyth, I. (1988). 'A psychoanalytic perspective on social institutions'. In E. Bott-Spillius (ed.), *Melanie Klein today, volume 2: Mainly practice* (pp. 284–99). London: Routledge.

Mercer, G. (2002). 'Emancipatory disability research'. In C. Barnes, M. Oliver and L. Barton (eds), *Disability studies today* (pp. 228–49). Cambridge: Polity Press.

Merleau-Ponty, M. (1962). *The phenomenology of perception*. New York: Humanities Press.

Michalko, R. (2002). *The difference that disability makes*. Philadelphia, PA: Temple University Press.

Miles, M. (2001). 'ICIDH meets postmodernism, or "Incredulity toward meta-terminology"'. *Disability World 7*. Available at: www.disabilityworld.org/03-04_01/resources/icidh.shtml (Accessed 15 July 2008).

Miller, E. J. and Gwynne, G. V. (1972). *A life apart: A pilot study of residential institutions for the physically handicapped and the young chronic sick*. London: Tavistock.

Miller, P. S. (2006). 'Toward truly informed decisions about appearance-normalising surgeries'. In E. Parens (ed.), *Surgically shaping children: Technology, ethics, and the pursuit of normality* (pp. 211–26). Baltimore, MD: Johns Hopkins University Press.

Mitchell, D. T. and Snyder, S. L. (1997). 'Introduction: Disability studies and the double bind of representation'. In D. T. Mitchell and S. L. Snyder (eds), *The body and physical difference: Discourses of disability* (pp. 1–31). Detroit: University of Michigan Press.

——(2001a). 'Representation and its discontents: The uneasy home of disability in literature and film'. In G. Albrecht, K. Seelman and M. Bury (eds), *Handbook of disability studies* (pp. 195–218). Thousand Oaks, CA: Sage.

——(2001b). *Narrative prosthesis: Disability and the dependencies of discourse*. Ann Arbor: University of Michigan Press.

Mitchell, J. (1974). *Psychoanalysis and feminism*. New York: Pantheon Books.

Morris, J. (1989). *Able lives*. London: The Women's Press.

——(1992). 'Personal and political: A feminist perspective on researching physical disability'. *Disability, Handicap and Society*, 7, 157–66.

——(1993). 'Prejudice'. In J. Swain, V. Finkelstein, S. French and M. Oliver (eds), *Disabling barriers – enabling environments* (pp. 101–6). London: Sage.

Morris, S. (2006). 'Twisted lies: My journey in an imperfect body'. In E. Parens (ed.), *Surgically shaping children: Technology, ethics, and the pursuit of normality* (pp. 3–12). Baltimore, MD: Johns Hopkins University Press.

Mouradian, W. E. (2006). 'What's special about the surgical context?' In E. Parens (ed.), *Surgically shaping children: Technology, ethics, and the pursuit of normality* (pp. 125–38). Baltimore, MD: Johns Hopkins University Press.

Murphy, R. (1987). *The body silent.* New York: Henry Holt.

——(1995). 'Encounters: The body silent in America'. In B. Ingstad and S. White (eds). *Disability and culture* (pp. 140–58). Los Angeles: University of California Press.

Murphy, R. F., Scheer, J., Murphy, Y. and Mack, R. (1988). 'Physical disability and social liminality: A study in the rituals of adversity'. *Social Science and Medicine*, 26(2), 235–42.

Murray, P. (2006). 'Being in school? Exclusion and the denial of psychological reality'. In D. Goodley and R. Lawthom (eds), *Disability and psychology: Critical introductions and reflections* (pp. 34–41). Basingstoke: Palgrave Macmillan.

Mutua, N. K. (2001). 'The semiotics of accessibility and the cultural construction of disability'. In L. J. Rogers and B. B. Swadener (eds), *Semiotics and dis/ability* (pp. 103–16). Albany: State University of New York Press.

Nagera, H. and Colonna, A. B. (1965). 'Aspects of the contribution of sight to ego and drive development: A comparison of the development of some blind and sighted children'. *Psychoanalytic Study of the Child*, 20, 267–87.

Niederland, W. (1965). 'Narcissistic ego impairment in patients with early physical malformations'. *Psychoanalytic Study of the Child*, 20, 518–34.

Norden, M. F. (1994). *The cinema of isolation: A history of physical disability in the movies.* New Brunswick, NJ: Rutgers University Press.

Obholzer, A. and Roberts, V. Z. (1994). *The unconscious at work.* London: Routledge.

Ogden, T. H. (1974). 'A psychoanalytic psychotherapy of a patient with cerebral palsy: The relation of aggression to self and body representations'. *International Journal of Psychoanalytic Psychotherapy*, 3, 419–32.

Ogden, T. K. (1979). 'On projective identification'. *International Journal of Psychoanalysis*, 60, 357–73.

Oliver, J. (1995). 'Counselling disabled people: A counsellor's perspective'. *Disability and Society*, 10, 261–79.

Oliver, M. (1986). 'Social policy and disability: Some theoretical issues'. *Disability, Handicap and Society*, 1, 15–17.

——(1990). *The politics of disablement.* London: Macmillan.

——(1993a). 'Redefining disability: A challenge to research'. In J. Swain, V. Finkelstein, S. French and M. Oliver (eds), *Disabling barriers – enabling environments* (pp. 61–67). London: Sage.

——(1993b). 'Disability and dependency: A creation of industrial societies?' In J. Swain, V. Finkelstein, S. French and M. Oliver (eds), *Disabling barriers – enabling environments* (pp. 49–60). London: Sage.

——(1996). *Understanding disability: From theory to practice.* New York: St. Martin's Press.

——(2001). 'Disability issues in the postmodern world'. In L. Barton (ed.), *Disability, politics, and the struggle for change* (pp. 149–59). London: David Fulton.

Oliver, M. and Barnes, C. (2008). '"Talking about us without us?" A response to Neil Crowther'. *Disability and Society*, 23(4), 397–99.

Olkin, R. (1999). *What psychotherapists should know about disability.* New York: Guilford Press.

Omwake, E. and Solnit, A. (1961). '"It isn't fair": The treatment of a blind child'. *Psychoanalytic Study of the Child*, 16, 352–404.

Orbach, S. (1994). 'Working with the false body'. In A. Erskine and D. Judd (eds), *The imaginative body: Psychodynamic therapy in health care* (pp. 165–78). London: Jason Aronson.

Palmer, B. (2002). 'The Tavistock paradigm: Inside, outside and beyond'. In R. D. Hinshelwood and M. Chiesa (eds), *Organisations, anxieties, and defences: Towards a psychoanalytic social psychology* (pp. 158–82). Philadelphia, PA: Whurr Publishers.

Parens, E. (2006). 'Introduction: Thinking about surgically shaping children'. In E. Parens (ed.), *Surgically shaping children: Technology, ethics, and the pursuit of normality* (pp. xiii–xx). Baltimore, MD: Johns Hopkins University Press.

——(2009). 'Respecting children with disabilities and their parents'. *Hastings Center Report*, 39(1), 22–23.

Parmenter, T. R. (2001). 'Intellectual disabilities – quo vadis?' In G. Albrecht, K. Seelman and M. Bury (eds), *Handbook of disability studies* (pp. 267–96). Thousand Oaks, CA: Sage.

Paterson, K. and Hughes, B. (1999). 'Disability studies and phenomenology: The carnal politics of everyday life'. *Disability and Society*, 14(5), 597–610.

Pernick, M. S. (1997). 'Defining the defective: Eugenics, aesthetics and mass culture in early-twentieth century America'. In D. T. Mitchell and S. L. Snyder (eds), *The body and physical difference: Discourses of disability* (pp. 89–110). Detroit: University of Michigan Press.

Peters, S. (1999). 'Transforming disability identity through critical literacy and the cultural politics of language'. In M. Corker and S. French (eds), *Disability discourse* (pp. 103–13). Philadelphia, PA: Open University Press.

Pfeiffer, D. (2000). 'The devils are in the details: The ICIDH2 and the disability movement'. *Disability and Society*, 15(7), 1079–82.

Phillips, M. J. (1985). '"Try harder": The experience of disability and the dilemma of normalisation'. *The Social Science Journal*, 22(4), 45–57.

Pinker, S. (2003). *The blank slate: The modern denial of human nature*. New York: Penguin.

Pinkerton, P. (1970). 'Parental acceptance of the handicapped child'. *Developmental Medicine and Child Neurology*, 12(2), 207–12.

Potgieter, C. (2006). 'The imagined future for gays and lesbians in South Africa: Is this it?' *Agenda*, 20(67), 4–8.

Preece, J. (1995). 'Disability and adult education: The consumer view'. *Disability and Society*, 10, 87–102.

Price, J. and Shildrick, M. (1998). *Vital signs: Feminist reconfigurations of the bio/logical body*. Edinburgh: Edinburgh University Press.

Priestley, M. (1998). 'Constructions and creations: Idealism, materialism and disability theory'. *Disability and Society*, 13(1), 75–94.

——(1999). 'Discourse and identity: Disabled children in mainstream high schools'. In M. Corker and S. French (eds), *Disability discourse* (pp. 92–102). Philadelphia, PA: Open University Press.

——(2005). 'We're all Europeans now! The social model of disability and European social policy'. In C. Barnes and G. Mercer (eds), *The social model of disability: Europe and the majority world* (pp. 17–31). Leeds: Disability Press.

——(2006). 'Disability and old age: Or why it isn't all in the mind'. In D. Goodley and R. Lawthom (eds), *Disability and psychology: Critical introductions and reflections* (pp. 84–93). Basingstoke: Palgrave Macmillan.

Pullin, G. (2009). *Design meets disability*. Cambridge, MA: MIT Press.

Ramlow, T. (2003). 'Bad boys: Abstractions of difference and the politics of youth "defiance"'. In R. McRuer and A. Wilkerson (eds), *Desiring disability: Queer theory meets disability studies*. Special issue, *Gay and Lesbian Quarterly*, 9(1–2), 107–32.

Raphael-Leff, J. (1994). 'Imaginative bodies of childbearing: Visions and revisions'. In A. Erskine and D. Judd (eds), *The imaginative body: Psychodynamic therapy in health care* (pp. 13–39). London: Jason Aronson.

Ravaud, J. F. and Stiker, H. J. (2001). 'Inclusion/exclusion: An analysis of historical and cultural meanings'. In G. Albrecht, K. Seelman and M. Bury (eds), *Handbook of disability studies* (pp. 490–512). Thousand Oaks, CA: Sage.

Read, J. (2000). *Disability, the family and society: Listening to mothers.* Buckingham: Open University Press.

Reeve, D. (2000). 'Oppression within the counselling room'. *Disability and Society*, 15(4), 669–83.

——(2002). 'Negotiating psycho-emotional dimensions of disability and their influence on identity constructions'. *Disability and Society*, 17(5), 493–508.

——(2004). 'Counselling and disabled people: Help or hindrance?' In J. Swain, V. Finkelstein, S. French and M. Oliver (eds), *Disabling barriers – enabling environments* (2nd edn) (pp. 233–38). London: Sage.

——(2006). 'Towards a psychology of disability: The emotional effects of living in a disabling society'. In D. Goodley and R. Lawthom (eds), *Disability and psychology: Critical introductions and reflections* (pp. 94–110). Basingstoke: Palgrave Macmillan.

Reich, W. (1945). *The sexual revolution.* New York: Orgone Institute Press.

——(1946). *The mass psychology of fascism.* New York: Orgone Institute Press.

Richards, B. (1986). 'Psychological practice and social democracy'. *Free Associations*, 5, 105–36.

——(1989). 'Introduction'. In B. Richards (ed.), *Crises of the self: Further essays on psychoanalysis and politics* (pp. 1–26). London: Free Association Books.

Richter, L. M. (2003). 'Baby rape in South Africa'. *Child Abuse Review*, 12(6), 392–400.

Rinck, C. and Calkins, F. (1996). 'Challenges across the lifespan for people with disabilities'. *Bioethics Forum*, 12(3), 37–46.

Rioux, M. H. (1994). 'New research directions and paradigms: Disability is not measles'. In M. Rioux and M. Bach (eds), *Disability is not measles: New research paradigms in disability* (pp. 1–8). Montreal: Roeher Institute.

——(2002). 'Disability, citizenship and rights in a changing world'. In C. Barnes, M. Oliver and L. Barton (eds), *Disability studies today* (pp. 210–27). Cambridge: Polity Press.

Rocque, B. (2010). 'Mediating self-hood: Exploring the construction and maintenance of identity by mothers of children labeled with autism spectrum disorder'. *Disability and Society*, 25(4), 485–97.

Rogers-Salyer, M., Jensen, A. G. and Barden, R. C. (1987). 'Effects of facial deformities and physical attractiveness on mother-infant bonding'. In D. Marchac (ed.), *Craniofacial surgery: Proceedings of the First International Congress of Cranio-Maxillo-Facial Surgery* (pp. 481–85). New York: Springer-Verlag.

Rose, N. (1989). *Governing the soul: The shaping of the private self.* London: Routledge.

Rossiter, J. C. (2001). 'Shareholder commentary'. In L. Rogers and B. Swadener (eds), *Semiotics and dis/ability* (pp. 97–99). Albany: State University of New York Press.

Roulstone, A., Thomas, P. and Balderston, S. (2011). 'Between hate and vulnerability: Unpacking the British criminal justice system's construction of disablist hate crime'. *Disability and Society*, 26(3), 351–64.

Rustin, M. (1991). *The good society and the inner world: Psychoanalysis, politics and culture.* London: Verso.

——(1996). 'Attachment in context'. In S. Kraemer and J. Roberts (eds), *The politics of attachment: Towards a secure society* (pp. 212–28). London: Free Association Books.

Ryan, S. and Runswick-Cole, K. (2008). 'Repositioning mothers: Mothers, disabled children and disability studies'. *Disability and Society*, 23(3), 199–210.

Ryan, W. (1971). *Blaming the victim.* Boston: Orbach and Chambers.

Samuels, A. (1993). *The political psyche.* London: Routledge.

Samuels, E. (2003). 'My body, my closet: Invisible disability and the limits of coming-out discourse'. In R. McRuer and A. Wilkerson (eds), *Desiring disability: Queer theory meets disability studies*. Special issue, *Gay and Lesbian Quarterly*, 9(1–2), 233–55.

Sandahl, C. (2003). 'Queering the crip or cripping the queer? Intersections of queer and crip identities in solo autobiographical performance'. In R. McRuer and A. Wilkerson (eds), *Desiring disability: Queer theory meets disability studies*. Special issue, *Gay and Lesbian Quarterly*, 9(1–2), 25–56.

Sanford, E. S. (2006). 'My shoe size stayed the same: Maintaining a positive sense of identity with achondroplasia and limb-lengthening surgeries'. In E. Parens (ed.), *Surgically shaping children: Technology, ethics, and the pursuit of normality* (pp. 29–42). Baltimore, MD: Johns Hopkins University Press.

Scheer, J. and Groce, N. (1988). 'Impairment as a human constant: Cross-cultural and historical perspectives on variation'. *Journal of Social Issues*, 44(1), 23–37.

Schriner, K. (2001). 'A disability studies perspective on employment issues and policies for disabled people: an international view'. In G. Albrecht, K. Seelman and M. Bury (eds), *Handbook of disability studies* (pp. 642–62). Thousand Oaks, CA: Sage.

Scotch, R. (1988). 'Disability as the basis for a social movement: Advocacy and the politics of definition'. *Journal of Social Issues*, 44(1), 159–72.

Scott, R. (1969). *The making of blind men: A study of adult socialisation*. New York: Russell Sage Foundation.

Scullion, P. (1999). 'Challenging discrimination against disabled patients'. *Nursing Standard*, 13(18), 37–40.

Scully, J. L. (2009). 'Disability and the thinking body'. In K. Kristiansen, S. Vehmas and T. Shakespeare (eds), *Arguing about disability: Philosophical perspectives* (pp. 57–73). London: Routledge.

Segal, H. (1973). *An introduction to the work of Melanie Klein*. London: Hogarth Press.

Shakespeare, T. (1994). 'Cultural representation of disabled people: Dustbins for disavowal?' *Disability and Society*, 9, 283–99.

——(1999). 'Art and lies? Representations of disability on film'. In M. Corker and S. French (eds), *Disability discourse* (pp. 164–72). Philadelphia, PA: Open University Press.

——(2006). *Disability rights and wrongs*. New York: Routledge.

——(2008). 'Debating disability'. *Journal of Medical Ethics*, 34, 11–14.

Shakespeare, T., Gillespie-Sells, K. and Davies, D. (1996). *The sexual politics of disability: Untold desires*. London: Cassell.

Shakespeare, T., Iezzoni, L. I. and Groce, N. E. (2009). 'The art of medicine: Disability and the training of health professionals'. *The Lancet*, 374, 1815–16.

Shakespeare, T. and Officer, A. (2011). 'Editorial'. *Disability and Rehabilitation*, 33(17–18), 1491–92.

Shakespeare, T. and Watson, N. (2001). 'Making the difference: Disability, politics and recognition'. In G. Albrecht, K. Seelman and M. Bury (eds), *Handbook of disability studies* (pp. 546–64). Thousand Oaks, CA: Sage.

Shaw, M. N. (2001). 'Personal assistance services and youth in transition'. In L. Rogers and B. Swadener (eds), *Semiotics and dis/ability* (pp. 165–85). Albany: State University of New York Press.

Sheldon, A. (2005). 'One world, one people, one struggle? Towards the global implementation of the social model of disability'. In C. Barnes and G. Mercer (eds), *The social model of disability: Europe and the majority world* (pp. 115–30). Leeds: Disability Press.

Shildrick, M. (2002). *Embodying the monster: Encounters with the vulnerable self*. London: Sage.

——(2004). 'Queering performativity: Disability after Deleuze'. *SCAN: Journal of Media Arts Culture*, 1(3), 1–6.

Siller, J. (1963). 'Reactions to physical disability by the disabled and the nondisabled'. *Rehabilitation Counselling Bulletin*, 7, 2–16.

Sinason, V. (1989). 'The psycholinguistics of discrimination'. In B. Richards (ed.), *Crises of the self: Further essays on psychoanalysis and politics* (pp. 217–28). London: Free Association Books.

——(1992). *Mental handicap and the human condition: New approaches from the Tavistock*. London: Free Association Books.

——(2002). 'Some reflections from twenty years of psychoanalytic work with children and adults with a learning disability'. *Disability Studies Quarterly*, 22(3), 38–45.

Singer, P. (1993). *Practical ethics* (2nd edn). Cambridge: Cambridge University Press.

Singh, V. and Ghai, A. (2009). 'Notions of self: Lived realities of children with disabilities'. *Disability and Society*, 24(2), 129–45.

Slack, S. (1999). 'I am more than my wheels'. In M. Corker and S. French (eds), *Disability discourse* (pp. 28–37). Philadelphia, PA: Open University Press.

Solnit, A. J. (1989). 'Preparing for uncertainty: Family reactions to a seriously impaired child'. In B. Heller, H. Flohr and L. Zegans (eds), *Psychosocial intervention with physically disabled persons*. New Brunswick, NJ: Rutgers University Press.

Solnit, A. J. and Stark, M. H. (1961). 'Mourning and the birth of a defective child'. *Psychoanalytic Study of the Child*, 12, 523–37.

Somers, R. (1994). 'The narrative construction of identity: A relational and network approach'. *Theory and Society*, 23, 605–49.

Sontag, S. (1991). *Illness as a metaphor*. London: Penguin.

——(1997). 'AIDS and its metaphors'. In L. Davis (ed.), *The disability studies reader* (pp. 232–40). New York: Routledge.

Sparrow, R. (2010). 'Implants and ethnocide: Learning from the cochlear implant controversy'. *Disability and Society*, 25(4), 455–66.

Stannett, P. (2006). 'Disabled and graduated: Barriers and dilemmas for the disabled psychology graduate'. In D. Goodley and R. Lawthom (eds), *Disability and psychology: Critical introductions and reflections* (pp. 71–84). Basingstoke: Palgrave Macmillan.

Stein, M. A. and Lord, J. E. (2010). 'Monitoring the Convention on the Rights of Persons with Disabilities: Innovations, lost opportunities, and future potential'. *Human Rights Quarterly*, 32(3), 689–728.

Stiker, H. J. (1982). *A history of disability*. (W. Sayers, Trans.). Ann Arbor: University of Michigan Press.

Swain, J., Finkelstein, V., French, S. and Oliver, M. (eds). (1993). *Disabling barriers – enabling environments*. London: Sage.

Swain, J. and French, S. (2000). 'Towards an affirmation model of disability'. *Disability and Society*, 15(4), 569–82.

——(2008). 'Affirming identity'. In J. Swain and S. French (eds), *Disability on equal terms* (pp. 65–78). London: Sage.

Swain, J., Griffiths, C. and French, S. (2006). 'Counselling with the social model: Challenging therapy's pathologies'. In D. Goodley and R. Lawthom (eds), *Disability and psychology: Critical introductions and reflections* (pp. 155–69). Basingstoke: Palgrave Macmillan.

Swartz, L. (1999). *Culture and mental health: A Southern African view*. Oxford: Oxford University Press.

Swartz, L. and Watermeyer, B. (2008). 'Cyborg anxiety: Oscar Pistorius and the boundaries of what it means to be human'. *Disability and Society*, 23(2), 187–90.

Tajfel, H. and Turner, J. (1979). 'An integrative theory of intergroup conflict'. In W. Austen and S. Worchel (eds), *The social psychology of intergroup relations* (pp. 33–47). Monterey, CA: Brooks/Cole.

Taussig, M. (1993). *Mimesis and alterity: A particular history of the senses*. London: Routledge.

Taylor, C. (1989). *Sources of the self: The making of modern identity*. Cambridge, MA: Harvard University Press.

Temperley, J. (1984). 'Our own worst enemies: Unconscious factors in female disadvantage'. *Free Associations (pilot issue)*, 23–38.

Thomas, C. (1999a). *Female forms: Experiencing and understanding disability*. Philadelphia, PA: Open University Press.

——(1999b). 'Narrative identity and the disabled self'. In M. Corker and S. French (eds), *Disability discourse* (pp. 47–55). Philadelphia, PA: Open University Press.

——(2001). 'Feminism and disability: The theoretical and political significance of the personal and the experiential'. In L. Barton (ed.), *Disability, politics, and the struggle for change* (pp. 48–58). London: David Fulton.

——(2002). 'Disability theory: Key ideas, issues and thinkers'. In C. Barnes, M. Oliver and L. Barton (eds), *Disability studies today* (pp. 38–57). Cambridge: Polity Press.

——(2007). *Sociologies of disability and illness: Contested ideas in disability studies and medical sociology*. London: Palgrave.

——(2010). 'Negotiating the contested terrain of narrative methods in illness contexts'. *Sociology of Health and Illness*, 32(4), 647–60.

Thomas, K. R. and Siller, J. (1999). 'Object loss, mourning, and adjustment to disability'. *Psychoanalytic Psychology*, 16(2), 179–97.

Thompson, N. (2003). *Promoting equality: Challenging discrimination and oppression* (2nd edn). New York: Palgrave Macmillan.

Todd, L. (2006). 'Enabling practice for professionals: The need for practical post-structuralist theory'. In D. Goodley and R. Lawthom (eds), *Disability and psychology: Critical introductions and reflections* (pp. 141–54). Basingstoke: Palgrave Macmillan.

Toombs, S. K. (1994). 'Disability and the self'. In T. Brinthaupt and R. Lipka (eds), *Changing the self: Philosophies, techniques and experiences* (pp. 337–57). Albany: State University of New York Press.

Treacher, A. (1989). 'Be your own person: Dependence/independence, 1950–85'. In B. Richards (ed.), *Crises of the self: Further essays on psychoanalysis and politics* (pp. 131–46). London: Free Association Books.

Tregaskis, C. (2004). *Constructions of disability: Researching the interface between disabled and nondisabled people*. London: Routledge.

——(2006). 'Parents, professionals and disabled babies: Personal reflections on disabled lives'. In D. Goodley and R. Lawthom (eds), *Disability and psychology: Critical introductions and reflections* (pp. 19–33). Basingstoke: Palgrave Macmillan.

Trent, J. W. (1994). *Inventing the feeble mind: A history of mental retardation in the United States*. Berkeley: University of California Press.

Turnbull, A. P. and Summers, J. A. (1987). 'From parent involvement to family support: Evolution to revolution'. In S. M. Pueschel, C. Tingey, C. Rynders, A. C. Crocker and D. M. Crutcher (eds), *New perspectives on Down syndrome* (pp. 289–306). Baltimore, MD: Brookes.

Turner, B. S. (2001). 'Disability and the sociology of the body'. In G. Albrecht, K. Seelman and M. Bury (eds), *Handbook of disability studies* (pp. 252–66). Thousand Oaks, CA: Sage.

Turner, V. (1969). *The ritual process structure and anti-structure*. Ithaca, NY: Cornell University Press.

United Nations. (2006). *Convention on the Rights of Persons with Disabilities*. Geneva: United Nations. Online. Available at: www.un.org/disabilities/convention/conventionfull.shtml (Accessed 20 November 2011).

US Department of Justice. (1990). *Americans with Disabilities Act*. Washington, DC: US Department of Justice.

Ussher, J. (1989). *The psychology of the female body*. London: Routledge.

Vash, C. and Crewe, N. M. (2004). *Psychology of disability* (2nd edn). New York: Springer.

Veck, W. (2002). 'Completing the story: Connecting relational and psychological processes of exclusion'. *Disability and Society*, 17(5), 529–40.

Vehmas, S. and Mäkelä, P. (2009). 'The ontology of disability and impairment: A discussion of the natural and social features'. In K. Kristiansen, S. Vehmas and T. Shakespeare (eds), *Arguing about disability: Philosophical perspectives* (pp. 42–56). London: Routledge.

Vernon, A. and Swain, J. (2002). 'Theorising divisions and hierarchies: Towards a commonality or diversity?' In C. Barnes, M. Oliver and L. Barton (eds), *Disability studies today* (pp. 77–97). Cambridge: Polity Press.

Wasserman, D. (2001). 'Philosophical issues in the definition and social response to disability'. In G. Albrecht, K. Seelman and M. Bury (eds), *Handbook of disability studies* (pp. 219–51). Thousand Oaks, CA: Sage.

Watermeyer, B. (2000). 'Psychoanalysis and disability: An exploration of the utility of psychoanalytic methods and analyses in the interrogation of social responses to impairment'. M.A. dissertation, University of Cape Town.

——(2002a). 'Blindness, attachment and self: Psychoanalysis and ideology'. *Free Associations*, 49, 335–52.

——(2002b). 'Disability and psychotherapy: An ideologically charged relationship in community mental health service provision'. In L. Swartz, K. Gibson and T. Gelman (eds), *Reflective practice* (pp. 85–98). Pretoria, South Africa: HSRC Press.

——(2006). 'Disability and psychoanalysis'. In B. Watermeyer, L. Swartz, M. Schneider, T. Lorenzo and M. Priestley (eds), *Disability and social change: A South African agenda* (pp. 31–43). Pretoria, South Africa: HSRC Press.

——(2009). 'Claiming loss in disability'. *Disability and Society*, 24(1), 91–102.

Watermeyer, B. and Swartz, L. (2006). 'Introduction and overview'. In B. Watermeyer, L. Swartz, M. Schneider, T. Lorenzo and M. Priestley (eds), *Disability and social change: A South African agenda* (pp. 1–6). Pretoria, South Africa: HSRC Press.

——(2008). 'Conceptualising the psycho-emotional aspects of disability and impairment: The distortion of personal and psychic boundaries'. *Disability and Society*, 23(6), 599–610.

Watson, N. (1998). 'Enabling identity: Disability, self and citizenship'. In T. Shakespeare (ed.), *The disability reader: Social science perspectives* (pp. 147–62). London: Cassell.

Wendell, S. (1996). *The rejected body: Feminist philosophical reflections on disability*. New York: Routledge.

——(1997). 'Toward a feminist theory of disability'. In L. Davis (ed.), *The disability studies reader* (pp. 260–78). New York: Routledge.

Wertz, D. C. (1995). *Geneticists' ethical views: A survey in 37 nations*. Paper presented to the European Society of Human Genetics, Berlin, 24–27 May.

White, P. (2003). 'Sex education: Or, how the blind become heterosexual'. In R. McRuer and A. Wilkerson (eds), *Desiring disability: Queer theory meets disability studies*. Special issue, *Gay and Lesbian Quarterly*, 9(1–2), 133–48.

WHO (World Health Organisation). (1980). *International classification of impairment, disability and handicap* (ICIDH). Geneva: World Health Organisation.

——(1999). *International classification of impairment, disability and handicap*. Revised version (ICIDH-2). Geneva: World Health Organisation.

——(2011). *World Report on Disability*. Geneva: World Health Organisation. Online. Available at: http://whqlibdoc.who.int/publications/2011/9789240685215_eng.pdf (Accessed 3 December 2011).

Whyte, S. R. (1995). 'Disability between discourse and experience'. In B. Ingestad and S. R. Whyte (eds), *Disability and culture* (pp. 267–92). Berkeley: University of California Press.

Williams, G. (2001). 'Theorizing disability'. In G. Albrecht, K. Seelman and M. Bury (eds), *Handbook of disability studies* (pp. 123–44). Thousand Oaks, CA: Sage.

Williams, S. J. (1999). 'Is anybody there? Critical realism, chronic illness and the disability debate'. *Sociology of Health and Illness*, 21(6), 797–819.

Wilson, S. (2003). *Disability, counselling and psychotherapy: Challenges and opportunities*. New York: Palgrave Macmillan.

Winnicott, D. W. (1947/1992). 'Hate in the countertransference'. In *Through paediatrics to psychoanalysis: Collected papers* (pp. 194–203). London: Karnac.

——(1960). 'Ego distortion in terms of true and false self'. In *The maturational process and the facilitating environment: Studies in the theory of emotional development* (pp. 140–52). New York: International Universities Press.

——(1963/1990). 'Communicating and not communicating leading to a study of certain opposites'. In *The maturational processes and the facilitating environment* (pp. 179–92). London: Karnac.

——(1965). *The maturational processes and the facilitating environment: Studies in the theory of emotional development*. London: Hogarth Press.

——(1974). *Playing and reality*. London: Tavistock.

Winzer, M. A. (1997). 'Disability and society before the eighteenth century: Dread and despair'. In L. Davis (ed.), *The disability studies reader* (pp. 75–109). New York: Routledge.

Wolfenstein, E. V. (1990). 'Group phantasies and "the individual": A critical analysis of psychoanalytic group psychology'. *Free Associations*, 20, 150–80.

Wright, K. (1991). *Vision and separation: Between mother and baby*. London: Free Association Books.

Yorke, C. (1980). 'Some comments on the psychoanalytic treatment of patients with physical disabilities'. *International Journal of Psycho-Analysis*, 61, 187–93.

Young, R. M. (1994). *Mental space*. London: Process Press.

Zizek, S. (1990). 'Eastern Europe's republics of Gilead'. *New Left Review*, 183, 50–62.

——(1991). *Looking awry*. Cambridge, MA: MIT Press.

——(2004). 'The structure of domination today: A Lacanian view'. *Studies in East Europen Thought*, 56, 383–403.

——(2008). *Violence*. London: Profile Books.

Zola, I. (1988). 'Policies and programs concerning ageing and disabilities: Towards a unifying agenda'. In S. Sullivan and M. Lewin (eds), *The economics and ethics of long term care and disability* (pp. 90–98). Lanham, MD: University Press of America.

——(1989). 'Toward the necessary universalising of disability policy'. *The Milbank Memorial Fund Quarterly*, 67(2), 401–28.

——(1994). 'Towards inclusion: The role of people with disabilities in policy and research in the United States – a historical and political analysis'. In M. H. Rioux and M. Bach (eds), *Disability is not measles: New research paradigms in disability* (pp. 49–66). North York, Ontario: Roeher.

Index

For Product Safety Concerns and Information please contact our EU representative GPSR@taylorandfrancis.com
Taylor & Francis Verlag GmbH, Kaufingerstraße 24, 80331 München, Germany

www.ingramcontent.com/pod-product-compliance
Lightning Source LLC
LaVergne TN
LVHW011124300926
849160LV00008B/501
* 9 7 8 1 1 3 8 7 8 1 2 1 4 *